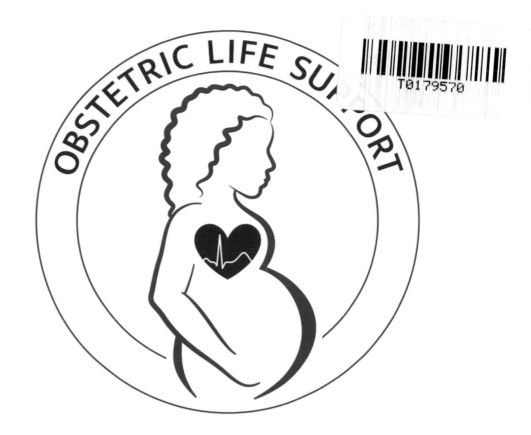

# Obstetric Life Support Manual

This text is a comprehensive review of normal and abnormal pregnancy physiology, the most common etiologies of maternal medical emergencies, recognition of maternal deterioration and pending cardiopulmonary arrest, modifications to cardiopulmonary resuscitation in pregnant and postpartum patients, special procedures that can assist in diagnosing and treating maternal medical emergencies tailored to the setting (e.g., point-of-care ultrasound, resuscitative cesarean delivery, extracorporeal cardiopulmonary resuscitation), treatment of trauma/stroke in pregnancy, and postpartum maternal medical emergencies. There are streamlined algorithms and cognitive aids designed to improve a team's ability to successfully implement techniques unique to treating maternal medical emergencies and cardiac arrest.

- Offers a practical guide to treating complex and challenging maternal medical emergencies
- Equips the entire team responding to a maternal cardiac arrest with the current evidence-based approaches and techniques
- Presents a thorough review, detailed algorithms, and a consolidated discussion of the practical aspects of implementation

The editors of this manual strive to use gender-inclusive language. However, in some instances, OBLS uses gender-specific language (e.g., pregnant women) to reference a study's findings. OBLS will periodically reassess this usage and make appropriate adjustments.

# Obstetric Life Support Manual

Etiology, prevention, and treatment of maternal medical emergencies and cardiopulmonary arrest in pregnant and postpartum patients

Edited by

## Andrea Shields, MD, MS
Principal Investigator, Associate Professor, University of Connecticut Health Center, Farmington, Connecticut

## Jacqueline Vidosh, MD
Co-Investigator, Assistant Professor, Department of Obstetrics and Gynecology
San Antonio Uniformed Services Health Education Consortium, San Antonio, Texas

## Laurie Kavanagh, MPH
Program Manager, Seattle, Washington

## Peter Nielsen, MD, MSS
Co-Investigator, Professor, Department of Obstetrics and Gynecology
University of Texas Health Science Center at San Antonio, San Antonio, Texas

## Brook Thomson, MD
Co-Investigator, Associate Professor, Department of Obstetrics and Gynecology
University of Texas Health Science Center at San Antonio, San Antonio, Texas

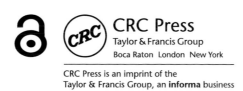

CRC Press
Taylor & Francis Group
Boca Raton London New York

CRC Press is an imprint of the
Taylor & Francis Group, an **informa** business

Designed cover image: OBLS Logo

First edition published 2024
by CRC Press
6000 Broken Sound Parkway NW, Suite 300, Boca Raton, FL 33487–2742

and by CRC Press
4 Park Square, Milton Park, Abingdon, Oxon, OX14 4RN

*CRC Press is an imprint of Taylor & Francis Group, LLC*

ISBN: 9781032289533 (hbk)
ISBN: 9781032289519 (pbk)
ISBN: 9781003299288 (ebk)

DOI: 10.1201/9781003299288

This manual is dedicated to all pregnant and postpartum people
who died from maternal cardiac arrest and Noah.

# Contents

*Acknowledgments*                                                                                    xi

**Obstetric Life Support Course Overview**                                                            1
0.1     Course Description                                                                            1
0.2     Course Objectives                                                                             1
0.3     Course Design                                                                                 2
0.4     Course Prerequisites                                                                          2
0.5     Successful Course Completion Requirement                                                      2
0.6     Course Materials                                                                              3
0.7     Manual Organization                                                                           3
0.8     Terminology                                                                                   3
0.9     Highlighted Boxes                                                                             3
0.10    OBLS Algorithms, Cognitive Aids, and Checklists                                               3

1  **Background on Maternal Cardiac Arrest**                                                          6
1.1     Introduction                                                                                  6
1.2     Learning Objectives                                                                           6
1.3     Maternal Mortality                                                                            6
1.4     Epidemiology of Maternal Cardiac Arrest                                                       8
1.5     The Role of Bias                                                                              9
1.6     Preventing Maternal Cardiac Arrest                                                           10
1.7     Planning and Preparation                                                                     11
Chapter 1. Practice Questions                                                                        12
Chapter 1. Answers                                                                                   13
Chapter 1. References                                                                                13

2  **Anatomic and Physiologic Adaptations of Pregnancy**                                             15
2.1     Introduction                                                                                 15
2.2     Learning Objectives                                                                          15
2.3     Cardiovascular Anatomic and Physiologic Adaptations in Pregnancy                             15
2.4     Respiratory Anatomic and Physiologic Adaptations in Pregnancy                                16
2.5     Neurophysiologic Adaptations in Pregnancy                                                    19
2.6     Hematologic Physiologic Adaptations in Pregnancy                                             20
2.7     Gastrointestinal Anatomic and Physiologic Adaptations in Pregnancy                           21
2.8     Genitourinary Anatomic and Physiologic Adaptations in Pregnancy                              21
2.9     Anatomic and Physiologic Impact on Medications in Pregnancy                                  22
2.10    Endocrine Anatomic and Physiologic Adaptations in Pregnancy                                  23
2.11    Immune System Adaptations in Pregnancy                                                       23
Chapter 2. Practice Questions                                                                        24
Chapter 2. Answers                                                                                   25
Chapter 2. References                                                                                25

3  **Prevention of Maternal Cardiac Arrest**                                                         27
3.1     Introduction                                                                                 27
3.2     Learning Objectives                                                                          27
3.3     Obstetric Early Warning Systems                                                              29
3.4     Institutional Planning for Critically Ill Pregnant and Postpartum Patients                   33
3.5     Communication                                                                                33
Chapter 3. Practice Questions                                                                        35

Chapter 3. Answers                                                                                    36
Chapter 3. References                                                                                 36

**4  Common Causes of Maternal Cardiac Arrest**                                                       **37**
4.1    Introduction                                                                                   37
4.2    Learning Objectives                                                                            37
4.3    BAACC TO LIFE: Bleeding                                                                        37
4.4    BAACC TO LIFE: Anesthesia                                                                      40
4.5    BAACC TO LIFE: Amniotic Fluid Embolism                                                         40
4.6    BAACC TO LIFE: Cardiovascular                                                                  43
4.7    BAACC TO LIFE: Peripartum Cardiomyopathy                                                       43
4.8    BAACC to LIFE: Clot/Cerebrovascular Pulmonary Embolism                                         44
4.9    BAACC TO LIFE: Trauma                                                                          47
4.10   BAACC TO LIFE: Overdose                                                                        48
4.11   BAACC TO LIFE: Acute Lung Injury/Acute Respiratory Distress                                    50
4.12   BAACC TO LIFE: Ions (Glucose, K⁺)                                                              51
4.13   BAACC TO LIFE: Fever                                                                           52
4.14   BAACC TO LIFE: Emergency Hypertension/Eclampsia                                                54
Chapter 4. Practice Questions                                                                         56
Chapter 4. Answers                                                                                    56
Chapter 4. References                                                                                 57

**5  Review of Cardiopulmonary Resuscitation Modifications for Pregnant Patients
in Basic Life Support**                                                                               **59**
5.1    Introduction                                                                                   59
5.2    Learning Objectives                                                                            59
5.3    Review of Basic Life Support                                                                   59
5.4    Basic Life Support Changes in Pregnancy                                                        61
5.5    Chest Compressions and Ventilation                                                             61
5.6    Automated Chest Compression Devices                                                            62
5.7    Defibrillation                                                                                 62
5.8    Left Uterine Displacement                                                                      62
5.9    Basic Life Support in the Reproductive-Age Female with Unknown Pregnancy Status                64
5.10   Vascular Access                                                                                64
5.11   Point-of-Care Ultrasound                                                                       64
Chapter 5. Practice Questions                                                                         67
Chapter 5. Answers                                                                                    68
Chapter 5. References                                                                                 68

**6  Review of Cardiopulmonary Resuscitation Modifications for Pregnant Patients in Advanced
Cardiac Life Support and Advanced Life Support**                                                      **69**
6.1    Introduction                                                                                   69
6.2    Learning Objectives                                                                            69
6.3    Review of Advanced Cardiac Life Support                                                        69
6.4    Interpretation of Cardiac Rhythms                                                              72
6.5    Shockable Rhythms: Ventricular Fibrillation and Pulseless Ventricular Tachycardia              72
6.6    Refractory Ventricular Fibrillation and Ventricular Tachycardia                                74
6.7    Nonshockable Rhythms: Pulseless Electrical Activity and Asystole                               74
6.8    Differential Diagnosis                                                                         75
6.9    Advanced Cardiac Life Support Changes in Pregnancy                                             75
6.10   Obstetric Life Support Cognitive Aid                                                           76
6.11   Airway Management: Basic                                                                       76
6.12   Airway Management: Advanced                                                                    76
6.13   Anti-Arrhythmic Drugs                                                                          78
6.14   Fetal Monitoring                                                                               78
6.15   Resuscitative Cesarean Delivery                                                                78
6.16   Vaginal Delivery                                                                               78

6.17    Factors That Could Decrease the Effectiveness of Advanced Cardiac Life Support and
         Cardiopulmonary Resuscitation in Pregnancy                                              79
6.18    Maternal Cardiac Arrest Team                                                             79
Chapter 6. Practice Questions                                                                    81
Chapter 6. Answers                                                                               82
Chapter 6. References                                                                            82

**7  Special Procedures in Obstetric Life Support**                                              **83**
7.1    Introduction                                                                              83
7.2    Learning Objectives                                                                       83
7.3    Resuscitative Cesarean Delivery                                                           83
7.4    OBLS in a Low-Resource Setting                                                            89
7.5    Point-of-Care Ultrasound                                                                  89
7.6    Obesity and Maternal Cardiac Arrest                                                       93
7.7    Extracorporeal Cardiopulmonary Resuscitation                                              94
7.8    Transport and Emergency Medical Staff Providers                                           95
Chapter 7. Practice Questions                                                                    96
Chapter 7. Answers                                                                               97
Chapter 7. References                                                                            97

**8  Traumatic Maternal Cardiac Arrest**                                                         **99**
8.1    Introduction                                                                              99
8.2    Learning Objectives                                                                       99
8.3    Traumatic Cardiac Arrest Review                                                           99
8.4    Approach to Reproductive-Age Females with Cardiac Arrest in Association with Trauma       100
Chapter 8. Practice Questions                                                                    104
Chapter 8. Answers                                                                               104
Chapter 8. Reference                                                                             105

**9  Postpartum Cardiac Arrest**                                                                 **106**
9.1    Introduction                                                                              106
9.2    Learning Objectives                                                                       106
9.3    Causes of Postpartum Maternal Cardiac Arrest                                              106
9.4    Management of Postpartum Cardiac Arrest by Cause                                          107
Chapter 9. Practice Questions                                                                    116
Chapter 9. Answers                                                                               117
Chapter 9. References                                                                            118

**10  Maternal Stroke and Acute Cerebrovascular Disease**                                        **120**
10.1    Introduction                                                                             120
10.2    Learning Objectives                                                                      120
10.3    Timing                                                                                   123
10.4    Recognizing Warning Signs and Symptoms of Maternal Stroke                                123
10.5    Out-of-Hospital Evaluation and Transport of Maternal Stroke                              124
10.6    Obstetric Stroke Protocol                                                                127
10.7    Maternal Stroke Team Composition                                                         128
10.8    Stroke Code                                                                              129
10.9    Intracranial Hemorrhage                                                                  133
10.10   Subarachnoid Hemorrhage                                                                  133
10.11   Reversal of Coagulopathy in Intracranial Hemorrhage and Subarachnoid Hemorrhage         133
10.12   Elevated Intracranial Pressure in Intracranial Hemorrhage and Subarachnoid Hemorrhage   134
10.13   Delivery in Intracranial Hemorrhage and Subarachnoid Hemorrhage                          134
10.14   Post-Stroke Care                                                                         135
10.15   Cerebral Venous Sinus Thrombosis                                                         137
Chapter 10. Practice Questions                                                                   138
Chapter 10. Answers                                                                              138
Chapter 10. References                                                                           139

**11  Post-Arrest Care**                                                                                      **140**
    11.1   Introduction                                                                                      140
    11.2   Learning Objectives                                                                               140
    11.3   Importance of Post-Arrest Care                                                                    140
    11.4   Standard Post-Return of Spontaneous Circulation Checklist after Maternal Cardiac Arrest           141
    11.5   <u>A</u>irway                                                                                     141
    11.6   <u>B</u>reathing                                                                                  141
    11.7   <u>C</u>irculation                                                                                141
    11.8   <u>D</u>isability                                                                                 142
    11.9   <u>E</u>xtracorporeal Cardiopulmonary Resuscitation                                               144
    11.10  <u>E</u>tiology                                                                                   144
    11.11  <u>F</u>etus                                                                                      144
    11.12  <u>G</u>ather                                                                                     145
    11.13  <u>H</u>ead                                                                                       145
    11.14  When to Cease Resuscitation Efforts                                                               146
    11.15  Determination of Death and Organ Procurement                                                      149
    Chapter 11. Practice Questions                                                                           150
    Chapter 11. Answers                                                                                      151
    Chapter 11. References                                                                                   151

**12  Communication during Maternal Cardiac Arrest**                                                          **154**
    12.1   Introduction                                                                                      154
    12.2   Learning Objectives                                                                               154
    12.3   Guiding Principles of Team-Based Care                                                             154
    12.4   Maternal Cardiac Arrest Team Structure                                                            156
    12.5   Situation, Background, Assessment, and Recommendation/Request                                     157
    12.6   Call-Outs                                                                                         157
    12.7   Check-Backs                                                                                       158
    12.8   Situation-Background-Assessment-Recommendation and Call-Outs for the Maternal Team
           Entering a Maternal Cardiac Arrest Event—The 5A's                                                 158
    12.9   Communication of Maternal Cardiac Arrest and Outcomes to the Family                               159
    12.10  Debriefing the Team after Maternal Cardiac Arrest                                                 161
    Chapter 12. Practice Questions                                                                           163
    Chapter 12. Answers                                                                                      164
    Chapter 12. References                                                                                   164

**13  Putting It All Together**                                                                               **165**
    13.1   Introduction                                                                                      165
    13.2   Scenario One                                                                                      165
    13.3   Scenario Two                                                                                      168
    13.4   Scenario Three                                                                                    170
    13.5   Scenario Four                                                                                     170
    Chapter 13. Reference                                                                                    172

Appendix A:  *Abbreviations*                                                                                 173
Appendix B:  *OBLS Mnemonics*                                                                                175
Appendix C:  *Resources*                                                                                     176
Appendix D:  *American Heart Association Opioid-Associated Emergency Algorithm for Healthcare Providers*      177
Appendix E:  *Post-ROSC Care Checklist IH*                                                                   178
Appendix F:  *Post-ROSC Care Checklist OH*                                                                   180
Appendix G:  *Venous Thromboembolism Prophylaxis Following Stroke*                                           181
Appendix H:  *Megacode Checklist OH Basic*                                                                   182
Appendix I:   *Megacode Checklist OH Advanced*                                                               184
Appendix J:  *Megacode Checklist IH*                                                                         186
Appendix K:  *Institutional Preparedness*                                                                    188
Appendix L:  *OBLS Drug List*                                                                                189

# Acknowledgments

*Obstetric Life Support* (OBLS) is made possible, and this project was funded by a generous grant from the Agency for Healthcare Research and Quality (AHRQ), U.S. Department of Health and Human Services (HHS). The editors and authors are solely responsible for this document's contents, findings, and conclusions, which do not necessarily represent the views of AHRQ. Readers should not interpret any statement in this report as an official position of AHRQ or of HHS. None of the editors or authors has any affiliation or financial involvement that conflicts with the material presented in this report.

Thank you to our main chapter author(s) who contributed their time and expertise to the manual:

Overview: *Laurie Kavanagh, Andrea Shields*; Chapter 1: *Lissa Melvin*; Chapter 2: *Peter Nielsen, Brook Thomson;* Chapter 3: *Andrea Shields;* Chapter 4: *Andrea Shields, Jacqueline Vidosh;* Chapter 5: *Jacqueline Vidosh;* Chapter 6: *Jacqueline Vidosh;* Chapter 7: *Andrea Shields;* Chapter 8: *Andrea Shields;* Chapter 9: *Jacqueline Vidosh;* Chapter 10: *Eliza Miller, Kara Shetler;* Chapter 11: *Jacqueline Vidosh;* Chapter 12: *Peter Nielsen;* Chapter 13: *Jacqueline Vidosh.* Thank you to the other content contributors: *Viviana de Assis, James Hill, Monica Lutgendorf, and Irene Stafford.*

Thanks to our expert panel members who graciously contributed their time and knowledge to this project:

*Elumalai Appachi, MBBS,* Baylor College of Medicine
*Julie Arafeh, RN, MSN,* Clinical Concepts in Obstetrics; Stanford School of Medicine, Department of Pediatrics, Division of Neonatal Medicine
*Les R. Becker, PhD, MS.MEdL, NRP, CHSE,* MedStar Institute for Innovation, MedStar Health and Georgetown University School of Medicine
*Utpal Bhalala, MD,* Driscoll Children's Hospital
*Rebecca Cypher, MSN, PNNP,* Maternal Fetal Solutions
*Shad Deering, MD,* Children's Hospital of San Antonio, CHRISTUS Health
*Sondie Epley, RN,* University of Texas Health Science Center at San Antonio
*Mary Ann Faucher, PhD, CNM, MPH,* Parkland Health and Hospital System
*Afshan Hameed, MD,* University of California, Irvine
*Heidi King, MS, FACHE, BCC, CMC, CPPS,* Uniformed Service University Department of Medicine Defense Health Agency
*Miranda Klassen,* Amniotic Fluid Embolism Foundation
*Monica Lutgendorf, MD,* Uniformed Services University of the Health Sciences
*David Markenson, MD,* American Red Cross

*Lissa Melvin, MD,* Baylor College of Medicine
*Eliza C. Miller, MD,* Columbia University
*Charles Minard, PhD,* Baylor College of Medicine
*Joshua Monson, MD,* Uniformed Services University of the Health Sciences
*Vincent N. Mosesso, Jr., MD, PHP,* University of Pittsburgh School of Medicine
*DeWayne M. Pursley, MD, MPH,* Harvard Medical Faculty Physicians at Beth Israel Deaconess Medical Center
*Jeffrey Quinlin, MD,* Roy J. and Lucille A. Carver College of Medicine, University of Iowa
*Stephen Rahm, NRP,* Centre for Emergency Health Sciences
*Carl Rose, MD,* Mayo Clinic
*P. James A. Ruiter, MD, MCFP*
*Cheryl K. Roth, PhD, WHNP-BC, RNC-OB, RN,* HonorHealth Scottsdale Shea & Osborn
*Brian Schaeffer,* International Association of Fire Chiefs
*Amir Shamshirsaz MD,* Baylor College of Medicine
*Paloma Toledo, MD, MPH,* Miller School of Medicine, University of Miami
*Fernando Stein, MD,* Texas Children's Hospital
*Carolyn Zelop, MD,* American Heart Association

Thank you to Stanford University for allowing use of "Obstetric Life Support," the American Heart Association for volunteering their algorithms, Laurie Kavanagh for her assistance with creating OBLS Figures 10.2, 10.6, 10.7, 12.2 and helping to draft our algorithms, Dr. Shad Deering for his assistance in developing the megacode checklists, and Elizabeth N. Weissbrod and Andrea McCulley for their drawings.

Many thanks to our partners—Baylor College of Medicine, the Children's Hospital of San Antonio, and Laerdal Medical—for collaborating with the OBLS team to create this product.

# Obstetric Life Support Course Overview

## 0.1 COURSE DESCRIPTION

The Obstetric Life Support (OBLS) course has been created for all healthcare providers who may encounter and participate in the management of maternal cardiopulmonary arrest or similar emergencies. Such personnel range from obstetricians and gynecologists (OB/GYNs), to emergency department (ED) providers, critical care providers, nurses, midwives, anesthesia providers, and all levels of emergency medical services (EMS) providers.

There are two broad areas of applicability of the OBLS course: in-hospital (IH) and out-of-hospital (OH). The IH applies to providers who care for pregnant people in clinics, urgent care and ED settings, and inpatient wards. The OH applies to EMS providers and has two arms: Advanced and Basic. Advanced OH OBLS is recommended for EMS providers who are required to be certified in Advanced Cardiac Life Support (ACLS).

The goal of this course is to improve maternal-fetal outcomes in the setting of maternal cardiac arrest (MCA) by increasing provider awareness and practice using the techniques specific to maternal cardiac arrest. By the end of this course, the learner will have improved knowledge of the unique modifications to Basic Life Support (BLS) and ACLS in pregnancy and will be better prepared to treat pregnant people in cardiac arrest.

## 0.2 COURSE OBJECTIVES

Upon completion of OBLS, learners should be able to do the following:

- Understand how to apply the differences in pregnancy-related changes to physiology and anatomy to the performance of BLS and ACLS during MCA.
- Demonstrate how to recognize pending cardiopulmonary arrest in the pregnant and postpartum patient by applying one of the early warning sign algorithms for pregnancy.
- Demonstrate effective OBLS with an emphasis on effective chest compressions with early activation of left uterine displacement (LUD) and automated external defibrillator (AED) use as indicated.
- In the setting of cardiac arrest in reproductive-age people (pregnancy status unknown), efficiently apply point-of-care ultrasound (POC-US), where applicable, to diagnose possible pregnancy and initiate required BLS/ACLS changes quickly and effectively.
- Efficiently apply pregnancy-specific changes to the ACLS algorithm, with an emphasis on early resuscitative cesarean delivery (RCD) within 5 minutes of arrest if pregnancy is suspected to be greater than 20 weeks or at the level of the maternal umbilicus and initial round of cardiopulmonary resuscitation (CPR) is ineffective at return of spontaneous circulation (ROSC).
- Apply unique modifications to the primary survey in a person of reproductive age undergoing trauma.
- Initiate immediate post-arrest care in the setting of ROSC, with special consideration to pregnancy/postpartum state.
- Consider extracorporeal cardiopulmonary resuscitation (ECPR) in those cases refractory to ROSC.
- Demonstrate clear and effective team communication using a TeamSTEPPS™ approach.
- Improve communication to the healthcare team and families in the setting of poor outcomes.
- Recognize proper disposition/transfer of care for a pregnant patient in cardiopulmonary arrest.
- Recognize and treat possible reversible causes of MCA.

DOI: 10.1201/9781003299288-1

# 0.3 COURSE DESIGN

## 0.3.1 Pre-Work

**Self-paced learning** using the OBLS Manual for personal study. Each chapter has practice questions to reinforce the learner's knowledge and skills.

## 0.3.2 OBLS Entry Exam

Learners are required to take and pass an entry exam covering the material in this manual. OBLS used an Angoff method to set the minimum passing scores for OH Basic, OH Advanced, and IH participants to ensure mastery of pre-work before the in-person training. A group of subject matter experts examined each question and predicted how many minimally qualified candidates would answer the question correctly. This method ensures that the passing grade of each of the three OBLS tracks is verifiable and determined empirically.

## 0.3.3 Instructor-Led, In-Person Course

Learners will participate in small-group, simulation-based course building on the foundations of OBLS learned in the pre-work. Instructors will lead groups in **rapid-cycle deliberate practice** on

- Team communication and dynamics management
- Leading and managing MCA
- Techniques such as chest compressions on a pregnant patient, LUD, and RCD
- Cardiac rhythm interpretation and vital sign management
- Application of ACLS drugs
- Debriefing for critical events
- Sharing difficult or serious news following MCA

Each scenario will take learners through situations they are going to experience when performing the OBLS Megacode. For both group practice and graded megacode, instructors will use a detailed scoring checklist as an objective grading system to ensure that learners have performed core concepts. Each concept is linked to a point system yielding a grade for each, and pass/fail criteria are based on this grade. Using this checklist helps to eliminate instructor subjectivity and provides a permanent record of the learner's performance.

## 0.3.4 Graded OBLS Megacode

Instructors will test each learner in how well they manage an OBLS megacode scenario. Learners may find the megacode checklists by which instructors will test them in Appendices H, I, and J.

# 0.4 COURSE PREREQUISITES

Learners must be proficient in BLS skills before taking OBLS; a basic understanding of ACLS is beneficial but not required.

The OBLS course does not review ACLS pharmacology or teach how to interpret cardiac rhythms. Learners may improve these skills by visiting the American Heart Association at www.aha.org.

# 0.5 SUCCESSFUL COURSE COMPLETION REQUIREMENT

To complete OBLS, the learner must complete and pass both a competency test based on the OBLS Manual and a team leader assessment during the in-person training megacode.

## 0.6 COURSE MATERIALS

Course materials include the OBLS Manual, the OBLS student website (www.obls.org), algorithms, cognitive aids, and checklists.

## 0.7 MANUAL ORGANIZATION

This manual provides an overview of the physiology and anatomy of pregnant patients, with each chapter building on the previous one. The physiology and anatomy of pregnant patients are drastically different from nonpregnant patients. Consequently, OBLS teaches how to modify BLS and ACLS in the setting of MCA. Understanding the impact of pregnancy on anatomy and physiology empowers providers to improve care and outcomes for their patients. The manual also highlights the common causes of MCA and introduces special procedures and effective team communication during MCA.

OBLS tools including the ALIVE @ 5™ Cognitive Aid, BAACC TO LIFE™ mnemonic, and the OBLS Master Algorithm are located following this introductory section. These aids are meant to accompany the learner throughout the course to remind the learner that many simultaneous steps must occur within the first 5 minutes of a maternal cardiac arrest. They also trigger a differential for causes of the arrest. This course does not include comprehensive treatment plans for each common cause of maternal cardiac arrest. It introduces them so that learners may improve overall resuscitation efforts by developing and considering differential diagnoses early in the case management.

## 0.8 TERMINOLOGY

- Abbreviations and acronyms are spelled out upon their first use per chapter, followed by an abbreviation in parentheses. See Appendix A for a full list of abbreviations and acronyms.
- See Appendix B for a list of mnemonics.
- Gender-neutral language:
  - In recognition of a nonbinary gender spectrum, we have incorporated gender-neutral language where appropriate, including using the term "patient" and the singular "they" instead of "he" or "she."
  - We continue to use gender-specific language to report most research and legal decisions.
- OBLS uses the term "resuscitative cesarean delivery" (RCD) instead of the previously common term "perimortem cesarean delivery" as it more accurately describes the procedure including the delivery of the fetus. See Chapter 7.

## 0.9 HIGHLIGHTED BOXES

OBLS highlights key concepts and differences critical to the success of the OBLS techniques with the following colors:

- **Key points** are denoted in purple. These focus on the critical knowledge and skills and their practical applications to successfully manage a maternal cardiac arrest.
- **Case vignettes** are in orange and allow the learner an opportunity to apply the concepts learned during the chapter.
- **Putting it all together** are in gray. These show how the OB-specific techniques work with each other to improve the efficient application of OBLS algorithms.

## 0.10 OBLS ALGORITHMS, COGNITIVE AIDS, AND CHECKLISTS

These quick-reference guides aid the proper application of OBLS and develop differential diagnoses for the causes of arrest and post-arrest care steps.

Following are algorithms, aids, and checklists with their corresponding manual location(s):

- ALIVE @ 5® Cognitive Aid (page after Introduction, and Chapter 6, Figure 6.8)
- BAACC TO LIFE™ Mnemonic (page after Introduction, and Chapter 4, Figure 4.1)
- OBLS Master Algorithm (page after Introduction, and Chapter 5, Figure 5.7)
- OBLS Algorithm with Modification of CPR, pregnancy known ≥20 weeks and unknown (Chapter 5, Figure 5.6)
- Traumatic Maternal Cardiac Arrest Algorithm (Chapter 8, Figure 8.1)
- Post-ROSC Checklist (Appendices E and F)
- ALIVE @ 5 Maternal Cardiac Arrest Debrief Tool (Chapter 12, Figure 12.5)
- SPIKES Protocol for Sharing Difficult or Serious News (Chapter 12, Figure 12.4)

Use the aids on the following pages as references while you complete your pre-work.

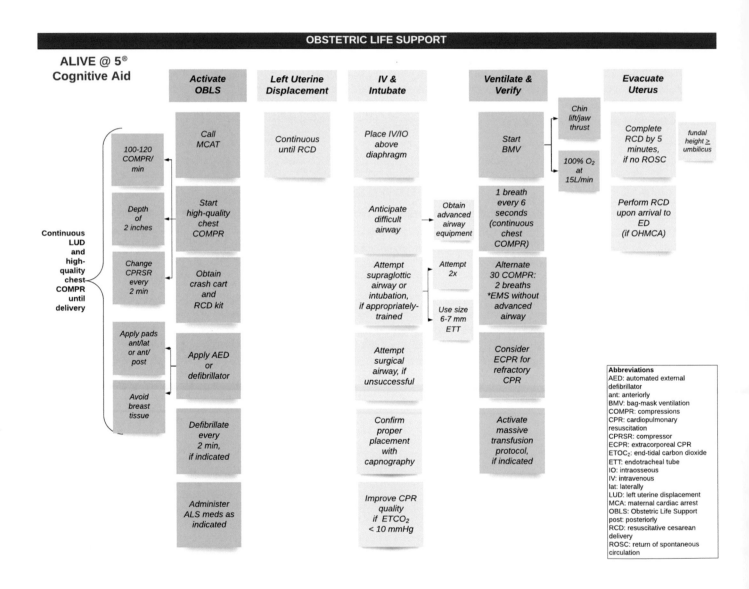

**BAACC**

**B**leeding

**A**nesthesia

**A**FE

**C**ardiovascular/cardiomyopathy

**C**lot/cerebrovascular

**TO**

**T**rauma

**O**verdose (magnesium sulfate/opioids/other)

**LIFE**

**L**ung injury/ARDS

**I**ons (glucose/K+)

**F**ever (sepsis)

**E**mergency hypertension/eclampsia

## OBSTETRIC LIFE SUPPORT

**Unconscious female, reproductive age.**
**No pulse, no or agonal breathing**
**OBLS should be done simultaneously with ongoing, high-quality CPR**

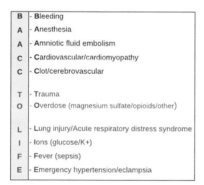

**Abbreviations**
ALS - Advanced Life Support
BDP - biparietal diameter
CPR - cardiopulmonary resuscitation
EGA - estimated gestational age
FL - femur length
LUD - left uterine displacement
OBLS - Obstetric Life Support
POC-US - point-of-care ultrasound
RCD - resuscitative cesarean delivery
ROSC - return of spontaneous circulation

| | |
|---|---|
| **B** | - Bleeding |
| **A** | - Anesthesia |
| **A** | - Amniotic fluid embolism |
| **C** | - Cardiovascular/cardiomyopathy |
| **C** | - Clot/cerebrovascular |
| **T** | - Trauma |
| **O** | - Overdose (magnesium sulfate/opioids/other) |
| **L** | - Lung injury/Acute respiratory distress syndrome |
| **I** | - Ions (glucose/K+) |
| **F** | - Fever (sepsis) |
| **E** | - Emergency hypertension/eclampsia |

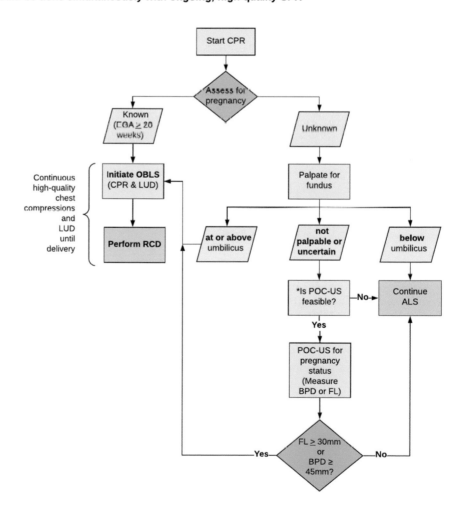

# Background on Maternal Cardiac Arrest

**1**

---

## 1.1 INTRODUCTION

---

This chapter provides the learner with a background on maternal cardiac arrest (MCA), introduces maternal mortality trends in the United States (U.S.), and discusses the epidemiology of MCA. It also discusses severe maternal mortality episodes and the importance of understanding how bias impacts patient care.

---

## 1.2 LEARNING OBJECTIVES

---

Learner will appropriately:

- Discuss the trends in pregnancy-related mortality ratio in the U.S. compared with the global maternal mortality ratio, including the leading causes of MCA and death.
- Describe the relationship between severe maternal morbidity (SMM) and maternal death, and the primary demographic risk factors for MCA and death.
- Discuss the potential role of implicit bias in reducing healthcare equity for all people.
- Describe current strategies being used to prevent MCA and death in the U.S.

---

## 1.3 MATERNAL MORTALITY

---

There has been a decreasing trend in maternal mortality for nations around the world. Although progress varies significantly by region and country, the global maternal mortality ratio decreased from 385 deaths per 100,000 live births in 1990 to 216 deaths per 100,000 live births in 2015.[1] Unlike the worldwide trend over past decades, the U.S. has seen an increase in the pregnancy-related mortality ratio (PRMR). This is an estimate of the number of pregnancy-related deaths for every 100,000 births. The PRMR is often used as an indicator of a nation's health. The Centers for Disease Control and Prevention (CDC) report that the PRMR in the U.S. has increased from 7.2 deaths per 100,000 live births in 1987 to 17.3 deaths per 100,000 live births in 2018.[2] In 2020, there were 861 reported maternal deaths in the U.S.[3] According to 2017–2019 data from the Maternal Mortality Review Committees, 80% of these deaths were determined to be preventable.[4] In 2021, there were a staggering 1,201 maternal deaths in the U.S., amounting to 33 deaths per 100,000 live births (Figure 1.1).[3] This 38% increase in maternal deaths from the previous year was largely attributed to Coronavirus Disease 2019.

Approximately 22% of maternal deaths occur antepartum, 25% on day of delivery or within 7 days after, and 53% occur between 7 days to 1 year after pregnancy.[4] Most maternal deaths within the first 7 days after delivery are due to postpartum hemorrhage, embolism, eclampsia and hypertensive disorders.[5]

Maternal mortality is a complex issue at the confluence of population health, access to healthcare, gaps in clinical care and team performance, and socioeconomic, racial, and ethnic inequalities[2–9]; each of these influencing health outcomes. Measuring pregnancy-related deaths is challenging due to incomplete and sometimes inaccurate vital statistics data.[10] The reasons for increasing PRMR in the U.S. are not entirely clear and are under investigation. An improvement in identifying deaths with the use of data linkages, changes in coding, and the addition of a pregnancy checkbox to the death certificate in 2003 may partly

DOI: 10.1201/9781003299288-2

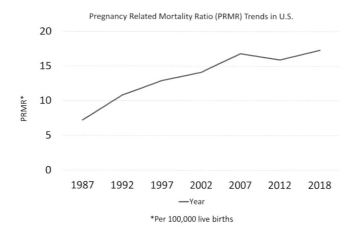

**FIGURE 1.1**   Pregnancy-related mortality ratio (PRMR) trends in the United States.

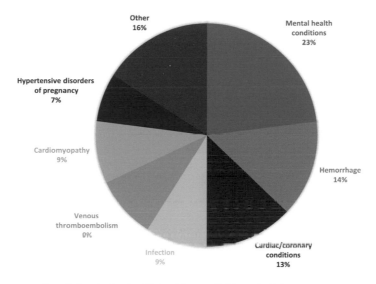

**FIGURE 1.2**   Causes of pregnancy-related deaths in the United States (2017–2019).[4]

explain the increasing numbers.[2,6,11] However, this improved system does not fully explain the rising trend.[7] The increase in chronic health conditions and obesity are likely contributing factors as well.[2,9]

The common causes of pregnancy-related deaths vary by region and patient demographics. Worldwide, hemorrhage is the number one cause for maternal mortality.[12] Causes and risk factors for pregnancy-related deaths in the U.S. have shifted over the years. Hemorrhage, hypertensive disorders, and anesthesia-related deaths have declined since 2006, while mental health and cardiovascular conditions have emerged as the leading cause of maternal mortality.[2,6,9] Cardiac and coronary conditions were the leading underlying cause of pregnancy-related deaths among non-Hispanic Black people, mental health conditions were the leading underlying cause for Hispanic and non-Hispanic White people, and hemorrhage was the leading underlying cause for non-Hispanic Asian people.[32] Based on a review of pregnancy-related deaths among AI/AN people, mental health conditions and hemorrhage were the most common underlying causes of death, accounting for 50% of deaths with a known underlying cause.[2] Other causes include amniotic fluid embolism, injury, cerebrovascular accident, cancer, metabolic/endocrine, and pulmonary conditions.[4] Figure 1.2 shows common causes of pregnancy-related death in the U.S.

**KEY POINTS**
- The PRMR in the U.S. has increased 50%, while the global maternal mortality ratio has decreased.
- Close to 1,200 people die from pregnancy-related complications each year in the U.S., and 80% of these deaths are preventable.
- Hemorrhage is the leading cause of maternal death worldwide, while cardiovascular and mental health conditions, including deaths to suicide and overdose/poisoning related to substance use disorder, have emerged as the leading causes of maternal mortality in the U.S.

# 1.4 EPIDEMIOLOGY OF MATERNAL CARDIAC ARREST

MCA occurs in one in 12,000 admissions for delivery in the U.S.[13] It is seen as the final common pathway for many critical illnesses and comorbidities similar to the ones that lead to maternal mortality, though with some key differences.[8,13] The most common potential etiology of cardiac arrest during hospitalization for delivery is hemorrhage followed by heart failure, AFE, then sepsis (Figure 1.3).[13] In contrast, the likelihood of MCA is highest for those diagnosed with AFE, followed by acute myocardial infarction, and venous thromboembolism (VTE) (Figure 1.4).[13] Heart disease, such as cardiomyopathy and cardiovascular disease, ultimately still results in the highest number of maternal mortalities.[13] Stroke is another major cause of maternal mortality, accounting for 40%–70% of deaths in people with preeclampsia, most of which are due to intracerebral hemorrhage.[14,15] Maternal survival to hospital discharge after cardiac arrest ranges from 40% to 60%, with survival depending on the underlying etiology of arrest.[8,13]

Like data for the maternal mortality ratio, there are gaps in reporting and processing data for MCA. The variation and inconsistencies of how information is collected make it challenging to assess the true prevalence of MCA. Researchers found that national databases and registries in the U.S. for out-of-hospital (OH) and in-hospital (IH) cardiac arrest did not consistently

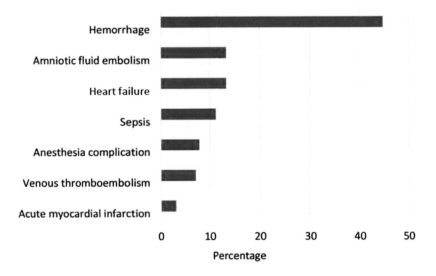

**FIGURE 1.3**   Proximate potential etiologies of maternal cardiac arrest during hospitalization for delivery in the United States (1998–2011).

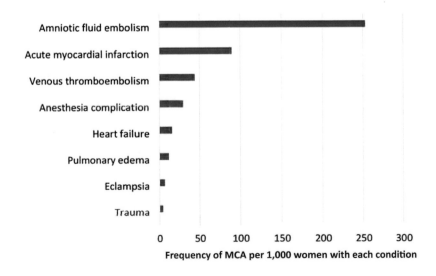

**FIGURE 1.4**   Cause-specific MCA frequency (per 1,000 women) during hospitalization for delivery in the United States (1998–2011).

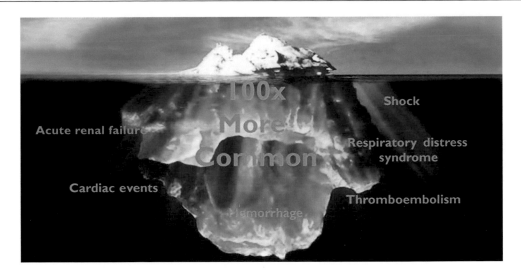

**FIGURE 1.5** Severe maternal morbidity iceberg.

account for pregnancy and the postpartum period.[16] These examples highlight the need for a mandatory national database for MCA.[7,16] Standardization and inclusion of pregnancy and postpartum status will better allow policymakers to assess trends, performance, and outcomes,[16,17] ultimately increasing survival and quality of life.

With rising rates of obesity, chronic diseases, and cesarean sections, SMM rates also increase.[18–20] Compared to MCA and death, it is necessary to highlight that SMM cases are far more common. Maternal deaths have been described as the "tip of the iceberg" with SMM the "rest of the iceberg"[20] below the surface (Figure 1.5). **For every maternal death, there are approximately 100 episodes of SMM each year.**[19] Many causes of SMM, including stroke and peripartum cardiomyopathy, may result in long-term permanent disability. This underscores the importance of systematic approaches to understand and prevent severe maternal morbidity.

**KEY POINTS**
- MCA is the final common pathway for many critical illnesses and comorbidities, like the ones that lead to maternal mortality.
- Hemorrhage is the most common potential etiology of cardiac arrest during hospitalization for delivery.
- AFE is the diagnosis most frequently complicated by cardiac arrest.
- For every maternal death, there are approximately 100 episodes of severe maternal morbidity scenarios each year.

# 1.5 THE ROLE OF BIAS

The lived experience of racism for specific racial and ethnic groups is a significant risk factor for maternal mortality and SMM. In the U.S., racial and ethnic disparities have persisted for decades and remain a national issue.[6,21–23] According to the CDC's Pregnancy-Related Mortality Surveillance System for 2016–2018, maternal mortality in the U.S. was more than three times higher in non-Hispanic Black (Black) people and almost two times higher in American Indian/Alaska Native (AI/AN) people when compared to non-Hispanic White (White) or Hispanic people (Figure 1.6).[2] This disparity increases with maternal age. Black and AI/AN people 30 years or older had a four to five times greater mortality compared to White, Hispanic, and Asian/Pacific Islander (A/PI) people, with the highest risk of maternal death seen in Black people aged 40 years or older. Higher socio-economic status and a greater level of education do not help to improve outcomes for Black people (data not available for AI/AN people). The PRMR for Black people with a college education or higher is more than three to five times greater than their White counterparts. And Black people with a college education or higher are two to three times as likely to die compared to White, Hispanic, and A/PI people who have less than a high school education.[21,22]

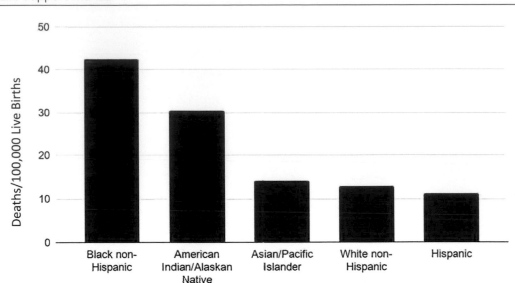

**FIGURE 1.6**    Deaths per live births by race/ethnicity.

Health disparities exist due to a complex interaction of components that occurs on many levels. Key factors include the patient/family (such as socioeconomic status, beliefs, biology, genetics), healthcare provider, clinical encounter, facility, community, and the healthcare system (including health insurance, distance from care, delivering hospital, and payment factors).[21–24]

Equally significant components contributing to healthcare disparities include social determinants of health, a deep-rooted history of injustice and discrimination, and the role of implicit bias.[23–25] Racial and ethnic disparities occur in many areas of American life, including healthcare.

Implicit bias refers to the attitudes and stereotypes that affect our understanding, actions, and decisions in an unconscious manner.[25] These actions are contrary to our stated conscious beliefs and are involuntary. They can lead to unequal treatment of patients based on race, ethnicity, sexual orientation, weight, language, income, and insurance status.

Implicit bias can perpetuate disparities and can directly lead to patient harm.[25] In times of stress and cognitive overload, memory is biased toward information that is consistent with stereotypes. Thus, the potential influence of implicit bias is especially pertinent in busy and stressful settings, such as in the field, emergency department (ED), or labor and delivery units.

---

**KEY POINTS**

- The lived experience of racism for specific racial and ethnic groups is a significant risk factor for maternal mortality and SMM.
- Black people are about three times, and AI/AN people are nearly two times, as likely as White people to die from a pregnancy-related cause.
- The highest risk of maternal death is seen in Black people 40 years of age or older.
- Implicit bias can lead to unequal treatment of patients based on race, ethnicity, sexual orientation, weight, language, income, and insurance status.

---

# 1.6 PREVENTING MATERNAL CARDIAC ARREST

Maternal morbidity and mortality are multifaceted issues. Therefore, actions to catalyze change must occur on multiple levels. Collaborative efforts should include the community, health facilities, patients and families, healthcare providers, and health systems.[26]

Comprehensive and systematic data collection is paramount when studying maternal deaths and near-death scenarios to understand how to prevent them. State-level maternal mortality review committees review cases of maternal deaths, outline contributing factors, and determine strategies to help avoid poor outcomes.[26] However, these valuable committees are not in all states and data collection is not consistent. Thus, an infrastructure for systematically assessing maternal deaths is needed. In December 2018, the U.S. Congress signed into law the Preventing Maternal Deaths Act (HR 1318). This legislation established and supports state Maternal Mortality Review Committees to review every pregnancy-related death and develop recommendations to prevent maternal deaths through federal funding and reporting of standardized data.[27]

To improve maternal outcomes, healthcare providers have implemented and are using a variety of practices and strategies, including improved education, early warning systems, team and simulation training, and the use of standardized protocols. The Alliance for Innovation on Maternal Health (AIM)[28] has provided sets of bundled guidance to provide standardized management of obstetric emergencies to improve safety in maternity care. The California Maternal Quality Care Collaborative (CMQCC) is an excellent example of the successful use of toolkits. These compendiums include best practice tools and articles, care guidelines, hospital-level implementation guide, and professional education slide sets. The aim of the toolkits is to improve the response to leading causes of preventable death among pregnant and postpartum people. The CMQCC has used data-driven, large-scale quality improvement projects that have resulted in a 58% decrease in maternal death between 2008 to 2016 (bringing deaths down to 5.9 per 100,000 live births) at a time when the U.S. continued to see an increase in maternal deaths.[29]

Outcomes are improved when patients at high risk deliver at hospitals that can appropriately care for them. Professional organizations have developed criteria for recommended Levels of Maternal Care (LoMC) for facilities to reduce maternal morbidity and mortality.[18] Additionally, recommendations and systems exist for the improvement of postpartum care and addressing critical factors, such as assistance with transitioning to a primary care physician or specialist, continued insurance coverage, and addressing the social factors that may limit access to care.[27] Last, while it is often uncomfortable for providers to accept and confront, prejudice and stereotyping exist in healthcare and contribute to the disproportionate outcomes seen in racial and ethnic minority individuals. In a step toward creating more significant health equity, the Alliance for Innovation on Maternal Health created a "Reduction of Peripartum Racial/Ethnic Disparity" bundle for healthcare providers and systems. This patient safety bundle offers insights into racial and ethnic disparities and mechanisms for safe and equitable healthcare. Recommendations include staff-wide education on implicit bias, training on the causes of racial and ethnic disparities, best practices for shared decision-making, and building of a culture of equity.[28]

**KEY POINTS**

- Comprehensive and systematic ways to collect data are paramount when studying maternal deaths and near-death scenarios to understand how to prevent them.
- The Preventing Maternal Deaths Act established and supports state Maternal Mortality Review Committees to review every pregnancy-related death and develop recommendations to prevent maternal deaths through federal funding and reporting of standardized data.
- A variety of practices and strategies, such as improved education, early warning systems, team and simulation training, and the use of protocols, have been implemented and are being used by providers to improve maternal outcomes.
- Safe and equitable healthcare for all includes staff-wide education on implicit bias, education on the causes of racial and ethnic disparities, best practices for shared decision-making, and building of a culture of equity.

## 1.7 PLANNING AND PREPARATION

The American Heart Association uses the Chain of Survival (Figure 1.7) to highlight the important steps that ultimately lead to successful resuscitation, and these can be applied to both the pre- and in-hospital settings. Although there is a high risk of maternal mortality after cardiac arrest, survival to hospital discharge for pregnant patients with IH cardiac arrest is higher when compared to nonobstetric populations. This higher survival rate may be due to different clinical risk factors between the two groups and/or differences in patient monitoring among hospital units.[13] Alternatively, this finding may illustrate that many arrests are reversible, representing an opportunity to optimize maternal survival with collaborative provider training and enhanced institutional preparation.[7] EMS providers play a crucial role given the potential for patient deterioration en route to the hospital. Additionally, most postpartum deaths occur more than 7 days after delivery, a time when most patients have been discharged from the hospital.[5]

It is challenging to maintain the skills and knowledge for extremely high-risk but rare events. Managing MCA demands simultaneous coordination of appropriate interventions, teamwork, clear communication, and confidence. Team practice is

**IHCA**

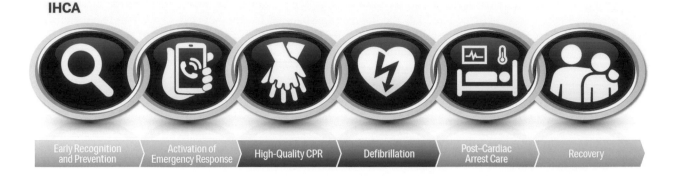

**OHCA**

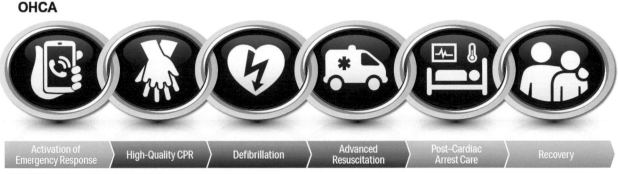

© 2020 American Heart Association

**FIGURE 1.7**   The American Heart Association Chain of Survival. Abbreviations: IHCA, in-hospital cardiac arrest; OHCA, out-of-hospital cardiac arrest.

necessary to reach this goal. Research shows that simulation is a valuable tool to educate providers in managing obstetric emergencies by improving competency in emergency decision-making, leadership skills, and individual and team performance. Specifically, simulation improves response time to starting cardiopulmonary resuscitation (CPR) and resuscitative cesarean delivery (RCD), airway management, better adherence to ACLS protocols, left uterine displacement (LUD), and identifying causes of arrest.[7,30] Additionally, simulation helps practitioners recognize local barriers, receive feedback, and correct mistakes in a nonthreatening environment.[31]

Regardless of the complex interplay of the many factors that exist for each maternal death, MCA is the final common pathway and represents the dividing line between survival and death.[7] OBLS recommends that all practitioners be prepared to respond and manage pregnant and postpartum patients who experience cardiac arrest.

**KEY POINTS**
- Survival to hospital discharge for pregnant populations with IH cardiac arrest is higher compared to non-obstetric populations.
- Team practice through simulation can help with simultaneous coordination of knowledge, teamwork, clear communication, and confidence when responding to an MCA.
- Simulation improves response time to starting CPR and RCD, airway management, better adherence to ALS protocols, LUD, and identifying the causes of arrest.

# CHAPTER 1. PRACTICE QUESTIONS

1. How many severe maternal morbidity cases occur for every maternal death in the U.S. each year?
   A. 10
   B. 50
   C. 100
   D. 200

2. Which racial/ethnic group has the highest risk of maternal death in the U.S.?
   A. Non-Hispanic Black (Black)
   B. Hispanic
   C. Native American
   D. White

3. According to the CDC, how many pregnancy-related deaths are preventable?
   A. 10%
   B. 25%
   C. 50%
   D. 80%

4. Since the 1980s, which cause of pregnancy-related death has been increasing over time?
   A. Hemorrhage
   B. Venous thromboembolism
   C. Cardiovascular disease
   D. Hypertensive disorders

5. Pregnancy-related deaths are most likely to occur at what point in pregnancy?
   A. Antepartum (prior to delivery)
   B. Peripartum (during admission for delivery and up to 6 days postpartum)
   C. Late Postpartum (between 7–365 days postpartum)
   D. Equally distributed throughout antepartum, peripartum, and late postpartum

# CHAPTER 1. ANSWERS

1. **ANSWER: C.** Compared to MCA and death, severe maternal morbidity cases are far more likely to occur. Maternal deaths have been described as the "tip of the iceberg," and severe maternal morbidity the "rest of the iceberg."[14] In fact, for every maternal death, there are approximately 100 episodes of severe maternal morbidity each year.
   These data underscore the importance of systematic approaches to understanding and preventing severe maternal morbidity.
2. **ANSWER: A.** Maternal mortality in the U.S. was more than three times higher in Black or African American people, and more than two times higher in A/AN people, when compared to White, Hispanic, and A/PI people.
3. **ANSWER: D.** In the U.S., maternal deaths have increased more than 50% of maternal deaths in the last three decades. That translates to 1,201 pregnancy-related maternal deaths in 2021. Eighty percent of these deaths are determined to be preventable.
4. **ANSWER: C.** Causes and risk factors for pregnancy-related deaths in the U.S. have shifted over the years. Hemorrhage, hypertensive disorders, and anesthesia-related deaths have declined since 2006, while cardiovascular conditions have emerged as the leading cause of maternal mortality. Collectively, cardiovascular conditions, cardiomyopathy, and cerebrovascular accidents accounted for more than 30% of pregnancy-related deaths from 2011 to 2016.
5. **ANSWER: C.** Twenty-two percent of maternal deaths occur antepartum, 25% on the day of delivery or within 7 days after, and 53% occur between 7 days to 1 year after pregnancy.

# CHAPTER 1. REFERENCES

1. Alkema L, Chou D, Hogan D, et al. Global, regional, and national levels and trends in maternal mortality between 1990 and 2015, with scenario-based projections to 2030: A systematic analysis by the UN maternal mortality estimation inter-agency group. *Lancet.* 2016;387:462.
2. Centers for Disease Control and Prevention. *Pregnancy mortality surveillance system.* Website. https://www.cdc.gov/reproductive health/maternal-mortality/pregnancy-mortality-surveillance-system.htm. Accessed March 16, 2023.

3. Centers for Disease Control and Prevention. *Maternal mortality rates in the United States, 2021*. Website. https://www.cdc.gov/nchs/data/hestat/maternal-mortality/2021/maternal-mortality-rates-2021.htm. Accessed March 17, 2023.

4. Centers for Disease Control and Prevention. *Four in 5 pregnancy-related deaths in the U.S. are preventable*. Website. https://www.cdc.gov/media/releases/2022/p0919-pregnancy-related-deaths.html. Accessed March 18, 2023.

5. The Commonwealth Fund. *Maternal mortality and maternity care in the United States compared with 10 other developed countries*. Website. https://www.commonwealthfund.org/publications/issue-briefs/2020/nov/maternal-mortality-maternity-care-us-compared-10-countries. Accessed March 19, 2023.

6. Creanga A, Syverson C, Seed K, Callaghan W. Pregnancy-related mortality in the United States. 2011–2013. *Obstet Gynecol*. 2017;130:366. doi: 10.1097/AOG.0000000000002114.

7. Zelop CM, Einav S, Mhyre JM, Martin S. Cardiac arrest during pregnancy: Ongoing clinical conundrum. *Obstet Gynecol*. 2018;219(1):52. doi: 10.1016/j.ajog.2017.12.232.

8. Zelop CM, Einav S, Mhyre JM, et al. Characteristics and outcomes of maternal cardiac arrest: A descriptive analysis of get with the guidelines data. *Resuscitation*. 2018;132:17.

9. Pregnancy and Heart Disease. ACOG Practice Bulletin No. 212. American College of Obstetricians and Gynecologists. *Obstet Gynecol*. 2019;133(5):320–356. doi: 10.1097/AOG.0000000000003243.

10. MacDorman MF, Declercq E, Cabral H, Morton C. Recent increases in the U.S. maternal mortality rate: Disentangling trends from measurement issues. *Obstet Gynecol*. 2016;128:447. doi: 10.1097/AOG.0000000000001556.

11. Davis NL, Hoyert DL, Goodman DA, et al. Contribution of maternal age and pregnancy checkbox on maternal mortality ratios in the United States 1978–2012. *Obstet Gynecol*. 2017;217:352.e1. doi: 10.1016/j.ajog.2017.04.042.

12. Say L, Chou D, Gemmill A, et al. Global causes of maternal death: A WHO systematic analysis. *Lancet Glob Health*. 2014;2. doi: 10.1016/S2214-109X(14)70227-X.

13. Mhyre JM, Tsen LC, Einav S, et al. Cardiac arrest during hospitalization for delivery in the United States, 1998–2011. *Anesthesiology*. 2014. doi: 10.1097/ALN.000000000000015.

14. Hasegawa J, Ikeda T, Sekizawa A, et al. Maternal death due to stroke associated with pregnancy-induced hypertension. *Circ J*. 2015;79(8):1835–1840. doi: 10.1253/circj.CJ-15-0297.

15. MacKay AP, Berg CJ, Atrash H. Pregnancy-related mortality from preeclampsia and eclampsia. *Obstet Gynecol*. 2001;97(4). doi: 10.1016/s0029-7844(00)01223-0.

16. Shields A, Battistelli J, Thomson B. Maternal cardiac arrest: Where is our data coming from. *Obstet Gynecol*. 2018;131:9S.

17. Shields A, Kavanagh L, Battistelli J. Leave no woman behind: A call to standardize and expand the Get with the Guidelines® Registry. *American Journal of Obstetrics and Gynecology* (2022), doi: https://doi.org/10.1016/j.ajog.2022.05.005.

18. American College of Obstetricians, Gynecologists, Society for Maternal-Fetal Medicine, Menard MK, Kilpatric S, Saade G, et al. Levels of maternal care. *Obstet Gynecol*. 2015;212:259–271. doi: 10.1016/j.ajog.2014.12.030. Epub 2015 January 22.

19. The Commonwealth Fund. *Severe maternal morbidity in the United States: A primer*. Website. https://www.commonwealthfund.org/publications/issue-briefs/2021/oct/severe-maternal-morbidity-united-states-primer. Accessed March 18, 2023.

20. Bryant A. Focusing on severe maternal morbidity (the rest of the iceberg). *NEJM J Watch Women's Health*. Waltham; 2014. doi: 10.1056/nejm-jw.NA34784.

21. Petersen EE, Davis NL, Goodman D, et al. Racial/ethnic disparities in pregnancy related deaths—United States, 2007–2016. *MMWR Morb Wkly Rep*. 2019;68:762. doi: 10.15585/mmwr.mm6835a3external icon.

22. The Council on Patient Safety in Women's Health Care. *Reduction of peripartum racial and ethnic disparities*. Website. https://safehealthcareforeverywoman.org/patient-safety-bundles/reduction-of-peripartum-racialethnic-disparities/#1472747274361-49911e4d-c2d60f3f-74eb.

23. Warnecke RB, Oh A, Breen N, Gehlert S, et al. Approaching health disparities from a population perspective: The National Institutes of Health Centers for Population Health and Health Disparities. *Am J of Public Health*. 2008;98(9):1608. doi: 10.2105/AJPH.2006.102525.

24. Institute of Medicine (US) Committee on Understanding and Eliminating Racial and Ethnic Disparities in Health Care. Unequal treatment: Confronting racial and ethnic disparities in health care. In: Smedley BD, Stith AY, Nelson AR, ed. *Unequal treatment: Confronting racial and ethnic disparities in health care*. National Academies Press; 2003.

25. Implicit Bias in Health Care. *Implicit bias in health care*. Website. https://www.jointcommission.org/-/media/tjc/documents/newsletters/quick-safety-issue-23-apr-2016-final-rev.pdf. Accessed March 18, 2023.

26. Petersen EE, Davis NL, Goodman D, et al. Vital signs: Pregnancy-related deaths, United States, 2011–2015, and strategies for prevention, 13 states, 2013–2017. *MMWR Morb Mortal Wkly Rep*. 2019;68:423–429. doi: 10.15585/mmwr.mm6818e1.

27. Kozhimannil KB, Backes K, Hernandez E, Mendez DD, et al. Beyond the Preventing Maternal Deaths Act: Implementation and further policy change. *Health Affairs Blog*. 2019. doi: 10.1377/hblog20190130.914004.

28. Alliance for Innovation on Maternal Health. *Patient safety bundles*. Website. https://saferbirth.org/patient-safety-bundles/#core-aim-psbs. Accessed March 2023.

29. CA-PMSS Surveillance Report: *Pregnancy-Related Deaths in California, 2008–2016*. Sacramento: California Department of Public Health, Maternal, Child and Adolescent Health Division. 2021.

30. Alimena A, Freret TS, King C, Lassey SC, Economy KE, Easter SR. Simulation to improve trainee knowledge and comfort in managing maternal cardiac arrest. *AJOG Global* Reports 2023;3(2). doi.org/10.1016/j.xagr.2023.100182.

31. Paige JT, Garbee DD, Brown KM, Rojas JD. Using simulation in interprofessional education. *Surg Clin North Am*. 2015 Aug;95(4):751–66. doi: 10.1016/j.suc.2015.04.004.

32. Trost SL, Beauregard J, Njie F, et al. Pregnancy-Related Deaths: Data from Maternal Mortality Review Committees in 36 US States, 2017–2019. Atlanta, GA: Centers for Disease Control and Prevention, US Department of Health and Human Services; 2022.

# Anatomic and Physiologic Adaptations of Pregnancy

# 2

## 2.1 INTRODUCTION

Understanding the anatomic and physiologic adaptations during pregnancy is critical to optimizing outcomes when responding to MCA. This chapter reviews the anatomy and physiology of the various systems in pregnancy compared to the nonpregnant adult and sets the stage for the recommended modifications of CPR in pregnancy.

## 2.2 LEARNING OBJECTIVES

Learner will appropriately

- Describe the variations in anatomy and physiology encountered during pregnancy.
- Discuss maternal vulnerabilities that result from changes in the cardiovascular, respiratory, hematologic, gastrointestinal, genitourinary, endocrinologic, and immunologic systems.

## 2.3 CARDIOVASCULAR ANATOMIC AND PHYSIOLOGIC ADAPTATIONS IN PREGNANCY

The cardiovascular adaptations encountered during pregnancy are significant and varied. Throughout pregnancy, the maternal heart rate increases by up to 20%, and maternal stroke volume increases by up to 30% by 32 weeks gestation, resulting in an increased maternal cardiac output of over 40%. These adaptations support the rapid changes occurring throughout the body, allowing adequate oxygen and nutrients to get to the placenta and the fetus(es). As a result, a normal grade 1–2 systolic ejection murmur due to increased blood flow across the left and right ventricular outflow tracts may appear in up to 90% of pregnant patients. Blood volume expands by 30% due to an increase in the plasma volume (just under a 50% increase). The red blood cell mass increases by approximately 18%, which leads to "hemodilution of pregnancy." The net result is that normal hemoglobin in pregnancy is around 11% lower than that of a nonpregnant female adult. Intravascular colloid oncotic pressure and albumin concentration both decrease (approximately 12%–18%) throughout the pregnancy as a result of hemodilution. A decline in colloid oncotic pressure, along with increased femoral venous pressure by uterine compression of the inferior vena cava, results in physiologic edema.

Even though blood volume is expanding throughout pregnancy, blood pressure remains normal in the first trimester. Blood pressure tends to decrease during the second trimester due to the decrease in systemic vascular resistance (up to 35%) in response to hormonally mediated vasodilation and the low resistance placental circuit. Blood pressure decreases to its lowest point in the second trimester, at times as early as 6–8 weeks gestation, with a gradual increase in the third trimester, reaching preconceptual levels by the postpartum period.[1] Measure a pregnant patient's blood pressure as you would with a nonpregnant adult: the patient sitting in a chair and with their arm resting at heart level.

Additional anatomic changes in the cardiovascular system have the greatest impact on CPR. The expanding uterine size impedes blood flow through the inferior vena cava and aorta due to direct compression by the uterus on the great vessels. Once

DOI: 10.1201/9781003299288-3

**TABLE 2.1**   Anatomic and Physiologic Cardiovascular Adaptations in Pregnancy

| PARAMETER | VALUES IN PREGNANCY |
|---|---|
| Heart rate (HR) | ↑ 20% |
| Stroke volume (SV) | ↑ 30% |
| Cardiac output (CO) | ↑ by more than 40%; can result in normal grade 1–2 systolic ejection murmur |
| Systemic vascular resistance (SVR) | ↓ by more than 30%, nadir at 32 weeks |
| Oncotic pressure | ↓ due to hemodilution and decreased serum albumin |
| Uterus | Palpable at the maternal umbilicus (generally corresponding to 20 weeks gestation with a single fetus), can ↓ preload and cardiac output |
| Breast tissue | Can be dense and enlarged, causing difficulty with hand placement and pad placement, and ↓ effectiveness of chest compressions |

the uterine size reaches the umbilicus (corresponding to approximately 20 weeks in a pregnancy with a single fetus), the gravid uterus can cause enough aortocaval compression to result in a 25% drop in cardiac output in the supine position. This can lead to significant hypotension and can negatively impact the success of CPR.

*There are several points to note:*
1. Aortocaval compression occurs at the umbilicus due to the location of the bifurcation of the great vessels. As such, it is the fundal height location in relation to the umbilicus, **not** strictly gestational age, that contributes to this hypotension.
2. A pregnancy with multiple fetuses (i.e., twins or triplets) often has a fundal height at or above the umbilicus prior to 20 weeks.
3. This effect may be more profound or occur more quickly as pregnancy advances.

From a clinical perspective, this compression of the inferior vena cava may keep fluids and medications from reaching the heart quickly and is why intravenous (IV) access is recommended above the level of the diaphragm.

While the anatomic location of the heart is unchanged, maternal breast tissue often expands and may interfere with hand placement during chest compressions. Table 2.1 summarizes the anatomic and physiologic cardiovascular changes that occur in pregnancy.

**KEY POINTS**
- An increased heart rate is normal in a pregnant person.
- Measure a pregnant patient's blood pressure as you would with a nonpregnant adult: the patient sitting in a chair and with their arm resting at heart level.
- Pregnancy is characterized by hemodilutional anemia due to an increase in the plasma volume as compared to the red blood cell mass.
- Many pregnant people experience physiologic edema due to decreased plasma oncotic pressure and an increased femoral venous pressure.
- Once the uterine size reaches the umbilicus, cardiac output can drop by 25% in the supine position. This may lead to significant hypotension and can compromise the success of CPR.
- Due to the expanding uterus and corresponding compression of the great vessels in supine position, place the IV above the level of the diaphragm.

# 2.4  RESPIRATORY ANATOMIC AND PHYSIOLOGIC ADAPTATIONS IN PREGNANCY

The respiratory adaptations encountered during pregnancy are substantially different from the nonpregnant state. These differences are not only physiologic and anatomic but also influenced by maternal habitus, including the body mass index (BMI).

During pregnancy, hormones such as progesterone, estrogen, and prostaglandin influence physiologic changes in the respiratory system.

Estrogen increases during pregnancy and results in an increase in the number and sensitivity of central progesterone receptors in the hypothalamus and medulla.[2] Estrogen also enhances the effects of progesterone.[3] Progesterone levels increase during pregnancy and peak at 37 weeks gestation. Progesterone increases the sensitivity of the respiratory center to carbon dioxide, relaxes airway smooth muscle tone (resulting in a bronchodilatory effect), and increases swelling and vascularity of mucosal surfaces resulting in increased nasal congestion[4] and decreased internal tracheal diameter. These effects result in decreased nasal patency and can lead to an increase in the Mallampati score.[5]

The Mallampati score, used by providers to assess the suspected difficulty of laryngoscopy, includes four classifications (Figure 2.1). Class I shows full visualization of the oropharynx (little or no anticipated difficulty), ranging to class IV, which corresponds to no visualization of the soft palate (significant anticipated difficulty). Multiple studies have shown an increase in Mallampati score to class IV at term in over 30% of patients. Labor can negatively impact the Mallampati score due to an increase in airway edema, leading to increased difficulty in airway management.[3,5]

Prostaglandins are present during all trimesters of pregnancy and increase during labor. Prostaglandin F2alpha (F2α) increases airway resistance through bronchial smooth muscle constriction. Prostaglandins E1 and E2 have bronchodilatory effects. It is for this reason that carboprost tromethamine, a synthetic analogue of prostaglandin F2α, commonly used to treat postpartum hemorrhage, is contraindicated in patients with asthma. Carboprost can exacerbate asthma by increasing airway resistance.

---

**KEY POINTS**

- Hormonal changes in pregnancy, mediated mainly through increased progesterone, can increase swelling of the mucosal surfaces of the airway, leading to an increase in nasal congestion.
- Pregnancy negatively impacts the Mallampati score, reflecting a progressively more difficult airway as pregnancy advances, especially in labor.
- Avoid using carboprost, a prostaglandin F2α analog, in treating postpartum hemorrhage in patients with asthma. Carboprost increases airway resistance through bronchial smooth muscle constriction.

---

Anatomic changes of pregnancy also contribute to respiratory changes. As the uterus grows, it elevates the diaphragm, ultimately leading to decreased functional residual capacity and total lung capacity. There is a significant increase in oxygen demand during normal pregnancy.[6] Combined with decreased functional residual capacity, this increased demand leads to overall lower oxygen reserves, putting a pregnant person at increased risk of oxygen desaturation much more rapidly than a nonpregnant person. The desaturation time is substantially shorter in pregnancy, at 3 minutes, compared to 9 minutes in nonpregnant adults. Normal maternal blood gases reflect a **mild respiratory alkalosis (pH = 7.4)**, which is higher than the nonpregnant population (pH = 7.35–7.45). Maternal $PaCO_2$ is also mildly decreased (28–32 mm Hg) compared to nonpregnancy values ($PaCO_2$ 35–45 mm Hg).[7] Table 2.2 compares normal arterial blood gas (ABG) values between pregnant and nonpregnant patients. The resultant effects of these hormonal and anatomic changes are summarized in Figure 2.2 and Table 2.3.[8]

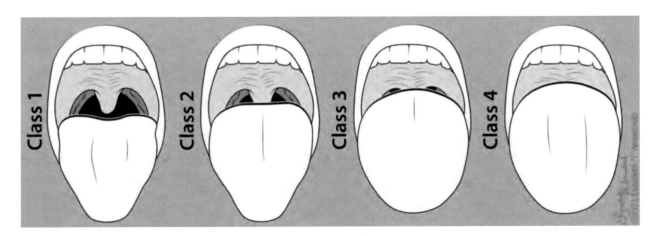

**FIGURE 2.1**   Mallampati scoring system.

**TABLE 2.2**  Arterial Blood Gas Values in Pregnant versus Nonpregnant Patients

| STATUS | pH | PaCO₂ | PaO₂ | HCO₃- |
|---|---|---|---|---|
| Pregnant | 7.40–7.45 | 28–32 mm Hg | >100 mm Hg | 22 mEq/L |
| Nonpregnant | 7.35–7.45 | 35–45 mm Hg | 75–100 mm Hg | 22–26 mEq/L |

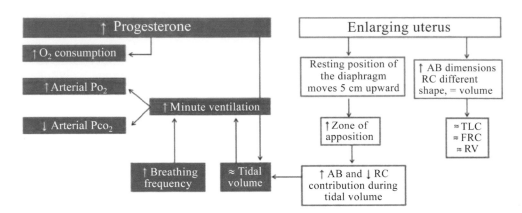

**FIGURE 2.2**  Flow diagram summarizing the most important effects of biochemical (left) and mechanical (right) pregnancy-induced factors on pulmonary function, ventilatory pattern, and gas exchange.[9] Abbreviations: ERV, expiratory reserve volume; FRC, functional residual capacity; IC, inspiratory capacity, PCO₂, carbon dioxide tension; PO₂, oxygen tension; TLC, total lung capacity; VC, vital capacity, AB, abdomen; RC, rib cage; ↑, increased; ↓, decreased; ≈, no change.[9]

**TABLE 2.3**  Anatomic and Physiologic Respiratory Adaptations in Pregnancy

| PARAMETER | VALUES IN PREGNANCY |
|---|---|
| Functional reserve capacity (FRC) | ↓ by 20% |
| Expiratory reserve volume (ERV) | ↓ by 15%–20% |
| Residual volume (RV) | ↓ by 20%–25% |
| Tidal volume (TV) | ↑ by 30%–40% |
| Minute ventilation | ↑ by 50% |
| Diaphragm | Elevated by gravid uterus resulting in ↓ FRC, ERV, RV, and total lung capacity |
| Progesterone | ↑ sensitivity of the respiratory center to carbon dioxide, relaxes airway smooth muscle tone (resulting in a bronchodilatory effect), and mediates hyperemia and edema of mucosal surfaces ↓ nasal patency |

The result of these normal physiologic adaptations in pregnancy is a more clinically challenging airway. Table 2.4 lists the anatomic and physiologic changes and clinical consequences of these adaptations (gastrointestinal adaptations and impact on the airway are also discussed later in this chapter). Providers must be aware of these adaptations and prevent avoidable complications. For example, preoxygenation is critical prior to the intubation of a pregnant patient due to the increased risks of desaturation. A pregnant patient who presents with respiratory distress and has PaCO₂ values >42 mm Hg should be immediately evaluated for respiratory decompensation, with a low threshold for intubation. The increase in PaCO₂ levels indicates a decrease in minute ventilation, signifying impending respiratory decompensation as respiratory fatigue results in decreased minute ventilation.

---

**KEY POINTS**
- An enlarged uterus decreases total lung capacity.
- Adaptations in the respiratory system during pregnancy lead to ↑ oxygen consumption, ↓ oxygen reserve, and ↑ vulnerability to earlier oxygen desaturation.
- Pregnancy is characterized with mild respiratory alkalosis, and normal ABG values for PaCO₂ are 28–32 mm Hg, lower than nonpregnant adults.
- Adaptations of the respiratory system are varied and result in a clinically challenging airway during pregnancy.
- A decreased lower esophageal sphincter tone increases the risk of aspiration during pregnancy.

**TABLE 2.4** Pregnancy-Related Maternal Anatomic and Physiologic Factors That May Contribute to Airway Difficulties and Adverse Airway-Related Events[10]

|  | *ANATOMIC AND PHYSIOLOGIC CHANGES* | *CLINICAL CONSEQUENCES* |
|---|---|---|
| Airway | • Weight gain in pregnancy<br>• Increased breast size<br>• Increased vascularity and edema of the airway mucosa | • Difficulty with positioning<br>• Difficulty with laryngoscope insertion<br>• Increased risk of airway bleeding and potential difficulty with endotracheal intubation |
| Respiratory | • Reduced functional residual capacity | • Increased rate of oxygen desaturation |
| Metabolic | • Increased oxygen consumption secondary to increased metabolic demand | • Increased rate of oxygen desaturation |
| Gastrointestinal | • Decreased lower esophageal sphincter tone<br>• Delayed gastric emptying | • Increased risk of gastric regurgitation and pulmonary aspiration |

# 2.5 NEUROPHYSIOLOGIC ADAPTATIONS IN PREGNANCY

Normal pregnancy results in several physiologic changes in the maternal nervous system. These changes can be categorized into central nervous system (CNS) changes, peripheral/autonomic nervous system (PANS) changes, and cerebrovascular adaptations (Table 2.5).

In the CNS, the normal hormonal changes of pregnancy have profound effects on neurotransmitters including oxytocin, prolactin, and dopamine, all of which play critical roles in pregnancy, birth, lactation, and maternal-infant bonding. Additional neurotransmitter changes, such as changes in the gamma-aminobutyric acid (GABA) receptor, can make the maternal brain more susceptible to seizure activity. In addition, pregnancy changes the maternal metabolism of medications that affect the CNS, such as anti-seizure medications, making people with epilepsy vulnerable to increased seizure activity. Of note, noneclamptic seizures are the leading cause of sudden cardiac death in pregnant people with epilepsy.

In the PANS, normal pregnancy increases sympathetic tone, decreases parasympathetic activity, and impairs baroreceptor activity, all factors that may affect a person's response to acute hypertension or hypotension, contributing to cardiac arrest risk. Preeclampsia is associated with an even greater increase in sympathetic hyperactivity, a factor that may contribute to cardiac arrhythmias, myocardial stunning, and coronary artery and/or cerebral artery vasospasm.

Pregnancy also has important effects on the cerebral vasculature. The brain requires a constant supply of energy and has no energy storage capacity. To address this, the cerebral vasculature dynamically adjusts to ensure constant cerebral blood flow at a wide range of blood pressures, a process known as cerebral autoregulation. Cerebral autoregulation appears to be enhanced during normal pregnancy but impaired during hypertensive pregnancy and in the postpartum period. In addition, the blood–brain barrier shows increased permeability in normal and especially in hypertensive pregnancy. Last, pregnancy-related hypercoagulability (see Chapter 10) can affect the cerebral veins and draining sinuses, leading to cerebral venous sinus thrombosis. These features likely contribute to increased risk of postpartum stroke, particularly in those with hypertensive disorders.

**TABLE 2.5** Maternal Central Nervous System Changes

| *SYSTEM* | *ANATOMIC AND PHYSIOLOGIC CHANGES* | *CLINICAL CONSEQUENCES* |
|---|---|---|
| Central nervous system (brain) | Changes in neurotransmitter levels and activity | Lowered seizure threshold |
| Metabolic | Changes in metabolism of anti-seizure medications | Increased risk of breakthrough seizures in people with epilepsy |
| Peripheral/Autonomic nervous system | Increased sympathetic activity<br>Decreased baroreceptor reflex | Increased risk of vasospasm and cardiac arrhythmias; impaired response to acute hypertension or hypotension |
| Cerebral vasculature | Changes in cerebral autoregulation, especially postpartum<br>Increased blood–brain barrier permeability<br>Hypercoagulability | Inability to compensate in brain for acute blood pressure changes<br>Increased risk of ischemic or hemorrhagic stroke<br>Increased risk of cerebral venous thrombosis |

**KEY POINTS**

- Normal pregnancy lowers the seizure threshold and alters maternal metabolism, increasing the risk of seizures, particularly for those with epilepsy.
- Pregnancy causes sympathetic nervous system activation, which is exaggerated in people with preeclampsia.
- Baroreceptor activity is altered in pregnancy; this may affect people's response to acute hypertension or hypotension.
- Changes in cerebral autoregulation and the blood–brain barrier may contribute to risk of pregnancy-associated stroke, especially in the postpartum period.

# 2.6 HEMATOLOGIC PHYSIOLOGIC ADAPTATIONS IN PREGNANCY

Significant hematologic adaptations occur during pregnancy. As previously mentioned, blood volume expands by 30% (approximately 1.5 L) due to a relative increase in the plasma volume compared to the red blood cell mass. It is normal to see an increased white blood cell (WBC) count in a pregnant person,[11] sometimes elevating as high as 29,000 cells per cubic milliliter during labor. Most pregnant people have a normal platelet count throughout pregnancy (150,000–400,000 per microliter). Lower platelet counts in pregnancy (as low as 70,000 per microliter) may be encountered due to gestational thrombocytopenia.[12] This is a benign, transient condition that improves after delivery. Table 2.6. summarizes hematologic adaptations during pregnancy.

Pregnancy also results in an increased risk of thrombosis due to its multiple effects on Virchow's triad (hypercoagulability, venous stasis, and vascular damage). There are significant increases in circulating estrogen and prothrombotic coagulation factors (such as fibrinogen, von Willebrand factor, and factors II, VII, VIII, and X). In addition, there is an acquired functional resistance to activated protein C and a 50%–60% reduction in protein S. Further derangements in coagulation hemostasis include a reduction in plasminogen activator and an increase in plasminogen activator inhibitors.[13] These changes result in a hypercoagulable state. Pressure on the pelvic vessels and inferior vena cava from the enlarging uterus increases venous stasis. These changes make a pregnant patient more susceptible to clot formation and pulmonary embolism.[13]

Normal values of fibrinogen in pregnancy are often higher (373–619 mg/mL) than those in nonpregnant patients (200–400 mg/dL). In the setting of active or recent bleeding, a fibrinogen level of 200–250 mg/dL may be an early indicator of significant hemorrhage and hypofibrinogenemia, prompting further evaluation. In the setting of significant bleeding (blood loss of ≥1,500 mL) or hypofibrinogenemia, administer blood products containing fibrinogen (such as fresh frozen plasma [FFP] or cryoprecipitate [cryo]).

**TABLE 2.6**  Physiologic Hematologic Adaptations in Pregnancy

| PARAMETER | VALUES IN PREGNANCY |
| --- | --- |
| Fibrinogen | Increases up to 600 mg/dL, average 400 mg/dL |
| Hemoglobin/Hematocrit | Decreases: average hemoglobin 11.2 g/dL |
| Platelets | No change: gestational thrombocytopenia can occur in 7%–12% at term[12], with platelet counts typically above 70,000 |
| Prothrombin time/Partial thromboplastin time | No change |
| WBC count | Slightly increased: as high as 25,000–29,000 in labor |

**KEY POINTS**

- It is normal for the WBC count to be elevated in pregnant people, and this does not necessarily suggest infection.
- Gestational thrombocytopenia may result in platelet counts as low as 70,000 per microliter in an otherwise normal pregnancy.
- Pregnancy causes an increased risk of developing blood clots due to hypercoagulability and venous stasis.
- A fibrinogen level of 200–250 is considered low for pregnancy and should prompt further workup for bleeding and consideration of blood products.

# 2.7 GASTROINTESTINAL ANATOMIC AND PHYSIOLOGIC ADAPTATIONS IN PREGNANCY

The gastrointestinal adaptations encountered during pregnancy result from both hormonal and anatomic causes. Increased saliva production in the oropharynx is common.[14,15] Gastric emptying is unchanged during pregnancy[16] but may be prolonged after giving opiates or sedatives (as may be seen during labor analgesia). The lower esophageal sphincter resting pressure is decreased secondary to progesterone effect. Increased progesterone and decreased motilin mutually contribute to lower motility of the small and large intestines. Combined with the compressive effects of the gravid uterus, this decreased intestinal motility leads to an increase in transit time, and constipation is common in pregnancy. Mechanical factors also cause the liver to shift upward from the abdominal cavity into the thoracic cavity. The gallbladder has decreased motility with a resultant increase in gallstone formation during pregnancy. Uterine distension, especially during the third trimester, can contribute to the increased incidence of hemorrhoids and urinary and renal incontinence.

The collective effect of increased saliva production, decreased lower esophageal sphincter resting pressure, and increased transit time through the intestines poses a significant risk for vomiting and aspiration during a maternal code (Table 2.7). In pregnancy, the airway may be obstructed and the vocal cords hard to see due to excessive oropharyngeal secretions. If possible, suction equipment should be immediately available during intubation given that liberal suctioning may be necessary. Early intubation will serve to secure the airway and protect against aspiration.

Injury to the liver during chest compressions may occur because the liver shifts upward from the abdominal cavity into the chest cavity under the ribs and sternum. Several reports document liver lacerations following maternal resuscitation.[17,18] It is unknown if these lacerations were a consequence of vigorous chest compressions or spontaneous rupture of the liver capsule due to pregnancy-specific causes such as preeclampsia. Changing hand placement will make chest compressions **less** effective and therefore decrease the likelihood of ROSC.[19] Current American Heart Association (AHA) guidelines recommend maintaining normal hand placement and performing an ultrasound to look for evidence of liver laceration/free fluid if ROSC is achieved and there is a suspicion for hypovolemia.

**TABLE 2.7**  Anatomic and Physiologic Gastrointestinal Adaptations in Pregnancy

| PARAMETER | VALUES IN PREGNANCY |
|---|---|
| Gallbladder | ↓ motility<br>↑ lithogenicity of bile/gallstones |
| Gastric emptying | Unchanged |
| Liver | Elevated into chest by growing uterus |
| Lower esophageal sphincter | ↓ pressure/tone |
| Rectum/anus | ↑ hemorrhoids, incontinence |
| Saliva | ↑ (ptyalism in up to 35%) |
| Small and large intestine | ↓ motility/↑ transit time<br>↑ constipation, bloating |

**KEY POINTS**
- There is a significant increase in the risk of vomiting and aspiration before and after a maternal code.
- Early intubation will serve to secure the airway and protect against aspiration.
- Injury to the liver during chest compressions may occur because the liver shifts upward from the abdominal cavity into the chest cavity under the ribs and sternum.

# 2.8 GENITOURINARY ANATOMIC AND PHYSIOLOGIC ADAPTATIONS IN PREGNANCY

Urinary tract adaptations encountered during pregnancy predispose people to infections and alter the metabolism or clearance of certain medications. The hormonal effect of increased progesterone, as well as compression of the ureters at the pelvic brim, lead to caliceal and renal pelvis dilation and may be considered hydronephrosis by radiologic standards in up to 80% of patients. The right side is affected more often due to dextrorotation of the uterus by the sigmoid colon, kinking of the ureter as it crosses the right iliac artery, and proximity to the right ovarian vein. Ureteral dilation also occurs due to progesterone relaxation of smooth muscle. Uterine growth may also create compression, causing the ureters to become elongated, tortuous, and displaced laterally with advancing gestational age. Superior and anterior displacement and compression by the enlarging uterus may further decrease bladder capacity.

The dilation of and decrease in peristalsis of the urinary collecting system, combined with intermittent vesicoureteral reflux due to increased intravesicular and decreased intraureteral pressure through an incompetent vesicoureteral valve,[20,21] lead to the collection of up to 300 mL of static urine in the pregnant bladder. This urinary stasis can serve as a reservoir for bacteria and lead to an increase in urinary tract infections including pyelonephritis and urosepsis. Urosepsis is a common cause of sepsis in pregnancy and should be considered in the setting of unstable maternal status and concern for infectious etiology.

Increased renal perfusion and glomerular filtration rate (GFR) are seen in pregnancy due to increased cardiac output and decreased systemic vascular resistance. GFR is also increased due to increased renal blood flow caused by pregnancy-related hormones. Reduced vascular responsiveness to vasopressors such as angiotensin II, norepinephrine, and antidiuretic hormone has also been shown.[22] Renal plasma flow (RPF) increases by 80% by the end of the first trimester, with a 50% increase in GFR. Both parameters decrease toward prepregnancy values near term with RPF returning to near preconception levels. GFR remains significantly elevated.

The physiologic increase in GFR during pregnancy results in a decrease in serum creatinine concentration to a normal range of 0.4–0.8 mg/dL and blood urea nitrogen to 8–10 mg/dL.[23] The plasma osmolality in normal pregnancy decreases to 270 mOsmol/kg from a nonpregnant level of 275–290 mOsmol/kg. Hyponatremia is also common in pregnancy with a decrease in plasma sodium concentration to 4–5 mEq/L below nonpregnant levels, with sodium levels remaining above 130 mEq/L.[24] The increased GFR also leads to increases in proteinuria and glucosuria in pregnancy. Urinary protein excretion rises from about 100 mg daily to about 150–200 mg daily in the third trimester, with values ≥300 mg per day considered an abnormal elevation.[25] Glucosuria (defined as glucose in the urine) is present in 50% of pregnant people and may occur independent of serum glucose levels.[26] Hypouricemia is also present with serum uric acid reaching a nadir of 2.0–4.0 mg/dL in the second trimester before slowly returning to baseline by term.[27]

The mild respiratory alkalosis that occurs in pregnancy results in a compensatory decrease in plasma bicarbonate levels from 26 mmol/L to approximately 22 mmol/L.[23] Second, the serum anion gap falls from 10.7 in the nonpregnant state to 8.5 during pregnancy.[28] This is likely due to the physiologic hypoalbuminemia of pregnancy, since negatively charged albumin is a major component of the anion gap.

Doubling of a patient's baseline creatinine, which is normally decreased to 0.4–0.6 mg/dL in pregnancy, to a value of 1.0 mg/dL or greater, usually indicates significant renal impairment in a patient with a normal baseline creatinine.

---

**KEY POINTS**

- Pregnant people are more prone to urinary tract infections and urosepsis due to urinary stasis.
- Pregnancy is characterized by respiratory alkalosis, decreased plasma bicarbonate levels to approximately 22 mmol/L, and a decreased serum anion gap to 8.5.
- Vesicoureteral reflux may make pregnant patients more susceptible to urinary tract infections and urosepsis.

---

# 2.9 ANATOMIC AND PHYSIOLOGIC IMPACT ON MEDICATIONS IN PREGNANCY

Common obstetric medications with renal clearance, such as magnesium sulfate, can rapidly increase to toxic levels and lead to ventricular arrhythmias and cardiac arrest if not carefully monitored and adjusted when decreased renal clearance/renal impairment is present.

Table 2.8 summarizes the resultant effects of these physiologic and anatomic changes. Medications such as digoxin, phenytoin, and midazolam are protein bound and can also lead to toxic levels more easily due to the low albumin levels in pregnancy combined with other physiologic changes, including increased tidal volume, partially compensated respiratory alkalosis, slowed gastrointestinal motility, and altered activity of hepatic drug-metabolizing enzymes.[29] Even though pregnancy can alter the pharmacokinetic properties of some drugs, it is still recommended to give the same medications and doses in MCA used in nonpregnant adult cardiac arrest.[30]

**TABLE 2.8**   Anatomic and Physiologic Genitourinary and Acid-Base Adaptations in Pregnancy

| PARAMETER | VALUES IN PREGNANCY |
| --- | --- |
| Acid-base balance | ↑ bicarbonate excretion[23] |
| Bladder/ureter | ↑ vesicoureteral reflux<br>↑ frequency, nocturia, urgency, dysuria, incontinence |
| Glomerular filtration rate/renal plasma flow | ↑ 50%[23]<br>↓ creatinine to <0.8 mg/dL<br>↑ excretion of glucose, protein, and amino acids[23] |
| Kidney size | ↑ 1–1.5 cm,[31] ↑ volume by 30% |
| Osmolality | ↓ threshold for thirst/vasopressin release<br>↑ vasopressin metabolism<br>Hyponatremia |
| Ureteral dilation | Resembles hydronephrosis[32] |

**KEY POINTS**

- Use all medications and their doses in CPR for MCA as you would for adult CPR. Do not change them based on the physiologic adaptations during pregnancy.
- High-risk medications with renal clearance, such as magnesium sulfate, can rapidly lead to cardiac arrest if not carefully monitored and adjusted when renal impairment is present.

# 2.10 ENDOCRINE ANATOMIC AND PHYSIOLOGIC ADAPTATIONS IN PREGNANCY

While the endocrine system undergoes various changes in pregnancy, these adaptations are relatively gradual and generally do not have a direct impact in a cardiac arrest scenario. Pregnancy may exacerbate some endocrine conditions, especially in the setting of noncompliance, and may predispose chronically ill people to cardiac arrest (e.g., diabetic ketoacidosis and thyroid storm). While this course does not cover the management of diabetic ketoacidosis (DKA), EMS and IH personnel caring for pregnant people should be aware that they are susceptible to DKA at much lower, and even normal, glucose thresholds. Thyroid storm in pregnancy may occur because of noncompliance with medications used to treat hyperthyroidism or unrecognized new-onset hyperthyroidism. Thyroid storm may be precipitated by stressors such as labor and delivery, surgical delivery (such as cesarean delivery), infection, and trauma. Early recognition and treatment of thyroid storm are critical to avoiding cardiovascular collapse. Thyroid storm can also be associated with preeclampsia, most commonly with severe features, and should be considered in the differential diagnosis of people with hypertension, especially with thyroid dysfunction.

**KEY POINTS**

- Pregnant patients are much more susceptible to DKA at lower and even normal glucose thresholds.
- In a pregnant patient with hyperthyroidism, early recognition of thyroid storm and appropriate treatment will help avoid cardiovascular collapse.

# 2.11 IMMUNE SYSTEM ADAPTATIONS IN PREGNANCY

Alterations of the immune system during pregnancy may help explain the altered susceptibility to and severity of infectious diseases during pregnancy. As pregnancy progresses, estrogen and progesterone levels progressively increase to supraphysiologic values. Whereas innate immunity is enhanced in pregnancy, cell-mediated and humoral immunity may be moderately suppressed, which may increase a pregnant person's susceptibility to certain infections such as influenza. Many infectious diseases will follow a similar course to that which occurs in a nonpregnant person, and the management in pregnancy will also be

**TABLE 2.9**   Anatomic and Physiologic Endocrinologic Adaptations in Pregnancy

| PARAMETER | NORMAL VALUES IN PREGNANCY |
|---|---|
| FT3 (free) | 2.4–4.4 pg/mL |
| FT4 (free) | 5.4–11.7 ng/dL |
| Glucose | <95 mg/dL fasting, <140 mg/dL 2-hour postprandial |
| TSH | 0.34–4.25 IU/mL |

Abbreviations: FT3, free triiodothyronine; FT4, free thyroxine; TSH, thyroid-stimulating hormone.

similar. Any infection that would lead to sepsis in nonpregnant patients can affect pregnant patients with risks for morbidity and mortality that are similar to or greater than nonpregnant patients. Although there is strong evidence for the increased severity of certain infections among pregnant people, the evidence regarding initial susceptibility to infection in pregnancy is weaker. Pregnancy physiologic changes may mask many of the signs and symptoms that would typically be used to identify a serious infection early in its course. See Chapter 3 for more details on how to recognize an unstable pregnant patient and manage sepsis.

**KEY POINTS**
- Alterations in cell-mediated and humoral immunity in pregnancy increase a pregnant person's susceptibility to certain infections, such as influenza.
- Pregnancy physiologic changes may mask many of the signs and symptoms that would typically be used to identify a serious infection early in its course.

# CHAPTER 2. PRACTICE QUESTIONS

1. A pregnant patient presents for their obstetric visit at 13 weeks and has a hemoglobin of 11.3%. You tell them that this value is normal and results from an increase in which of the following?
   A. Oncotic pressure relative to systemic vascular resistance
   B. Glomerular filtration rate relative to blood volume
   C. Plasma volume relative to red blood cell mass
   D. Red blood cell mass relative to blood volume

2. Which of the following BEST reflects the normal acid-base status in pregnancy?
   A. Mild respiratory acidosis
   B. $PaCO_2$ between 28 and 32 mm Hg
   C. Compensatory respiratory acidosis
   D. pH of 7.35

3. An increase in the Mallampati score during pregnancy leads to difficulty with airway management. During a maternal cardiac arrest, a change in the size of which of the following MOST significantly impacts the Mallampati score?
   A. Neck
   B. Breasts
   C. Oropharynx
   D. Nasal passage

4. Which of the following normal physiologic responses results in a GREATER risk of aspiration during pregnancy?
   A. Decrease in motility of the gallbladder
   B. Decrease in Mallampati score
   C. Increase in biliary sludge
   D. Decrease in lower esophageal sphincter tone

5. Which of the following reasons accounts for people being more susceptible to urinary tract infections and urosepsis during pregnancy?
   A. Increased vesicoureteral reflux
   B. Increased peristalsis of the ureters
   C. Decreased intravesical pressure
   D. Decreased glucosuria

# CHAPTER 2. ANSWERS

1. **ANSWER: C.** Blood volume expands by 30% due to an increase in the plasma volume (just under a 50% increase). The red blood cell mass increases by approximately 18%, leading to hemodilution. The net result is that normal hemoglobin in pregnancy is around 11%, lower than that of a nonpregnant female adult. Intravascular colloid oncotic pressure and albumin concentration (12%–18%) both decrease throughout the pregnancy as a result of hemodilution.

2. **ANSWER: B.** Maternal blood gases typically reflect a mild respiratory alkalosis (pH = 7.4), which is different from the nonpregnant population (pH = 7.35–7.45). Maternal $PaCO_2$ is also mildly decreased (28–32 mm Hg) due to an increase in minute ventilation. This is also different in the nonpregnant population, where normal ABG values for $PaCO_2$ are 35–45 mm Hg.

3. **ANSWER: C.** An increase in oropharyngeal edema, especially during labor, significantly impacts the Mallampati score. Multiple studies have shown an increase in Mallampati score to class IV at term in over 30% of patients, largely due to an increase in oropharyngeal edema.

4. **ANSWER: D.** The collective effect of increased saliva production and transit time through the intestines, potentially prolonged gastric emptying, and decreased lower esophageal sphincter resting pressure poses a significant risk for vomiting and aspiration during a maternal code. Suction equipment should be immediately available given that liberal suctioning may be necessary. Early intubation will serve to secure the airway and protect against aspiration.

5. **ANSWER: A.** The dilation of and decrease in peristalsis of the urinary collecting system, combined with **increased vesicoureteral reflux** due to increased intravesicular and decreased intraureteral pressure through an incompetent vesicoureteral valve, lead to the collection of up to 300 mL of static urine. This urinary stasis can serve as a reservoir for bacteria and lead to a urinary tract infection including pyelonephritis and potential for urosepsis.

# CHAPTER 2. REFERENCES

1. Sanghavi M, Rutherford JD. Cardiovascular physiology of pregnancy. *Circulation*. 2014;130:1003–1008. doi: 10.1161/CIRCULATIONAHA.114.009029.

2. Weinberger SE, Weiss ST, Cohen WR, Weiss JW, Johnson. Pregnancy and the lung. *Am Rev Respir Dis*. 1980 Mar;121(3):559–81. doi: 10.1164/arrd.1980.121.3.559.

3. Boutonnet M, Faitot V, Katz A, Salomon L, Keita H. Mallampati class changes during pregnancy, labour, and after delivery: can these be predicted? *Br J Anaesth*. 2010;104(1):67–70. doi: 10.1093/bja/aep356.

4. Lyons HA, Antonio R. The sensitivity of the respiratory center in pregnancy and after administration of progesterone. *Trans Assoc Am Physicians*. 1959;72:173–180.

5. Pilkington S, Carli F, Dakin MJ, et al. Increase in Mallampati score during pregnancy. *British Journal of Anaesthesia*. 1995;74(6): 638–642. doi: 10.1093/bja/74.6.638.

6. Crapo RO. Normal cardiopulmonary physiology during pregnancy. *Clin Obstet Gynecol*. 1996;39(1):3–16. doi: 10.1097/00003081-199603000-00004.

7. Arterial Blood Gas (ABG) interpretation for medical students, OSCEs and MRCP PACES. Oxford Medical Education. Website. http://www.oxfordmedicaleducation.com/abgs/abg-interpretation/. Accessed March 11, 2023.

8. Antony KM, Racusin DA, Aagaard K, Dildy GA. Maternal Physiology. In Gabbe S, Niebyl J, Simpson J, et al. ed. *Obstetrics: Normal and Problem Pregnancies*. Elsevier; 2016:46.

9. LoMauro A, Aliverti A. Respiratory physiology of pregnancy. Physiology masterclass. *Breathe*. 2015;11(4):297–301. doi: 10.1183/20734735.008615.

10. Bordoni L, Parsons K, Rucklidge MWM. Obstetric Airway Management. *Obstetric Anesthesia* Tutorial 393. ATOTW 393 (14 December 2018).

11. Abbassi-Ghanavati M, Greer L, Cunningham F. Pregnancy and laboratory studies: A reference table for clinicians. *Obstet Gynecol*. 2009;114(6):1326–1331. doi: 10.1097/AOG.0b013e3181c2bde8.

12. Boehlen F, Hohlfeld P, Extermann P, Perneger TV, de Moerloose P. Platelet count at term pregnancy: a reappraisal of the threshold. *Obstet Gynecol*. 2000;95(1):29–33. doi: 10.1016/s0029-7844(99)00537-2.

13. Ye Y, Vattai A, Zhang X, Zhu J, Thaler CJ, Mahner S, Jeschke U, Von Schönfeldt V. Role of plasminogen activator inhibitor type 1 in pathologies of female reproductive diseases. *International Journal of Molecular Sciences*. 2017;18(8):1651. https://doi.org/10.3390/ijms18081651.

14. Thaxter Nesbeth KA, Samuels LA, Nicholson Daley C, et al. Ptyalism in pregnancy—a review of epidemiology and practices. *Eur J Obstet Gynecol Reprod Biol*. 2016;198:47. doi: 10.1016/j.ejogrb.2015.12.022.

15. Nazik E, Eryilmaz G. Incidence of pregnancy-related discomforts and management approaches to relieve them among pregnant women. J Clin Nurs 2014;23:1736. doi:10.1111/jocn.12323.

16. Whitehead EM, Smith M, Dean Y, O'Sullivan G. An evaluation of gastric emptying times in pregnancy and the puerperium. *Anaesthesia* 1993;48:53.

17. Shinohara S, Uchida Y, Kasai M, Ogawa T, Hirata S. Liver injury after cardiopulmonary resuscitation for cardiac arrest during cesarean delivery. *Int J Obstet Anesth.* 2017 Feb;29:86–87. doi: 10.1016/j.ijoa.2016.09.007.

18. Cox TR, Crimmins SD, Shannon AM, Atkins KL, Tesoriero R, Malinow AM. Liver lacerations as a complication of CPR during pregnancy. *Resuscitation.* 2018 Jan;122:121–125. doi: 10.1016/j.resuscitation.2017.10.027.

19. Callaway CW, Soar J, Aibiki M, Böttiger BW, Brooks SC, Deakin CD, Donnino MW, Drajer S, Kloeck W, Morley PT, Morrison LJ, Neumar RW, Nicholson TC, Nolan JP, Okada K, O'Neil BJ, Paiva EF, Parr MJ, Wang TL, Witt J; on behalf of the Advanced Life Support Chapter Collaborators. Part 4: Advanced life support: 2015 International Consensus on Cardiopulmonary Resuscitation and Emergency Cardiovascular Care Science with Treatment Recommendations. *Circulation.* 2015;132(suppl 1):S84–S145. doi.org/10.1161/CIR.0000000000000273.

20. Mattingly RF, Borkowf HI. Clinical implications of ureteral reflux in pregnancy. *Clin Obstet Gynecol.* 1978;21(3):863. doi: 10.1097/00003081-197809000-00022.

21. Heidrick WP, Mattingly RF, Amberg JR. Vesicoureteral reflux in pregnancy. *Obstet Gynecol.* 1967;29(4):571.

22. Gant NF, Chand S, Whalley PJ, MacDonald PC. The nature of pressor responsiveness to angiotensin II in human pregnancy. *Obstet Gynecol.* 1974;43(6):854.

23. Cunningham F, Leveno KJ, Bloom SL, Dashe JS, Hoffman BL, Casey BM, Spong CY (Eds). Maternal physiology. *Williams Obstetrics, 25e.* McGraw-Hill; 2018. https://accessmedicine.mhmedical.com/content.aspx?bookid=1918&sectionid=144754618. Accessed March 12, 2023.

24. Lindheimer MD, Barron WM, Davison JM. Osmoregulation of thirst and vasopressin release in pregnancy. *Am J Physiol.* 1989;257(2 Pt 2):F159.

25. Kattah A, Milic N, White W, Garovic V. Spot urine protein measurements in normotensive pregnancies, pregnancies with isolated proteinuria and preeclampsia. *Am J Physiol Regul Integr Comp Physiol.* 2017;313:R418. doi: 10.1152/ajpregu.00508.2016.

26. Alto WA. No need for glycosuria/proteinuria screen in pregnant women. *J Fam Pract.* 2005;54:978.

27. Lind T, Godfrey KA, Otun H, Philips PR. Changes in serum uric acid concentrations during normal pregnancy. *Br J Obstet Gynaecol.* 1984;91(2):128. doi: 10.1111/j.1471-0528.1984.tb05895.x.

28. Akbari A, Wilkes P, Lindheimer M, Lepage N, Filler G. Reference intervals for anion gap and strong ion difference in pregnancy: A pilot study. *Hypertens Pregnancy.* 2007;26(1):111.

29. Costantine MM. Physiologic and pharmacokinetic changes in pregnancy. *Front Pharmacol.* 2014;5(65). doi: 10.3389/fphar.2014.00065.

30. Jeejeebhoy F, Zelop C, Lipman S, Carvalho B, Joglar J, Mhyre J, Katz V, Lapinsky S, Einav S, Warnes C, Page R, Griffin R, Jain A, Dainty K, Arafeh J, Windrim R, Koren G, Callaway C and on behalf of the American Heart Association Emergency Cardiovascular Care Committee, Council on Cardiopulmonary, Critical Care, Perioperative and Resuscitation, Council on Cardiovascular Diseases in the Young, and Council on Clinical Cardiology. Cardiac Arrest in Pregnancy. *Circulation.* 2015;132:1747–1773. https://doi.org/10.1161/CIR.0000000000000300.

31. Bailey RR, Rolleston GL. Kidney length and ureteric dilatation in the puerperium. *Obstet Gynaecol Br Commonw.* 1971;78:55. doi: 10.1111/j.1471-0528.1971.tb00191.x.

32. Rasmussen PE, Nielsen FR. Hydronephrosis during pregnancy: A literature survey. *Eur J Obstet Gynecol Reprod Biol.* 1988;27:249.

# Prevention of Maternal Cardiac Arrest

3

## 3.1 INTRODUCTION

A 2022 CDC report suggested that more than 80% of maternal mortalities following MCA could have been prevented. Most of the causes of MCA will result in demonstrable changes in symptoms and vital signs prior to the development of cardiac arrest. This chapter reviews the following:

- How vital signs can be used with tools such as maternal early warning systems to assist with detecting the deteriorating maternal status.
- Examples of scoring systems that can be integrated into clinical practice for early detection of deteriorating maternal status.
- Management strategies and escalation protocols that have been utilized in response to change in status.
- How to recognize the presenting symptoms and signs of the most common causes leading to maternal cardiac arrest.

## 3.2 LEARNING OBJECTIVES

Learner will appropriately

- Identify specific trigger thresholds for responding to changes in the patient's vital signs and clinical condition.
- Describe a plan for and implementation of diagnostic workup.
- Describe at least two different tools available for early recognition of unstable pregnant patients.
- Describe management strategies and escalation protocols.

### 3.2.1 Normal and Abnormal Maternal Vital Signs and Symptoms

Normal physiologic changes in pregnancy may mask maternal deterioration in the critically ill patient at different times in pregnancy. Recognizing a critically ill pregnant person requires an understanding of the normal physiologic changes in pregnancy, which are covered in previous chapters and are reviewed here (Table 3.1). External factors that influence maternal physiology are covered next.

Because pregnancy generally occurs in a younger and fitter population, lower baseline and mean arterial blood pressure are common as is mild maternal tachycardia. In nonpregnant patients, vital sign changes (such as hypotension and tachycardia) are some of the earliest indicators of deteriorating status. However, waiting for vital sign changes to indicate maternal deterioration is not always reliable, as these warning signs may be masked or may not appear until the moment of impending respiratory or cardiovascular collapse (such as maternal hypotension or tachycardia during acute blood loss). A comprehensive understanding of normal physiology in pregnancy and its impact on vital signs is critical to the accurate and timely interpretation of vital signs and symptoms and recognition of maternal deterioration. Tables 3.2 and 3.3, respectively, outline the common symptoms and conditions and the normal physiologic changes throughout pregnancy that may mask serious conditions.

DOI: 10.1201/9781003299288-4

**TABLE 3.1**    Impact of Normal Physiologic Changes in Pregnancy on Maternal Condition

| SYSTEM | CHANGES | EFFECT |
|---|---|---|
| Blood | ↑ plasma volume<br>↑ red cell volume | Dilutional anemia<br>Greater reduction of oxygen supply to tissues |
| Cardiovascular | ↓ peripheral vascular resistance<br>↑ heart rate<br>↓ arterial pressure<br>↑ cardiac output | Masks initial signs of sepsis and increased hypoperfusion |
| Coagulation | ↑ factors VII, VIII, IX, X, XII, von Willebrand and fibrinogen<br>↓ protein S<br>↓ fibrinolytic activity | ↑ risk of thrombotic events<br>↑ risk of disseminated intravascular coagulation |
| Gastrointestinal | ↓ muscle tone across the digestive tract<br>Delayed gastric emptying<br>Diaphragm elevation by the pregnant womb<br>Changes in bile composition<br>↑ production of pro-inflammatory cytokines by Kupffer cells | ↑ risk of bacterial translocation<br>↑ risk of aspiration pneumonia<br>↑ risk of cholestasis, hyperbilirubinemia, and jaundice |
| Genital | ↓ vaginal pH<br>↑ glycogen in vaginal epithelium | ↑ risk of chorioamnionitis |
| Renal | Ureteropelvic dilation and<br>↓ ureteral pressure due to smooth muscle relaxation<br>Flaccid bladder<br>↑ intravesical pressure due to the pregnant uterus weight<br>↑ vesicoureteral reflux<br>↑ renal plasma flow<br>↑ glomerular filtration rate<br>↓ urea and creatinine average values | Asymptomatic bacteriuria<br>Delayed identification of renal injury secondary to sepsis<br>↑ risk of pyelonephritis and urosepsis |
| Respiratory | ↑ tidal volume<br>↓ residual volume<br>↑ minute ventilation by 30%–40%<br>↑ respiratory center stimulation<br>↑ respiratory rate<br>↓ $PaCO_2$ | Impaired oxygenation<br>Delayed physiologic response to metabolic acidosis |

**TABLE 3.2**    Common Changes and Symptoms in Pregnancy That May Mask Serious Conditions

| MOST COMMON SYMPTOMS | NORMAL PHYSIOLOGIC CHANGES | SERIOUS CONDITIONS MASKED |
|---|---|---|
| Headache | Tension, migraine, rebound, postdural puncture | Stroke, cerebral venous sinus thrombosis |
| Heartburn | Gastroesophageal reflux | Myocardial infarction, preeclampsia, HELLP syndrome, pancreatitis |
| Shortness of breath | Dyspnea of pregnancy, asthma | Pulmonary embolism, cardiomyopathy/heart failure |
| Nausea and vomiting | Nausea and vomiting of pregnancy | Preeclampsia, HELLP syndrome, pancreatitis, myocardial infarction |
| Swollen ankles/feet | Gestational edema, prior injury | Preeclampsia, deep venous thrombosis, cardiomyopathy/heart failure |
| Palpitations/Chest pain | Anemia, anxiety, thyroid disorder | Myocardial infarction, cardiac arrythmia, cardiomyopathy/heart failure |

Abbreviation: HELLP, hemolysis, elevated liver enzymes, and low platelets.

**TABLE 3.3**  Conditions Masked by Normal Physiologic Changes during Pregnancy

| TIME IN PREGNANCY | NORMAL PHYSIOLOGIC CHANGES | CONDITIONS MASKED |
|---|---|---|
| **Antepartum** | | |
| | • Gestational edema<br>• Shortness of breath<br>• Mild tachycardia<br>• Predisposition to asymptomatic bacteriuria | • Cardiomyopathy, cardiovascular disease, cerebral edema, stroke<br><br>• Pyelonephritis and/or sepsis (e.g., urinary tract infection can rapidly progress in susceptible pregnant patients, especially those with diabetes or sickle cell disease) |
| **Intrapartum** | | |
| Fluid administration | • Temporary increase in blood pressure<br>• Dilution of coagulation factors | • Predisposed to pulmonary edema with infection, and disseminated intravascular coagulation in hemorrhage |
| Labor pain | • Increased blood pressure<br>• Mild to moderate tachycardia<br>• Shortness of breath | • Infection/sepsis, pulmonary embolism, preeclampsia, abruption |
| Pain medications | • Blunts pain response<br>• Alters mental status | • Sepsis, intra-abdominal hemorrhage |
| Regional anesthesia | • Decrease in mean arterial pressure<br>• Low-grade fever<br>• Blunts pain response | • Intra-abdominal hemorrhage, infection |
| Hemorrhage medications (e.g., misoprostol) | • Low-grade fever | • Infection/sepsis |
| **Early postpartum** | | |
| | • Maternal tachycardia<br>• Baseline low blood pressure<br>• Increased blood volume<br>• Increased coagulation factors<br>• No clear portal of entry for genitourinary infections | • Postpartum hemorrhage (may not see changes until after a quantitative blood loss of 1,500 mL)<br><br>• Puerperal sepsis caused by group A streptococcus |
| **Late postpartum** | | |
| | • Exhaustion from lack of sleep<br>• Postpartum blues | Major depression, suicidal ideation |

**KEY POINTS**
- Normal physiologic changes in pregnancy may mask maternal deterioration in the critically ill patient.
- Clinical factors such as normal physiologic changes of pregnancy, fluid administration, anesthesia, and medications may alter maternal vital signs and mask clinical deterioration until the moment of impending respiratory or cardiovascular collapse.

# 3.3 OBSTETRIC EARLY WARNING SYSTEMS

There are several obstetric early warning systems (EWS) to detect changes in maternal vital signs that precede critical illness and identify patients who may need rapid escalation of care. While most of these systems are applied to the in-hospital setting, there are a few out-of-hospital warning systems for sepsis.[1] An EWS functions as a screening and communication tool and contains two essential components:

- The maternal early warning criteria
- An effective escalation policy

Current warning systems can be divided into single-parameter scoring systems and aggregate-weighted scoring systems. **Single-parameter** systems evaluate individual vital sign parameters, and an evaluation is triggered if any **single** parameter is abnormal.

**Aggregate-weighted** scoring systems use a combination of maternal parameters (e.g., temperature, blood pressure, pulse, respiratory rate, oxygen saturation, level of consciousness, pain level, proteinuria, discharge/lochia) to arrive at an aggregate clinical score, which triggers an evaluation. Single-parameter systems are simpler and more **specific**, meaning they are more likely to identify risk of death. In comparison, aggregate-weighted scoring systems are more complex and more **sensitive**. A more sensitive test will detect multiple minor changes in vital signs earlier than those using a single parameter.

The increased specificity of the single-parameter systems will increase the positive predictive value (PPV) of the test. The PPV indicates how likely it is that a patient with a positive screening test truly has the disease. In this case, a flag in an EWS will identify a critically ill mother. Additionally, the prevalence of the disease (critical illness) in the population being tested will affect the PPV of the test. In populations with a higher prevalence of the condition, the PPV will be higher than in lower-prevalence populations.

Current limitations include their relatively low PPV, with many suffering from a high false trigger rate, which can contribute to what is known as trigger fatigue, especially in high-volume, high-acuity units.[2] Systems with higher specificity, lower sensitivity, and higher predictive value may be ideal for these units, to help minimize the false trigger rate. It should be noted that no one system is universally applicable to all healthcare settings.

Facilities should choose a system that best meets their needs and balances the trade-offs between sensitivity and specificity. Table 3.4 lists current early warning systems, and Table 3.5 outlines their predictive values.

Effective escalation algorithms consist of guidance on communication including when and how to call for help (activate the rapid response team) and how providers will respond (come to the patient's bedside for evaluation), guidance on initial diagnostic evaluation and treatment, and timing of repeat observations.

**TABLE 3.4**   Proposed Early Warning Systems for Predicting Adverse Obstetric Outcomes[3]

| IN-HOSPITAL | OUT-OF-HOSPITAL |
|---|---|
| Confidential Enquiry into Maternal and Child Health (CEMACH) Modified Early Obstetric Warning System | Quick Sequential Organ Failure Assessment Score (qSOFA)[1] |
| CRADLE Vital Signs Alert Early Warning System | Red Flag Sepsis[4] |
| Preeclampsia Integrated Estimate of RiSk (PIERS; fullPIERS and miniPIERS models) | |
| Intensive Care National Audit & Research Centre (ICNARC) Modified Early Obstetric Warning System | |
| Irish Maternity Early Warning System (IMEWS) | |
| Maternal Early Warning Criteria (MEWC) | |
| Maternal Early Warning Trigger (MEWT) tool | |
| Modified Early Obstetric Warning System (MEOWS) | |
| Modified Early Warning System (MEWS) | |
| National Early Warning System (NEWS) | |
| Sepsis in Obstetrics Score (S.O.S.) | |
| CMQCC Maternal Sepsis Evaluation Flow Chart | |

**TABLE 3.5**   Predictive Values of Early Warning Systems

| TOOL | IN-HOSPITAL | OUT-OF-HOSPITAL | PARAMETER | POSITIVE PREDICTIVE VALUE | NEGATIVE PREDICTIVE VALUE |
|---|---|---|---|---|---|
| MEOWS | X | | Aggregate | 41%–54% | 97%–98% |
| MEWC | X | | Single | | |
| MEWS | X | | | 5.4% | |
| MEWT | X | | Aggregate | 12%–95% | 77%–99% |
| Red Flag Sepsis | | X | Aggregate | | |
| S.O.S. | X | | Aggregate | | 98.6% |
| CMQCC* | X | | Aggregate | 97% | 99% |

*CMQCC undergoing validation trials with anticipated sensitivity and specificity values based on clinical practice data sets.[5]

## 3.3.1 Examples of Obstetric Early Warning Systems

This section introduces examples of early warning systems and how providers may implement them for prompt recognition of the critically ill pregnant patient. Institutions adopting an EWS for identification of the critically ill pregnant patient should tailor it to their specific needs and unique unit considerations. Reviewed are two selected examples of maternal EWS: the Maternal Early Warning Trigger (MEWT) and the S.O.S. OBLS do **not** endorse any specific EWS.

---

**KEY POINTS**

- An obstetric EWS uses a combination of maternal parameters (e.g., temperature, blood pressure, pulse, respiratory rate, oxygen saturation, level of consciousness, pain level, proteinuria, discharge/lochia) to arrive at a clinical score, and the clinical score is used to trigger an escalation algorithm.
- An EWS is limited by a low PPV resulting in a high false alarm rate. This can contribute to trigger fatigue, especially in high-volume, high-acuity units.
- Adoption of an EWS for identification of the critically ill pregnant patient should be specific and modified to an institution/unit's needs.

---

## 3.3.2 MEWT

The MEWT tool has been shown to reduce maternal morbidity in the U.S.[6] It is designed to address the four most common causes of maternal morbidity: infection-sepsis, cardiopulmonary dysfunction, hypertension, and obstetric hemorrhage. The MEWT tool provides criteria for the assessment of vital signs and management recommendations.[6] The MEWT tool contains parameters for maternal status, or "maternal triggers," which include changes in vital signs (temperature, oxygen saturation, heart rate, respiratory rate, blood pressure), any altered mental status, and/or the presence of fetal tachycardia. The MEWT tool includes nurses' concerns about the patient, with suggested pathways leading to expanded evaluation and an escalation algorithm. Laboratory and radiologic evaluation are also recommended within the primary categories as part of the algorithm (Figure 3.1).

## 3.3.3 S.O.S.

S.O.S. is used to predict the need for an intensive care unit (ICU) admission in pregnant people presenting with signs and symptoms concerning for sepsis.[7] This validated scoring system uses physiologic and laboratory parameters to arrive at a clinical score (Table 3.6). A prospective validation trial of the S.O.S. on 1,250 pregnant or postpartum people presenting to the emergency department who met criteria for systemic inflammatory response syndrome revealed that 425 (34%) had a clinical

**TABLE 3.6**  S.O.S.[7]

| VARIABLE | HIGH ABNORMAL RANGE | | | | NORMAL | LOW ABNORMAL RANGE | | | |
|---|---|---|---|---|---|---|---|---|---|
| Score | +4 | +3 | +2 | +1 | 0 | +1 | +2 | +3 | +4 |
| Temperature (°C) | >40.9 | 39–40.9 | | 38.5–38.9 | 36–38.4 | 34–35.9 | 32–33.9 | 30–31.9 | <30 |
| Systolic blood pressure (mm Hg) | | | | | >90 | | 70–90 | | <70 |
| Heart rate (beats per minute) | >179 | 150–179 | 130–179 | 120–129 | ≤119 | | | | |
| Respiratory rate (breaths per minute) | >49 | 35–49 | | 25–34 | 12–24 | 10–11 | 6–9 | | ≤5 |
| SpO$_2$ (%) | | | | | ≥92% | 90%–91% | | 85%–89% | <85% |
| White blood cell count (/µL) | >39.9 | | 25–39.9 | 17–24.9 | 5.7–16.9 | 3–5.6 | 1–2.9 | | <1 |
| % Immature neutrophils | | ≥10% | | | <10% | | | | |
| Lactic acid (mmol/L) | | ≥4 | | | <4 | | | | |

Used with permission from Dr. Catherine Albright.

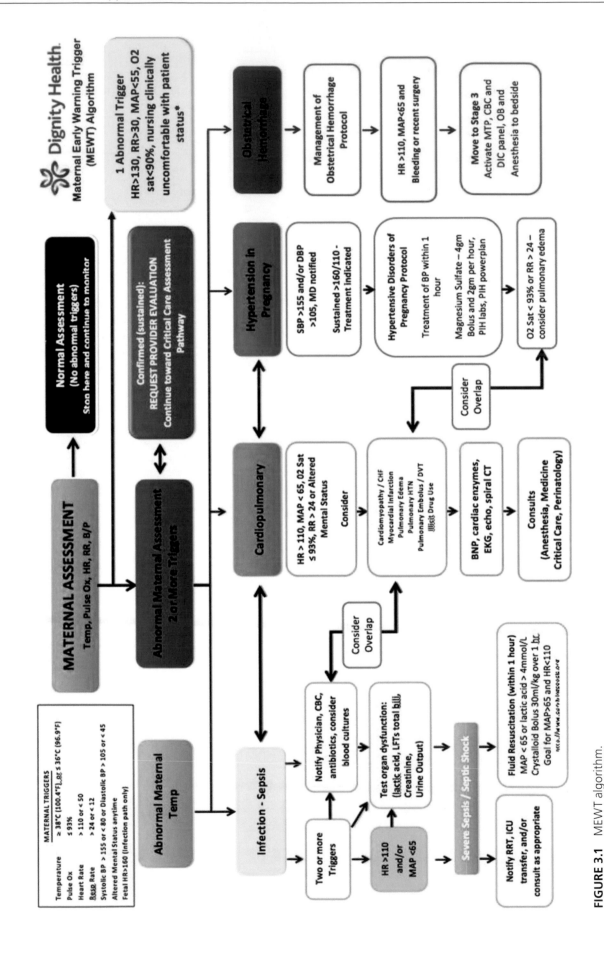

**FIGURE 3.1**   MEWT algorithm.

Used with permission from Dr. Laurence Shields.

suspicion or diagnosis of infection, with 14 (3.3%) admitted to the ICU. A score less than six had a negative predictive value of 98.6% and ruled **out** the need for ICU admission.[7] Those with a score of six or higher were more likely to be admitted to the ICU, admitted to a telemetry unit, and have antibiotic therapy initiated. This is one of the only validated scoring systems specific to the detection of septic shock in pregnancy. More research is needed to determine if this scoring system reduces maternal morbidity and mortality.

# 3.4 INSTITUTIONAL PLANNING FOR CRITICALLY ILL PREGNANT AND POSTPARTUM PATIENTS

Prevention of MCA is multifactorial, and access to and compliance with prenatal and postpartum care are essential. Additionally, all hospitals caring for obstetric patients must have a written policy in place to identify and evaluate critically ill pregnant or postpartum patients and ensure that they have adequate resources to care for these types of patients. Designating a team to respond to MCA ensures a unified call to action for obstetric/gynecologic providers, and the code and neonatal/pediatrics teams. Chapter 6 reviews MCA teams (MCATs) in more detail.

Hospitals with limited resources should institute a maternal transport policy, allowing efficient transfer of patients to the proper maternal care facility.

**KEY POINTS**
- All hospitals caring for obstetric patients must have a written policy in place to identify and evaluate critically ill pregnant or postpartum patients and ensure that they have adequate resources to care for these types of patients.
- S.O.S. is the only validated scoring system for predicting ICU admission in maternal sepsis and uses physiologic and laboratory parameters to arrive at a clinical score. An S.O.S. score less than 6 **rules out** the need for ICU admission.
- The CMQCC two-step flow chart for diagnosis and treatment of maternal sepsis is currently undergoing validation trials.

# 3.5 COMMUNICATION

Timely and accurate communication between the nurse and clinician is vital, especially with the escalation of care. There are numerous recommendations to improve initial communication of early warning signs, proper escalation of care, and ongoing communication about changes in the patient status to prevent delays and potential patient harm.

Chapter 12 reviews effective communication styles to address these issues. An established, supported, and transparent chain of command policy can help to alleviate tension that may occur when escalating care.

The following clinical vignette presents how the MEWT and S.O.S. tools can be implemented for earlier recognition of a critically ill pregnant patient.

**Case Vignette**

An 18-year-old multiparous person at 16 weeks gestation with a twin pregnancy presents to the ED, reporting the presence of fever, pain with urination, and back pain. In addition, the patient describes feeling short of breath and appears lethargic.

Admission vital signs are temperature 101.5°F, blood pressure 90/60, pulse 130, respiratory rate 30, and pulse oximetry of 88% on room air. Chest radiographs, a complete blood count, a comprehensive metabolic panel, blood and urine cultures, and lactic acid are ordered. After diagnosing pyelonephritis, the team gives IV fluid boluses and 2 L of oxygen by nasal cannula, orders antibiotics, and calls for an obstetric consult. They administer antibiotics 1.5 hours after the patient's arrival at the ED. During this time they also administer 2.5 L of IV fluids.

Two hours after initial presentation to the ED, the patient reports worsening shortness of breath and chest tightness, and passes out. The patient is unresponsive and without a pulse. The team calls a maternal code and starts OBLS. The cardiac rhythm is noted to be pulseless electrical activity (PEA). The team palpates the uterus at the umbilicus, continues high-quality cardiopulmonary resuscitation (CPR) and left uterine displacement, and administers epinephrine.

After 4 minutes of CPR, the rhythm check continues to show PEA. While intubating, the team notices a frothy ooze from the endotracheal tube. The OB/GYN performs a resuscitative cesarean delivery, and the neonatal team provides comfort care to the nonviable neonates. After 2 more minutes of CPR, a rhythm check demonstrates ventricular fibrillation, and shock is applied. The patient has return of spontaneous circulation and is sent to the ICU for post-arrest management of presumed urosepsis with respiratory failure due to acute respiratory distress syndrome. Care includes mechanical ventilation and high positive end-expiratory pressure.

## REVIEW QUESTIONS

**Q.** What are abnormal vital sign parameters in pregnancy?
**A.** Based on MEWT, abnormal vital signs include the following:

1.  Maternal heart rate >110 or <50
2.  Temperature >100.4°F or <96.9°F
3.  Respirations: >24 or <12
4.  Blood pressure: systolic >155 or <80 **or** diastolic >105 or <45
5.  Pulse ox: ≤93%
6.  Any altered mental status
7.  Fetal heart rate >160 (infection concern)

While each reporting system varies slightly, these are reflective of the generally accepted abnormal parameters in pregnancy.

**Q.** According to the MEWT tool and based on the presenting symptoms and signs, which major category would this patient correspond to—cardiovascular, infection-sepsis, hypertension, or obstetric hemorrhage?
**A.** Based on the presenting vital signs, the MEWT tool would be triggered via maternal fever, abnormal heart rate (>110), elevated respiratory rate (>24), and low pulse ox reading (<93%). Based on MEWT, the presence of greater than two triggers should prompt immediate provider evaluation as well as activation of the "infection-sepsis" tree.

**Q.** What scoring systems can be applied to the pregnant patient to screen for risk for adverse outcome or admission to the ICU?
**A.** There are multiple different warning systems, and no one system is perfect. Following are the warning systems currently available. See Tables 3.3 and 3.4 for more information.

1. MEWT      4. MEWS      7. CRADLE      10. PIERS
2. MEOWS     5. S.O.S.    8. ICNARC      11. CMQCC
3. MEWC      6. NEWS      9. CEMACH

**Q.** What is the treatment for a pregnant patient with suspected sepsis?
**A.** Following the MEWT protocol, promptly evaluate a patient with suspected sepsis. Follow with labs (complete blood count, cultures, comprehensive metabolic panel, lactic acid) and prompt administration of broad-spectrum antibiotics and IV fluids with fluid resuscitation. Ideally, antibiotics are started within the "golden hour" of presentation. Each patient's clinical presentation and score (based on MEWT or S.O.S., for instance) will prompt where the patient should be admitted (i.e., floor or ICU). Closely monitor the patient's response to resuscitation and treatment to ensure therapies are working and that end organ damage/injury is avoided or contained.

Applying the MEWT to our clinical vignette, a provider would be directed to the following:

1.  The major category of "infection-sepsis" based on maternal fever and four abnormal triggers (pulse oximetry, temperature, heart rate, and respiratory rate), then to

2. The "sepsis-septic shock" category based on heart rate, then
3. Triggered to notify the rapid response team, ICU transfer, and/or consult as appropriate, then
   • Obtain complete blood count, start antibiotics, and consider blood cultures
   • Test for organ dysfunction (e.g., lactic acid, liver function tests, total bilirubin, creatinine, and urine output)
4. Start fluid resuscitation.

Applying the S.O.S. system, a provider would recognize the following:

1. Preliminary S.O.S. is 9 before lab results, which would alert the provider to suspect sepsis that will likely require ICU admission.
2. Administer broad-spectrum antibiotics within 1 hour of suspected sepsis to comply with the surviving sepsis campaign bundle and reduce maternal morbidity and mortality.
3. Administer IV fluids and closely monitor inputs and outputs, as patients with urosepsis in pregnancy are at increased risk of lung injury, pulmonary edema, and acute respiratory distress syndrome.

# CHAPTER 3. PRACTICE QUESTIONS

1. The **priority** goal of the obstetric EWS is to identify patients who may need which of the following?
   A. Rapid escalation of care
   B. Immediate cesarean delivery
   C. The MCAT
   D. CPR

2. Which of the following signs or symptoms requires an escalation of care in a patient in labor?
   A. White blood cell count of 20,000/mm
   B. Fetal heart rate of 160 beats per minute
   C. Shortness of breath during pushing attempts
   D. Altered mental status

3. Which of the following statements BEST reflect current obstetric emergency warning systems?
   A. Can use same vital sign parameters as nonpregnant patients
   B. Their use may decrease maternal morbidity
   C. Have high positive predictive value, with low false-positive trigger rates
   D. Do not require a process for escalation of care

4. A nulliparous person at 16 weeks gestation presents to the emergency department with reports of shortness of breath and chest pain. Pulse is 120 and pulse oximeter is 90%. The patient is afebrile. Which of the following laboratory and imaging examinations would be the BEST next step in management according to the MEWT protocol?
   A. B-type natriuretic peptide (BNP), cardiac enzymes, electrocardiogram (ECG), echo, and spiral computed tomography
   B. Lactic acid, liver function tests (LFTs), total bili, and creatinine
   C. Complete blood count (CBC), disseminated intravascular coagulation (DIC) panel
   D. Random glucose, hemoglobin A1c, comprehensive metabolic panel (CMP)

5. Which of the following validated EWS predicts the need for admission to the ICU from sepsis in pregnancy?
   A. MEWT
   B. MEOWS
   C. S.O.S.
   D. CEMACH Modified Early Obstetric Warning System

# CHAPTER 3. ANSWERS

1. **ANSWER: A.** Obstetric emergency warning systems have been proposed to detect changes in maternal vital signs that precede critical illness and **identify patients who may need rapid escalation of care**. Warning systems use a combination of maternal parameters (such as temperature, blood pressure, pulse, respiratory rate, oxygen saturation, level of consciousness, pain level, proteinuria, discharge/lochia) to arrive at a clinical score, and the clinical score is used to trigger an escalation algorithm. Escalation algorithms guide the timing of repeat observations, when and how to call for help (e.g., call the provider about the patient's status, call the provider to the bedside, and/or activate the rapid response team), and initial diagnostic evaluation and treatment. While patients who trigger rapid escalation of care based on an EWS may ultimately need the MCAT, immediate cesarean delivery, or CPR, the most correct answer is A.

2. **ANSWER: D.** Warning systems use a combination of maternal parameters (such as temperature, blood pressure, pulse, respiratory rate, oxygen saturation, level of consciousness, pain level, proteinuria, discharge/lochia) to arrive at a clinical score, which then triggers an escalation algorithm. Most warning systems include any mental status change as a significant maternal trigger that requires escalation of care. While a white blood cell count of 20,000 is abnormal in the nonpregnant population, this may be normal for a patient in labor. Similarly, it is normal for a patient to have shortness of breath with pushing efforts. A fetal heart rate of 160 bpm can be a sign for fetal distress (such as in the setting of infection) however is not as concerning as maternal altered mental status. Also, as a single indicator, it would not trigger immediate escalation of care.

3. **ANSWER: B.** Normal physiologic changes in pregnancy may mask maternal deterioration in the critically ill patient. EWS use a combination of maternal parameters to arrive at a clinical score, which then triggers an escalation algorithm. The MEWT tool has been shown to **reduce maternal morbidity** in the U.S.

4. **ANSWER: A.** The MEWT tool is designed to address the four most common causes of maternal morbidity: infection-sepsis, cardiopulmonary, hypertension in pregnancy, and obstetric hemorrhage. MEWT provides criteria for the assessment of vital signs and management recommendations. According to the MEWT algorithm, this patient has two or more abnormal vital signs concerning for cardiovascular disease. The proposed evaluation based on the tool and category (cardiovascular) is a BNP, cardiac enzymes, ECG, echo, and spiral computed tomography to evaluate for some of the common etiologies of cardiovascular disease in pregnancy (e.g., pulmonary embolism, pulmonary hypertension, pulmonary edema, myocardial infarction, cardiomyopathy/congestive heart failure, and arrhythmia).

5. **ANSWER: C.** The only validated scoring system for the detection of sepsis during pregnancy that will likely require ICU admission is the S.O.S. This scoring system was developed to predict the need for ICU admission in pregnant people presenting with signs and symptoms concerning for sepsis. The scoring system uses physiologic and laboratory parameters to arrive at a clinical score. A score less than 6 has a negative predictive value of 98.6% and rules out the need for ICU admission.

# CHAPTER 3. REFERENCES

1. Shu E, Tall CI, Frye W, et al. Pre-hospital qSOFA as a predictor of sepsis and mortality. *Am J Emerg Med.* 2019 Jul;37(7):1273–1278. doi: 10.1016/j.ajem.2018.09.025. Epub 2018 September 18.

2. Blumenthal E, Hooshvar N, McQuade M, McNulty J. A validation study of maternal early warning systems: A retrospective cohort study. *Am J Perinatol.* 2019 Sep;36(11):1106–1114. doi: 10.1055/s-0039-1681097.

3. Umar A, Ameh CA, Muriithi F, Mathai M. Early warning systems in obstetrics: A systematic literature review. *PLoS One.* 2019;14(5):e0217864. doi: 10.1371/journal.pone.0217864.

4. Seymour CW, Cooke CR, Heckbert SR, Spertus JA, Callaway CW, Martin-Gill C, Yealy DM, Rea TD, Angus DC. Prehospital intravenous access and fluid resuscitation in severe sepsis: An observational cohort study. *Crit Care.* 2014 September 27;18(5):533. doi: 10.1186/s13054-014-0533-x.

5. Gibbs R, Bauer M, Olvera L, Sakowski C, Cape V, Main E. *Improving Diagnosis and Treatment of Maternal Sepsis: A California Maternal Quality Care Collaborative Quality Improvement Toolkit.* 2022. Available at https://www.cmqcc.org/resources-toolkits/toolkits/improving-diagnosis-and-treatment-maternal-sepsis-errata-712022. Accessed March 18, 2023.

6. Shields LE, Wiesner S, Klein C, Pelletreau B, Hedriana HL. Use of maternal early warning trigger tool reduces maternal morbidity. *Am J Obstet Gynecol.* 2016;21(4):527.e1–527.e6. doi: 10.1016/j.ajog.2016.01.154.

7. Albright CM, Has J, Rouse L, Hughes L. Internal validation of the Sepsis in Obstetrics Score to identify risk of morbidity from sepsis in pregnancy. *Obstet Gynecol.* 2017 October;13(4):747–755. doi: 10.1097/AOG.0000000000002260.

# Common Causes of Maternal Cardiac Arrest

# 4

## 4.1 INTRODUCTION

Maternal cardiac arrest (MCA) results from etiologies which are substantially different and more broadly diverse than those etiologies associated with cardiac arrest in the nonpregnant patient. This chapter highlights some of the most common causes of MCA, reviews presenting symptoms and signs, and introduces initial steps to prevent the progression from symptoms to full arrest. Additionally, we review the immediately reversible causes of MCA that providers must recognize and treat quickly for optimal recovery. Finally, we introduce the mnemonic and post-arrest aid **BAACC TO LIFE** to help recall the common etiologies of MCA (Figure 4.1 and Appendix D, respectively).

## 4.2 LEARNING OBJECTIVES

Learner will appropriately

- Review the most common etiologies of MCA.
- Recognize the presenting symptoms and signs of the etiologies that may lead to MCA.
- Discuss the treatment of the most common etiologies leading to MCA.
- Recognize and understand treatments for the leading immediately reversible causes of MCA, including hypoglycemia, high spinal, and lidocaine and magnesium sulfate toxicity.
- Describe the major causes of MCA using the mnemonic BAACC TO LIFE.

## 4.3 BAACC TO LIFE: BLEEDING

Maternal hemorrhage is the leading cause of maternal morbidity and mortality worldwide.[1] Bleeding following delivery, known as postpartum hemorrhage (PPH), accounts for approximately three-quarters of these cases.[1] More than 50% of maternal deaths from PPH happen within the first 24 hours of delivery.[2] Delayed PPH is defined as bleeding occurring more than 24 hours after delivery and less than 6 weeks postpartum. Uterine atony is the most common cause of PPH, occurring in approximately 70%–80% of cases.[3] A uterus at term receives 500–800 mL of blood per minute; thus, uterine atony can result in rapid loss of large amounts of blood. Other causes of maternal hemorrhage are listed in Table 4.1. Due to how common and severe PPH can be, it is essential that all patients are closely monitored for bleeding during the first 24–48 hours after delivery.

PPH is a symptom. Once identified, providers should search for the cause (diagnosis), while simultaneously transfusing blood products as necessary. If concerned about excessive bleeding following delivery, providers should perform a detailed examination for, and control, the source of bleeding. Further laboratory evaluation includes a complete blood count and coagulation studies, although providers should not wait on these results to begin medical treatment of obstetric hemorrhage. Laboratory assessments during PPH are helpful to monitor trends, though values in acute hemorrhage often lag. As PPH is the most common cause of uterine atony, Table 4.3 describes the treatment options for uterine atony. If medical treatment is

DOI: 10.1201/9781003299288-5

BAACC
- **B**leeding
- **A**nesthesia
- **A**FE
- **C**ardiovascular/cardiomyopathy
- **C**lot/cerebrovascular

TO
- **T**rauma
- **O**verdose (magnesium sulfate/opioids/other)

LIFE
- **L**ung injury/ARDS
- **I**ons (glucose/K+)
- **F**ever (sepsis)
- **E**mergency hypertension/eclampsia

**FIGURE 4.1**  Etiologies for maternal cardiac arrest, the BAACC TO LIFE mnemonic.

**TABLE 4.1**  Maternal Hemorrhage: Major Causes throughout Pregnancy

| TIME PERIOD | MAJOR CAUSES OF HEMORRHAGE |
| --- | --- |
| Antepartum | • Placental abnormalities (abruption, previa, accreta spectrum)<br>• Trauma<br>• Uterine rupture<br>• Coagulation defects (inherited, acquired) |
| Intrapartum or immediate postpartum (within 24 hours of delivery) | • Uterine atony<br>• Uterine inversion<br>• Coagulation defects (inherited or acquired)<br>• Vaginal/cervical lacerations<br>• Episiotomy<br>• Retained conception products or retained placenta, placental abnormalities (abruption, previa, accreta spectrum)<br>• Amniotic fluid embolism (AFE)<br>• Uterine rupture<br>• Bleeding surgical sites/pedicles |
| Delayed postpartum (>24 hours after delivery, <6 weeks postpartum) | • Retained products of conception/placenta<br>• Infection |

unsuccessful, proceed with tamponade balloon placement, vacuum-induced hemorrhage control, or laparotomy (surgery) with the potential need for a hysterectomy to control the bleeding.

Pregnant people can lose up to 1,500 mL of blood before showing changes in vital signs. Thus, maternal vital sign changes in the setting of bleeding are an ominous sign, and providers should promptly activate the massive transfusion protocol and rapid response teams. Rapid volume repletion with IV fluid and blood products, as well as identification and correction of the source of bleeding, will reduce the likelihood of significant maternal morbidity or mortality. Table 4.2 outlines a stage-based response to obstetric hemorrhage.

Delayed hemorrhages (≥24 hours and <6 weeks from delivery) can also occur. Provide all postpartum patients with detailed discharge instructions that include when to seek medical care for excessive bleeding.

**KEY POINTS**

- Maternal hemorrhage is the leading cause of maternal morbidity and mortality worldwide. Postpartum hemorrhage from uterine atony accounts for approximately three-quarters of these cases.
- Pregnant people can lose up to 1,500 mL of blood before showing vital sign changes. If vital sign changes are present, prompt activation of the massive transfusion protocol and rapid response team is indicated.
- Time and indecision kill. Do **not** delay treatment during maternal hemorrhage. Ongoing hemorrhage with or without maternal vital sign changes requires swift activation of the massive blood transfusion protocol and rapid response team. Refractory hemorrhage requires surgery, with possible hysterectomy to control the bleeding.

**TABLE 4.2**   Stage-Based Hemorrhage Management

| STAGE | DEFINITION | ACTION |
|---|---|---|
| Identify Hemorrhage Risk on Admission | | |
| Stage 0 | • Active management with oxytocin infusion | • Quantitative blood loss (QBL) assessment (1 g = 1 mL)<br>• Ongoing evaluation of vital signs |
| Stage 1 | • Continued bleeding and blood loss<br>• >1,000 mL vaginal or cesarean<br>• Early vital sign changes (15%)<br>• Increased bleeding in recovery period | • Notify obstetric (OB) and anesthesia providers<br>• Establish IV<br>• Massage fundus<br>• Administer second uterotonic<br>• Empty bladder<br>• Type and cross for 2 units packed red blood cells (PRBC)<br>• Consider potential etiologies<br>• Cumulative QBL |
| Stage 2 | • Continued bleeding with QBL <1,500 mL | • OB provider to bedside<br>• Administer a third uterotonic<br>• Start second IV<br>• Administer tranexamic acid<br>• Uterine balloon tamponade or vacuum-induced hemorrhage control<br>• Move to operating room, prepare for procedural interventions<br>• B-Lynch<br>• Interventional radiology<br>• Transfuse 2 units PRBC (do not wait for lab results)<br>• Order STAT labs (complete blood count, comprehensive metabolic panel, prothrombin time/partial thromboplastin time, fibrinogen)<br>• Cumulative QBL<br>• Announce vital signs |
| Stage 3 | • QBL ≥1,500 mL or maternal tachycardia, hypotension, or vital sign changes<br>• Or >2 units PRBC administered<br>• Or suspect disseminated intravascular coagulation (DIC) | • Activate Massive Transfusion Protocol<br>• Transfuse 1:1:1 (PRBC:fresh frozen plasma:platelets) or whole blood, if available<br>• Notify second surgeon or gynecology/oncology surgeon, if available<br>• Consider hysterectomy if still bleeding<br>• Keep patient warm<br>• Use fluid warmer/rapid infuser<br>• Repeat labs every 30–60 minutes<br>• Postpartum intensive care unit management |
| Stage 4 | • Cardiac arrest | • Obstetric life support |

**TABLE 4.3**  Medical Treatment of Postpartum Hemorrhage Due to Uterine Atony

| MEDICATION | DOSE | SIDE EFFECTS | CONTRAINDICATIONS |
|---|---|---|---|
| Oxytocin | 10–40 units in 500–1,000 mL IV continuous infusion | Nausea, vomiting, hyponatremia due to antidiuretic effect, cardiac arrhythmia | Hypersensitivity to oxytocin |
| 15-Methyl prostaglandin F2α | 250 mcg intramuscular or intramyometrial every 15 minutes for 8 doses | Nausea, vomiting, diarrhea, bronchospasm | Asthma, history of allergy to prostaglandins, hypertension (use with caution) |
| Methylergonovine maleate | 200 mcg intramuscular every 2–4 hours | Hypertension, seizure, headache, abdominal pain, nausea, and vomiting | Hypertension, preeclampsia, cardiovascular disease |
| Misoprostol | 600–1,000 mcg rectal, oral, or sublingual, single dose | Fever, diarrhea, nausea, vomiting, stomach cramps, gas, constipation, headache | Allergy to prostaglandins |
| Tranexamic acid (TXA) | 1-g IV infusion or slow push over 10 minutes; may repeat 1 dose in 30 minutes | Nausea, vomiting, diarrhea, allergic dermatitis, and hypotension observed when IV injection is too rapid | Active intravascular clotting (e.g., deep vein thrombosis or pulmonary embolism), subarachnoid hemorrhage, acquired defective color vision |

# 4.4  BAACC TO LIFE: ANESTHESIA

Maternal deaths can occur from complications due to intrapartum regional and general anesthesia. In a series of maternal deaths in Michigan between 1985 and 2003, anesthesia-related deaths contributed to 1.7% of maternal deaths.[4] These cases often result from the presence of other comorbidities, such as preeclampsia with severe features or extreme obesity, where the presence of oropharyngeal edema complicates airway management. Risk factors for anesthesia-related maternal deaths are listed in Table 4.4.

Providers should be aware of potential anesthetic complications, such as high spinal or lidocaine toxicity, which can occur in pregnant people with few risk factors. These immediately reversible causes of MCA require prompt recognition and treatment.

A pregnant patient with a high spinal will frequently report feeling anxious; have difficulty breathing, nausea, and numbness or weakness of the arms; and may develop hypotension and bradycardia. Symptoms may proceed to loss of consciousness and respiratory arrest. Treatment for high spinal consists of supportive care with 100% oxygen application for ventilation, IV fluid bolus, and possible intubation. Other actions include activation of the rapid response team, and administering lipid emulsion, and peripheral vasoconstrictors (alpha 1-antagonist) such as phenylephrine for hypotension and atropine for bradycardia. Other vasoconstrictors that may be used include ephedrine and low doses of dilute adrenaline solution.

A pregnant person with acute local anesthetic systemic toxicity during placement of the epidural or repair of a perineal laceration may present with circumoral numbness, facial tingling, restlessness, vertigo, tinnitus, slurred speech, tonic-clonic seizures, and cardiac arrest. Figure 4.2 reviews the treatment of acute local anesthetic systemic toxicity.

# 4.5  BAACC TO LIFE: AMNIOTIC FLUID EMBOLISM

AFE is a rare and catastrophic complication of pregnancy with a comparatively high mortality rate. The incidence of AFE is low, between 1.9 and 6.1 per 100,000 births, and with a mortality rate as high as 60%. AFE is thought to be an immune-mediated response to amniotic fluid and debris circulating in the maternal bloodstream. Though AFE typically occurs during labor or shortly after birth, it can be associated with trauma and prolonged rupture of membranes. Consider AFE in the differential diagnosis of sudden cardiovascular collapse of a laboring or recently delivered person.

AFE often presents with cardiac arrest, thus the initial response should be high-quality CPR. AFE occurs in two stages. The first stage consists of a **respiratory arrest phase**, and the second phase consists of a **hemorrhagic phase**, which quickly develops into DIC.

**TABLE 4.4**  Risk Factors for Anesthesia-Related Maternal Deaths[4]

| | |
|---|---|
| Airway obstruction | Lived experience of anti-Black racism |
| Emergence and recovery from general anesthesia | Obesity |
| Lack of clinical protocols and safety measures in delivering anesthetic care | Perioperative hypoventilation |

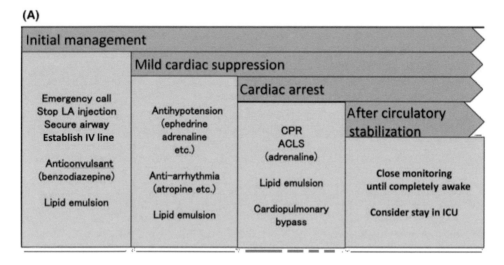

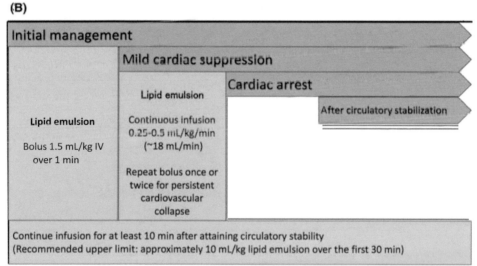

**FIGURE 4.2**  Management of acute local anesthetic toxicity. (A) Sequence of symptoms and required treatments. (B) Sequence of symptoms and program of lipid emulsion (20%) infusion. Abbreviations: ACLS, advanced cardiovascular life support; CPR, cardiopulmonary resuscitation; ICU, intensive care unit; LA, local anesthetic.

Signs and symptoms might include the following:

- Acute-onset chest pain
- Shortness of breath
- Nausea and/or vomiting
- Tachypnea, tachycardia, and hypotension
- Patient report of feeling an impending sense of doom
- Rapid deterioration into respiratory arrest

The respiratory arrest phase includes increased levels of pulmonary vasoconstrictors and mechanical obstruction that lead to respiratory failure and severe hypoxemia and severe acute right heart failure. These lead to hemodynamic collapse,

**TABLE 4.5**   Recommended Medication Doses to Treat Acute Right Ventricular Failure

| AGENT | DOSE |
|---|---|
| Dobutamine | 2.5–5.0 mcg/kg per minute. Higher doses may compromise right ventricular filling time caused by tachycardia |
| Inhaled nitric oxide | 5–40 ppm. Follow methemoglobin levels every 6 hours, and avoid abrupt discontinuation |
| Inhaled prostacyclin | 10–50 ng/kg per minute |
| IV prostacyclin | Start at 1–2 ng/kg per minute through a central line and titrate to desired effect. Side effects include systemic hypotension, nausea, vomiting, headache, jaw pain, and diarrhea |
| Milrinone | 0.25–0.75 mcg/kg per minute. Most common side effect is systemic hypotension |
| Norepinephrine | 0.05–3.3 mcg/kg per minute |
| Sildenafil | 20 mg three times a day by mouth or through nasogastric or orogastric tube |

decreased left-sided cardiac output, and late-onset left ventricular failure. These ultimately lead to cardiogenic pulmonary edema and systemic hypotension. Please see Table 4.5 for medications that can be considered in the treatment of right heart failure.

Airway management with immediate intubation is crucial during the respiratory arrest stage. Current recommended treatment for the respiratory phase of AFE includes pulmonary vasodilators, prostaglandins, and sympathomimetics to address right ventricular failure. Norepinephrine and inotropes are used to maintain hemodynamics and address left ventricular failure. The hemorrhagic phase consists of activation of factor VII and platelets with DIC. Inflammation further activates the clotting cascade, and ongoing hemorrhage contributes to hemodynamic instability.[5] During the hemorrhagic phase, early and aggressive utilization of the massive transfusion protocol with goal-directed transfusion will improve the patient's chances of survival.

If AFE results in cardiac arrest, perform RCD as indicated (subsequent chapters review RCD in detail). While treatment for AFE is mostly supportive, consider using the **A-OK** protocol[6] as soon as suspicion for AFE is raised. This consists of:

- 1 mg **A**tropine
- 8 mg **O**ndansetron
- 30 mg **K**etorolac

Supportive post-arrest care often occurs in the intensive care unit and consists of vasopressors, medications, and transfusion if indicated. Successful treatment of AFE with cardiopulmonary bypass and exchange transfusions has also been described.

**KEY POINTS**
- AFE has a high mortality rate and is usually seen with cardiac arrest.
- AFE should be suspected in a patient with acute development of hypoxia, hypotension, and coagulopathy.
- Upon recognizing AFE, perform high-quality CPR, supportive care, and consider the A-OK protocol.
- AFE requires aggressive supportive management utilizing massive transfusion protocol, rapid intubation, and delivery.
- Recommendations for treating the respiratory phase of AFE consist of pulmonary vasodilators, prostaglandins, and sympathomimetics.
- Right ventricular failure should be treated with inotropic agents and pulmonary vasodilators.

# 4.6 BAACC TO LIFE: CARDIOVASCULAR

The mean age of first-time mothers has been steadily climbing for the past 50 years and is currently 26 years of age.[7] Compared to their historical counterparts, pregnant patients also tend to have more comorbidities, with cardiovascular disease currently complicating approximately 4% of all pregnancies in the U.S.[7] Cardiovascular disease is also responsible for more than a third of U.S. maternal mortalities, with the vast majority of these due to acquired cardiovascular disease.[8] This section reviews peripartum cardiomyopathy and acute coronary syndrome. The following red flags require prompt evaluation, hospitalization, and consultation with cardiology and maternal-fetal medicine for acute symptoms of cardiovascular disease[9]:

- Shortness of breath at rest
- Severe orthopnea four or more pillows
  - Orthopnea: shortness of breath when lying down
  - Four or more pillows: the number of pillows needed to prop the patient to improve their breathing
- Resting heart rate ≥120 bpm
- Resting systolic blood pressure ≥160 mm Hg
- Resting respiratory rate ≥30
- Oxygen saturations ≤94% with or without personal history of cardiovascular disease

# 4.7 BAACC TO LIFE: PERIPARTUM CARDIOMYOPATHY

Peripartum cardiomyopathy (PPCM) is the most common cardiomyopathy diagnosed in pregnancy[10] and is the leading cause of late postpartum maternal mortality.[3] PPCM is an idiopathic disorder defined as heart failure occurring during the last month of pregnancy and up to 5 months postpartum, and more rare, 1 year postpartum.[3] A person with PPCM will typically present with increasing shortness of breath upon exertion (dyspnea on exertion), at rest (dyspnea), or while lying down (orthopnea).

Excessive weight gain and peripheral edema can be seen from fluid retention, especially with advanced disease. On physical exam, patients can have mild tachycardia, hypertension, and hypoxia (oxygenation saturations <94% on room air). On physical exam, bibasilar crackles of the lungs may be heard, and jugular venous distention (JVD) may be present. People with PPCM will also have a decreased ejection fraction on echocardiogram and a B-type natriuretic peptide ≥100 pg/mL. Prompt evaluation and treatment are important to improve maternal outcomes. Although many patients will experience recovery of cardiac function in the first 3–6 months postpartum, some may experience irreversible cardiac dysfunction, and there is a high rate of recurrence in subsequent pregnancies.

## 4.7.1 Cardiovascular: Other

Based on guidance from the American College of Obstetricians and Gynecologists, any pregnant patient presenting with chest pain (either typical or atypical) should be evaluated for acute coronary syndrome. Typical symptoms include chest pain, shortness of breath, radiating left arm pain, and/or palpitations. Atypical chest pain includes nausea/vomiting, epigastric, and abdominal pain. Evaluation is like the workup for nonpregnant patients and should include an electrocardiogram and laboratory evaluation with cardiac enzymes such as troponins. **While evaluating and treating, place pregnant patients in full left lateral tilt to improve venous return to the heart**.

Obstetric Life Support otherwise recommends following the same guidelines as for nonpregnant patients: administer oxygen, aspirin, nitroglycerin, and a beta-blocker (unless the patient has asthma), and use IV heparin and interventional cardiac catheterization if there is concern for acute coronary syndrome. To reduce fetal exposure to radiation, shield the pregnant abdomen during the cardiac catheterization.

**KEY POINTS**

- When evaluating patients for acute cardiac concerns, place them in a left lateral tilt. Initial treatment is the same as for nonpregnant adults.
- Perform interventional cardiac catheterization if there is concern for acute coronary syndrome in a pregnant patient. Shield the abdomen to reduce fetal radiation exposure.
- A person with PPCM will typically present with increasing shortness of breath, excessive weight gain, and ankle swelling.

# 4.8  BAACC TO LIFE: CLOT/CEREBROVASCULAR/ PULMONARY EMBOLISM

Pulmonary embolism (PE) is a life-threatening condition that has been associated with severe maternal morbidity and mortality. Injuries to vascular structures (from an injury or surgery), increased venous stasis (from pregnancy or immobilization), and increased hypercoagulability (due to increased circulating estrogen and increased clotting factors) all increase a pregnant person's chances of developing a blood clot.

Patients with PE typically present with acute-onset shortness of breath, tachycardia, and/or chest pain. Initial evaluation consists of an electrocardiogram and chest radiography. Historically, D-dimer testing has not been clinically useful during pregnancy as increased D-dimer concentrations are found in a normal pregnancy, resulting in a high rate of false-positive D-dimer tests.[11] New evidence suggests that a pregnancy-adapted YEARS criteria with D-dimer testing helps to rule out pulmonary embolism in pregnant patients.[12] This algorithm uses the assessment of the following three clinical criteria for pulmonary embolism (YEARS criteria):

- Clinical signs of deep vein thrombosis (DVT)
- Hemoptysis
- PE as the most likely diagnosis

In patients with clinical signs of DVT based on the YEARS criteria, a lower extremity compression ultrasound is performed on the symptomatic leg(s). If the ultrasound is abnormal, anticoagulation is initiated. If the ultrasound is negative, a D-dimer is sent, with further evaluation based on positive YEARS criteria and D-dimer levels.[12] Table 4.6 summarizes the recommended evaluation strategy based on YEARS criteria and D-dimer levels.

While most accurate in the first trimester, use of the YEARS criteria resulted in a reduced number of patients who had CT angiograms of the chest, thus reducing radiation exposure during pregnancy. While further studies may be required, the pregnancy YEARS algorithm using D-dimers with the YEARS clinical criteria can be used to evaluate for PE in all trimesters of pregnancy.[12]

If clinical suspicion is high for PE, start therapeutic anticoagulation therapy empirically with heparin or low-molecular-weight heparin while pursuing further evaluation with either CT angiogram of the chest, or ventilation-perfusion scan. Shield the pregnant person's abdomen when performing a CT angiogram. Fetal anomalies, growth restriction, and pregnancy loss have not been reported with radiation exposure of less than 50 milligray (mGy).[13] The risk of carcinogenesis because of in utero exposure

**TABLE 4.6**  Pregnancy YEARS Evaluation[12]

| POSITIVE YEARS CRITERIA | D-DIMER LEVELS | EVALUATION AND RECOMMENDATIONS |
|---|---|---|
| None | <1,000 ng/mL | PE ruled out, no anticoagulation |
| None | ≥1,000 ng/mL | Computed tomography (CT) pulmonary angiography, with anticoagulation if positive CT angiography |
| One to three | <500 ng/mL | PE ruled out, no anticoagulation |
| One to three | ≥500 ng/mL | CT pulmonary angiography, with anticoagulation if positive CT angiography |

to radiologic procedures is unclear, but probably rare,[13] and necessary diagnostic imaging for maternal indications should not be withheld.

Treating PE in pregnancy includes therapeutic anticoagulation consisting of unfractionated or low-molecular-weight heparin with possible transition to warfarin in the postpartum patient. Heparin or low-molecular-weight heparin are preferred anticoagulants in pregnancy as neither cross the placenta. Generally, low-molecular-weight heparin is preferred due to more predictable anticoagulant effect and lower risk of developing heparin-induced thrombocytopenia. However, in unstable patients or where surgical intervention is necessary, unfractionated heparin is preferred due to the ease of monitoring levels and reversibility. If the patient is receiving unfractionated heparin, obtain a complete blood count 4–5 days after starting heparin to assess for thrombocytopenia indicative of heparin-induced thrombocytopenia. Oral anticoagulation with non–vitamin K antagonist is not recommended in pregnant or postpartum nursing mothers. Warfarin is also not recommended in pregnancy due to its teratogenic potential, though it may be used in postpartum nursing mothers.

Case reports describe treatment for massive/saddle PE leading to MCA. Patients have been successfully treated with both thrombolytic therapy and embolectomy with favorable maternal and fetal outcomes. Emerging data show improved maternal outcomes using ECPR in this patient population and should also be considered. These patients will require a large multidisciplinary team (such as maternal-fetal medicine, pulmonologist, and vascular or cardiothoracic surgery specialists), and consideration should be given to transporting them to an ECPR-capable facility. These patients will often undergo RCD and may be at higher risk for bleeding complications. Thus, consider this complication in the decision to initiate thrombolytic therapy.

## 4.8.1 Cerebrovascular (Stroke)

While stroke is a rare cause of sudden cardiac death, it is a leading cause of severe maternal morbidity and mortality, particularly in those with preeclampsia.[8,14] Stroke can be either ischemic, due to blockage of a cerebral artery or vein, or hemorrhagic, due to rupture of blood vessels in or around the brain. Importantly, ischemic and hemorrhagic strokes can present with similar symptoms, so a rapid head CT is always needed to exclude hemorrhage. Stroke can occur at any time in pregnancy but is most common in the first 2 weeks postpartum. All types of stroke can cause death directly due to swelling and herniation of the brain, or indirectly as a result of poststroke complications such as aspiration or pulmonary embolism. Failure to recognize stroke signs and symptoms and act promptly can lead to devastating consequences, since "Time Is Brain."[15] Common stroke syndromes are reviewed in Table 4.7. A few stroke types have extremely high morbidity and mortality and are reviewed here.

**Large vessel occlusion** (LVO) is the occlusion of large arteries supplying blood to the brain, including the carotid, middle cerebral, or vertebrobasilar arteries. This is most commonly caused by a blood clot embolizing from the heart. This can occur in the setting of heart failure, arrhythmia, or so-called paradoxical embolism from a DVT in a person with a patent foramen ovale. Treatment for LVO may include IV thrombolysis or mechanical thrombectomy. While strokes due to LVO can cause severe disability and death, treatment has been revolutionized due to the success of thrombectomy trials.[16] Pregnancy is not a contraindication to thrombolysis or mechanical thrombectomy, and stroke protocols should be followed as usual, with close involvement of the obstetrics and neurology team. Importantly, a basilar artery occlusion may present with sudden loss of consciousness and convulsive activity and should always be considered in an unresponsive patient.

**Subarachnoid hemorrhage** (SAH) occurs most commonly when an artery ruptures on the surface of the brain causing arterial hemorrhage into the subarachnoid space. This can be due to a ruptured intracranial aneurysm, or to other causes. The

**TABLE 4.7** Stroke Causes, Signs, and Symptoms

| STROKE CAUSE | SIGNS AND SYMPTOMS |
|---|---|
| Left carotid or middle cerebral artery occlusion | Left gaze deviation, aphasia, right hemiparesis, hemiplegia<br>Right mouth/facial droop and right hemineglect |
| Right carotid or middle cerebral artery occlusion | Right gaze deviation, left hemineglect, left hemiparesis<br>Left mouth/facial droop and left hemiplegia |
| Basilar artery occlusion | Headache; loss of vision; loss of consciousness, posturing, convulsive activity |
| Subarachnoid hemorrhage | "Thunderclap" headache, neck stiffness, vomiting, loss of consciousness |
| Intracerebral hemorrhage | Headache, vomiting, focal neurologic deficits (depending on location of bleed), seizure |

presenting symptom is most commonly a sudden "thunderclap" headache. SAH can result in an overwhelming sympathetic nervous system surge, leading to neurogenic myocardial stunning and cardiac arrest.[17] For this reason, we recommend that all patients with cardiac arrest have prompt brain imaging prior to initiation of cooling protocols.

The management of SAH is complex and should be done in close consultation with neurocritical care specialists, vascular neurologists, or neurosurgeons, in a neurocritical care unit, if possible.

**Intracerebral hemorrhage** (ICH) is a leading cause of death and disability in people with preeclampsia.[18] Patients may present with headache, focal neurologic deficits (similar to ischemic stroke), seizure, or loss of consciousness, and may mimic eclampsia, making prompt brain imaging critical. Antithrombotic medications should be reversed, and immediate lowering of the blood pressure (BP) to below systolic BP of 140 is recommended, as well as elevation of the head of the bed.[19] Like SAH, ICH requires multidisciplinary management, ideally in a neurocritical care unit. Different hemorrhagic and ischemic strokes are illustrated in Figure 4.3. Table 4.7 outlines the type of stroke and the corresponding signs and symptoms teams should be aware of.

The out-of-hospital and in-hospital acute management of maternal stroke are reviewed in more detail in Chapter 10.

---

**KEY POINTS**

- PE is a frequent cause of MCA and should be suspected in the setting of acute maternal shortness of breath, hypoxia, and tachycardia. Evaluate promptly with a computed tomography (CT) angiogram of the chest, shielding the abdomen.
- Treat PE in pregnancy with therapeutic anticoagulation with heparin or low-molecular-weight heparin. Consider either thrombolytics, such as recombinant tissue plasminogen activator (rtPA) or catheter/surgical thrombectomy, for PE and a hemodynamically unstable patient. However, use thrombolysis with caution in patients in cardiac arrest who are candidates for RCD or who have undergone surgery within a 2-week window.
- ECPR is emerging as a possible therapy of choice for massive PE resulting in maternal cardiac arrest. Limited data also support the use of thrombolytics for thrombectomy in pregnant patients with massive PE.
- In acute stroke, follow "Time Is Brain" and institutional stroke protocols (Code Stroke).
- Pregnancy is not a contraindication to acute therapies for ischemic stroke such as IV thrombolysis and mechanical thrombectomy. Multidisciplinary consultation is recommended including obstetrics and neurology.
- SAH can cause cardiac arrest due to neurogenic myocardial stunning.
- ICH and basilar artery occlusion can both present with loss of consciousness and/or convulsions. Brain imaging is recommended in all unresponsive patients.

---

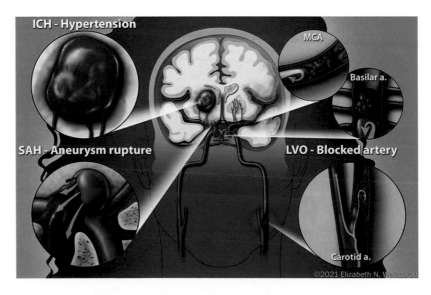

**FIGURE 4.3**   Ischemic and hemorrhagic strokes.

From www.strokeinfo.org/stroke-facts-statistics/.

# 4.9 BAACC TO LIFE: TRAUMA

Trauma is damage to the body caused by an external force. This force can come in many different forms, from falls to intimate partner violence (IPV). This section reviews causes of unintentional (such as low-speed motor vehicle collisions or falls) and intentional (such as IPV) trauma in pregnancy, as well as commonly seen consequences of trauma that can lead to MCA (such as tension pneumothorax and cardiac tamponade).

## 4.9.1 Unintentional Trauma: Motor Vehicle Collision

Even seemingly minor trauma, such as a low-speed motor vehicle collision, can lead to devastating consequences. Therefore, it is critical to closely monitor pregnant patients following a traumatic incident.

Motor vehicle collisions are the most common cause of trauma in pregnancy, followed by falls.[20] Approximately one in 12 pregnancies will be affected by some form of trauma.[21] Trauma is the leading cause of nonobstetric, or indirect, mortality in pregnant patients. Adverse pregnancy outcomes can occur even after seemingly minor trauma.

Blunt abdominal trauma, occurring during falls or motor vehicle collisions, can result in significant injuries and increase a pregnant patient's risk for placental abruption (where the placenta separates from the uterine wall).[21] In early pregnancy, the uterus is small and protected by the maternal pelvis. After 12 weeks of gestation, the uterus becomes an intra-abdominal organ, and there is an increased risk for direct injury with trauma.

Placental abruption occurs when trauma to the abdomen and uterus results in shearing forces between the elastic uterine wall and the inelastic placenta. These forces result in premature separation of the placenta and bleeding. Placental abruptions are typically associated with abdominal pain, contractions, and vaginal bleeding. Some abruptions are concealed, with the bleeding remaining within the uterus and without any visible vaginal bleeding. Bleeding from placental abruptions can be severe and catastrophic, leading to hypovolemic shock, fetal death, and DIC. More insidious presentations of abruptions can occur, especially in the setting of concealed hemorrhages, where there may be minimal changes in maternal vitals with significant intra-abdominal bleeding that can quickly lead to hemodynamic instability, and cardiac arrest.

Evaluate patients involved in motor vehicle collisions and falls according to Advanced Trauma and Life Support protocols.[22] Prompt maternal evaluation and treatment are key. Therefore, do not delay necessary diagnostic imaging and treatments due to pregnancy. For more minor trauma, evaluate patients with fetal and contraction monitoring after the event. In patients with no clinical evidence of abruption (no abdominal pain, vaginal bleeding, or contractions) and no evidence of abruption on ultrasound, monitor for a minimum of 6 hours. Monitor the following patients for a minimum of 24 hours:

- Patients experiencing abdominal pain, vaginal bleeding, or four or more contractions per hour
- Patients with an ultrasound showing possible abruption
- Patients who experienced significant falls or motor vehicle collisions

## 4.9.2 Intentional Trauma: Assault, Intimate Partner Violence, Suicide

IPV is a serious public health issue. In the U.S., the rates of IPV are between 4% and 20% during pregnancy.[23] Pregnancy is linked to an increased risk of intimate partner homicide.[24,25] Nearly half of female homicide victims are killed by a current or former male intimate partner, and approximately 15% of female homicide victims of reproductive age (18–44 years) were pregnant or postpartum.[26] Of those who reported violence during pregnancy, a majority report a history of abuse by the same partner prior to pregnancy, and half report being assaulted for the **first** time during pregnancy.[23] Prevention is paramount to halting the cycle of IPV. Obstetric Life Support recommends universal screening for IPV of pregnant patients at the first prenatal visit and at least once each trimester and postpartum.[27] Private screening and referral to services for those experiencing IPV allow people to leave abusive relationships. These are the first steps to breaking the cycle of violence and reducing maternal morbidity and mortality from IPV.

## 4.9.3 Suicide

Suicide attempts are a significant cause of maternal cardiac arrest, both in pregnancy and within the first year postpartum.[28] A 2017 study revealed that almost 5% of MCAs occurred as a result of suicide, most of these hanging, jumping, or intentionally falling.[29]

These methods differ from those used by nonpregnant people, which typically involve overdose or poisoning. Another study revealed that almost one-third of pregnancy-related deaths resulted from self-harm, although most of these occurred in the postpartum period (2004–2012).[30]

Universal mental health screenings should be performed at the initiation of prenatal care, at 28 weeks, and at postpartum visits. The American College of Obstetricians and Gynecologists advocates for increased visits in the postpartum period to improve maternal well-being, including an early postpartum (within 1–3 weeks) and a late postpartum (up to 12 weeks) visit. Access to appropriate mental health treatment and therapies are also important.

## 4.9.4 Tamponade, Cardiac

There are multiple causes of cardiac tamponade, but the most common cause is trauma to the heart (such as gunshot wounds or blunt trauma). Other causes include pericarditis (infection of the pericardium), ruptured aortic aneurysm, myocardial infarction, invasive cancer, or iatrogenic injury such as from cardiac catheterization or central line placement. Blood or fluid builds up between the heart and the pericardial sac. As the sac fills, it restricts the heart's ability to pump blood effectively, which can lead to cardiac arrest. Patients with cardiac tamponade will often present with severe chest pain, tachycardia, muffled heart sounds, low blood pressure, and increased jugular venous distention.

Treat cardiac tamponade with a pericardiocentesis, which drains the fluid in the sac. This releases the pressure from the pericardial fluid. Pericardiocentesis can be performed initially with needle decompression; however, in the setting of major trauma and a large effusion, a thoracotomy may be required. POC-US is especially helpful in this situation, as it can both diagnose a cardiac tamponade and help guide needle placement during pericardiocentesis.

**KEY POINTS**
- Trauma is the leading indirect, or nonobstetric, cause of maternal mortality.
- Minor trauma in pregnancy can lead to devastating consequences. If patients have evidence of vaginal bleeding, contractions or abdominal pain, monitor for a minimum of 24 hours.
- Trauma from motor vehicle collision is the most common form of trauma seen in pregnancy.
- Pregnant people are at high risk for IPV and suicide.
- Pregnancy and postpartum may be associated with more violent means of suicide, such as hanging, jumping, or intentional falling.
- Cardiac tamponade is typically associated with the classic triad of hypotension, muffled or distant heart sounds, and jugular venous distention. Early decompression of the pericardium via needle pericardiocentesis is recommended.

# 4.10  BAACC TO LIFE: OVERDOSE

Accidental and intentional overdose can occur in both in-hospital and out-of-hospital settings. In the labor and delivery suite, anesthesia complications or iatrogenic overdoses from IV magnesium sulfate can lead to MCA. In out-of-hospital settings, opioid overdose is the most common cause of accidental overdose leading to MCA. If suspected and treated early, these causes of MCA are easily reversed and treated. Reversible causes and treatments of overdose leading to maternal respiratory and cardiac arrest are reviewed in Table 4.8 and are discussed in more detail in the following sections. Of note, lidocaine toxicity was previously reviewed in the Anesthesia section earlier in this chapter but is included in Table 4.8 as it falls into the category of a reversible cause of MCA.

## 4.10.1 Overdose: Magnesium Toxicity

In pregnancy, magnesium sulfate is used for seizure prevention in preeclampsia with severe features or eclampsia, or for fetal neuroprotection in preterm labor. Magnesium sulfate is usually given intravenously, although it can also be given intramuscularly in the setting of a patient with eclampsia (seizures) without IV access. Magnesium toxicity may result from errors such as inappropriate mixing or bolusing or may occur due to decreased magnesium sulfate clearance in patients with renal insufficiency. Conditions such as preexisting renal disease or preeclampsia can affect the kidneys' ability to clear magnesium, which can lead

**TABLE 4.8**   Reversible Causes and Treatments of Overdose Leading to Maternal Respiratory and Cardiac Arrest

| CAUSE OF OVERDOSE | TREATMENT |
|---|---|
| Benzodiazepine overdose | • Overdose within 1–2 hours: gastric lavage<br>• Overdose within 4 hours: activated charcoal<br>• Severe overdose (including respiratory or cardiac arrest): Flumazenil 0.2 mg IV × 1, wait 30 seconds, then 0.3 mg ×1 as required, wait 30 seconds, then 0.5 mg IV every minute as required up to six times for maximum of 5 mg total[b] |
| Local anesthetic systemic toxicity (see the Anesthesia section) | • Lipid emulsion: bolus 1.5 mL/kg IV over 1 minute, then continuous infusion 0.25–0.5 mL/kg/min with repeat bolus up to two times for persistent cardiovascular collapse<br>• Continue infusion for approximately 10 minutes following cardiovascular stability<br>• Upper limit of 10 mL/kg over the first 30 minutes of administration |
| Magnesium toxicity | • 10 mL of 10% calcium gluconate given intravenously over 3 minutes[a] |
| Opioid overdose | • Naloxone 2 mg intranasal or 0.4 mg intramuscular, repeat after 4 minutes if necessary |

[a] If not readily available, pharmacy may need to mix.
[b] Patients receiving flumazenil must be closely monitored as it can cause withdrawal and seizures in patients with chronic benzodiazepine abuse.

to a buildup of toxic magnesium levels over time. Monitor patients receiving IV magnesium sulfate with periodic assessments for clinical signs of magnesium toxicity. Signs of magnesium toxicity include the loss of deep tendon reflexes and decreased respiratory rate which can lead to respiratory depression and cardiac arrest. Development of these symptoms should alert the provider to the possibility of magnesium toxicity. Treatment includes the prompt discontinuation of magnesium sulfate while a STAT serum magnesium level is obtained. Administer calcium gluconate if significant magnesium toxicity is suspected, and intubate the patient if respiratory depression is present. Magnesium sulfate levels of >25 mEq/L may result in maternal cardiac arrest. Table 4.9 reviews serum magnesium levels and the corresponding physical exam findings.

If the patient receiving IV magnesium sulfate has acute or chronic renal insufficiency, periodically monitor for clinical signs of magnesium toxicity. Consider using serum magnesium levels in addition to lower magnesium infusion rates. Target magnesium levels are typically in the range of 4–6 mEq/L. Recommendations include stopping the magnesium infusion at levels of 8 mEq/L and monitoring serum magnesium values every 2 hours to ensure resolution. For levels >10 mEq/L, administer calcium gluconate and consider intubation if respiratory depression is present.

**KEY POINTS**
- Magnesium toxicity—either as a medication error or unrecognized toxic buildup in patients with acute or chronic renal insufficiency—can lead to maternal respiratory or cardiac arrest in pregnant patients with receiving treatment for preeclampsia or preterm labor.
- Deep tendon reflexes and respiratory exam should be periodically monitored to identify and prevent magnesium toxicity.
- Treat magnesium toxicity promptly with IV calcium gluconate and supportive care with intubation in the setting of respiratory depression.

**TABLE 4.9**   Magnesium Serum Levels (mEq/L) and Corresponding Physical Exam Findings

| mEq/L | FINDINGS |
|---|---|
| <7 | Normal findings |
| 7–9 | Loss of deep tendon reflexes |
| 10–24 | Respiratory depression |
| >25 | Cardiac arrest |

## 4.10.2 Overdose: Opioids

Between 2000 and 2009, there was a fivefold increase in the rate of opioid abuse during pregnancy.[31] Maternal deaths from opioid overdose are also increasing in the postpartum period. Studies show that one in 300 people who have a cesarean delivery become addicted to opioids.[32] Cesarean delivery is the most common surgical procedure performed in the U.S., and most of these patients are being given opioids at the time of surgery. Cesarean delivery therefore represents a common source of initial exposure to opioids. OBLS recommends using protocols such as enhanced recovery after surgery (ERAS) to reduce or limit the number of pills prescribed at the time of discharge from a hospitalization for delivery.

Signs and symptoms of opioid toxicity include respiratory depression, pinpoint pupils, clammy and/or cold skin, and unresponsiveness. Risk factors for opioid toxicity or overdose include a history of opioid use or abuse, recent major surgery or accident, untreated mental health disorders, and socioeconomic factors associated with substance use.

The treatment for opioid overdose is naloxone, which is safe for use in pregnancy and the postpartum period. The dose for naloxone is 2 milligrams administered intranasally or 0.4 milligrams intramuscularly. If the initial dose proves ineffective, a second dose can be administered after 4 minutes.

## 4.10.3 Overdose: Other

Approximately 5% of pregnancies are complicated by at least one form of drug abuse, including benzodiazepine abuse.[33,34] While less commonly a sole cause of overdose, benzodiazepine use is seen more frequently in patients with mental health conditions, including anxiety and post-traumatic stress disorder. Benzodiazepine abuse can have detrimental effects on both the mother and the fetus, especially when used in conjunction with narcotics and/or alcohol.[35] These combinations increase the drug's sedative effects, thereby increasing the patient's risk of respiratory collapse and arrest. Presenting symptoms of benzodiazepine overdose include excessive sedation, difficult arousal, and sluggish speech.

Signs include shallow breathing, clammy skin, bluish lips, dilated pupils, weak or rapid pulse, low blood pressure, and depressed reflexes. Patients may also present in a coma and/or cardiopulmonary arrest. Treatment of benzodiazepine overdose depends on the timing of the overdose and the severity of the presentation. If the benzodiazepine overdose occurs within 1–2 hours of presentation, gastric lavage may be adequate. If the overdose occurs within 4 hours of presentation, activated charcoal should be used. Administer flumazenil if the patient presents with a severe overdose with coma and/or cardiac arrest. This should be carefully monitored, as flumazenil can precipitate withdrawal and/or seizures in patients who chronically abuse benzodiazepine.

**KEY POINTS**
- The incidence of opioid overdose is rising in pregnant and postpartum patients.
- In the U.S., one in 300 patients who undergoes a cesarean delivery develops an opioid addiction.
- If cardiac arrest is due to opioid overdose, start high-quality CPR and consider administering naloxone.
- If cardiac arrest is due to benzodiazepine overdose, start high-quality CPR and consider flumazenil as an antidote.

# 4.11  BAACC TO LIFE: ACUTE LUNG INJURY/ ACUTE RESPIRATORY DISTRESS

Acute lung injury (ALI) and acute respiratory distress syndrome (ARDS) are clinical syndromes of acute respiratory failure with substantial morbidity and mortality. ALI and ARDS can be caused by lung infection, sepsis, aspiration, multiple trauma/shock, and other insults, such as transfusion-related acute lung injury. These are reviewed in Table 4.10.

Symptoms of ALI and ARDS include shortness of breath, hypoxemia, and reduced breath sounds or bibasilar crackles. Confirm the diagnosis with imaging studies such as chest radiography or CT scan. Do not withhold such procedures from a pregnant patient due to concern for radiation exposure.[36] Promptly evaluate for intubation any pregnant person presenting with respiratory distress and hypoxemia (oxygen <90%) with hypercapnia (elevated $PaCO_2$).

**TABLE 4.10**  Pregnancy-Associated Direct and Indirect Causes of Acute Lung Injury/Acute Respiratory Distress Syndrome

|  | INDIRECT | DIRECT |
|---|---|---|
| Aspiration | Cesarean delivery<br>Intubation |  |
| Asthma | Iatrogenic—secondary to administration<br>of Hemabate<br>Exacerbation due to infection/exercise/<br>smoking | Asthma exacerbation/attack |
| DIC | Inherited coagulopathy | Retained products of<br>conception<br>AFE |
| Massive transfusion | Multiple trauma | Postpartum hemorrhage |
| Pancreatitis | Gallstones, hypertriglyceridemia, alcoholism | Pregnancy-associated pancreatitis |
| Pneumonia | Pneumonia<br>Influenza<br>Varicella<br>Coccidioidomycosis | Pulmonary edema<br>Preeclampsia<br>Tocolysis |
| Sepsis | Pyelonephritis<br>*Listeria bacteremia* | Chorioamnionitis<br>Missed abortion |
| Trauma | Tension pneumothorax<br>Hemothorax |  |

## 4.11.1 BAACC TO LIFE: Acute Lung Injury: Tension Pneumothorax/Hemothorax

Early recognition of injuries such as tension pneumothorax leads to timely treatment and prevention of cardiac arrest. Tension pneumothorax or hemothorax is typically caused by a punctured lung, typically from trauma (from fractured rib[s], gunshot or stabbing injuries, or following chest surgery). A spontaneous pneumothorax can occur in patients with a history of tobacco abuse or those with underlying lung disease (such as cystic fibrosis or apical blebs) and can progress in a tension pneumothorax. Decompress a tension pneumothorax or hemothorax in the field by inserting a large-bore (14- or 16-gauge) needle into the fourth intercostal space in the midaxillary line. Follow this with more definitive treatment with a chest tube when the patient arrives at the hospital.

See Chapter 8 for more details on managing traumatic MCA.

**KEY POINTS**
- Common causes for ALI in pregnancy include sepsis, pneumonia, trauma, DIC, and massive transfusion.
- If in the field, decompress a tension pneumothorax with the lateral insertion of large-bore needle at the fourth intercostal space in the midaxillary line. Once the patient arrives at the hospital, follow with more definitive treatment with a chest tube.

## 4.12 BAACC TO LIFE: IONS (GLUCOSE, K⁺)

Acidosis rarely causes MCA; however, there are important factors that can increase the risk for electrolyte abnormalities to cause cardiac arrest in pregnancy. For example, pregestational diabetes may result in an increased risk for hypoglycemia in the first trimester, precipitated by pregnancy-related nausea and vomiting (hyperemesis gravidarum). In diabetic people with significant nausea and vomiting, hypoglycemia can lead to mental confusion, seizures, arrhythmias, a hypoglycemic coma, and cardiac arrest. Obtain a point-of-care glucose value for any pregnant or postpartum person in cardiac arrest. When the patient is unconscious and/or in cardiac arrest, treat severe hypoglycemia with an IV bolus of 20–50 mL of 50% glucose solution or a subcutaneous or intramuscular (IM) injection of glucagon 0.5–1.0 mg.

While a relatively rare cause of maternal cardiac arrest, DKA affects up to 5%–10% of pregnancies complicated by insulin-dependent diabetes, most commonly in the setting of type 1 diabetes mellitus. DKA can occur in the setting of lower or normal blood glucose levels and is often precipitated by hyperemesis in early pregnancy, infections, lack of compliance with insulin, new onset of the diagnosis in pregnancy, and prenatal steroid use. With appropriate management, maternal mortality is rare in the setting of DKA. These patients improve rapidly with identification and correction of the underlying cause and aggressive IV fluid hydration, insulin, electrolyte repletion, and subsequent improvements in acidosis.

As chronic comorbidities such as cardiac disease, long-standing pregestational diabetes, and renal disease increase in the pregnant population, electrolyte abnormalities may become more common etiologies of maternal cardiac arrest. The most concerning electrolyte abnormalities include hypo- and hyperkalemia, both of which may precede cardiac arrest. Manage patients with high-risk conditions for electrolyte abnormalities (pregnant patients receiving dialysis) with a multidisciplinary team composed of specialists in maternal-fetal medicine, cardiology, and nephrology. This team can coordinate care to prevent dangerous electrolyte abnormalities from occurring during pregnancy and postpartum.

**KEY POINTS**
- In a pregnancy complicated by insulin-dependent diabetes, DKA may be diagnosed with low or normal glucose values.
- Obtain a point-of-care glucose value for any pregnant or postpartum person in cardiac arrest.
- Patients with DKA improve rapidly with aggressive IV fluid hydration, insulin, electrolyte repletion, and subsequent improvement in acidosis.

# 4.13  BAACC TO LIFE: FEVER

According to the CDC, infection or sepsis is responsible for approximately 12.4% of maternal deaths.[8] Sepsis is the third leading all-cause of cardiac arrest in the U.S., accounting for 13% of these events.[35] Clinical signs and symptoms of sepsis in pregnancy include the following:

- Body temperature changes (e.g., hypothermia and hyperthermia)
- Tachycardia (heart rate >120)
- Changes in white blood cell (WBC) count (e.g., high or low WBC count)
- Hypotension (systolic BP <90, diastolic BP <60, mean arterial pressure <60–65)

Recognizing sepsis in a pregnant person can be challenging due to the physiologic changes in pregnancy that may mask early clinical signs of sepsis. For example, 25% of pregnant people who died from sepsis never develop a fever.[37] WBC counts are commonly elevated in pregnancy, and intrapartum levels may be as high as 29,000 per microliter. Lower blood pressure is common in healthy, pregnant persons due to the vasodilatory effects of progesterone, especially in the second trimester. Additionally, infectious sources may not be obvious because the portal of entry may be the genitourinary tract, such as seen with group A streptococcal infection.

The S.O.S.[38] is the only validated scoring system for identifying patients with sepsis in pregnancy who may require admission to the intensive care unit. Please see Chapter 3 for more details on this early warning system. The dysregulated host response to infection can affect any organ system in the body. Table 4.11 summarizes common dysfunctions seen in various organ systems during sepsis.

Obstetric causes of infection during pregnancy include septic abortions, chorioamnionitis, endometritis, and wound infections. Nonobstetric causes include urinary tract infections, appendicitis, and pneumonia. Based on the most recent Surviving Sepsis Campaign recommendations for adults with suspected sepsis or septic shock include obtaining blood cultures and serum lactate. Other markers of inflammation such as C-reactive protein and procalcitonin may also be considered. Sepsis or septic shock should be aggressively treated with broad-spectrum antibiotics (tailored toward the most likely source) and balanced crystalloid solutions within 1 hour of presentation with abnormal vital signs and/or documentation of clinical concern.[39] Patients with refractory hypotension or evidence of end organ hypoperfusion should be started on vasopressors such as norepinephrine, with a search for the cause of the underlying infection, and therapies aimed at source control. In the absence of sepsis treatment data in pregnancy, experts recommend adoption of these guidelines for treatment of sepsis in pregnancy.[39]

**TABLE 4.11**   Organ Systems Affected by Sepsis

| ORGAN SYSTEM | PRESENTATION |
|---|---|
| Cardiovascular | Hypotension, myocardial dysfunction |
| Central nervous | Altered mental status |
| Endocrine | Adrenal dysfunction and increased insulin resistance |
| Gastrointestinal | Paralytic ileus |
| Hepatic | Hepatic failure or transaminitis |
| Hematologic | Thrombocytopenia or DIC |
| Pulmonary | ARDS |
| Urinary | Oliguria, acute kidney injury |

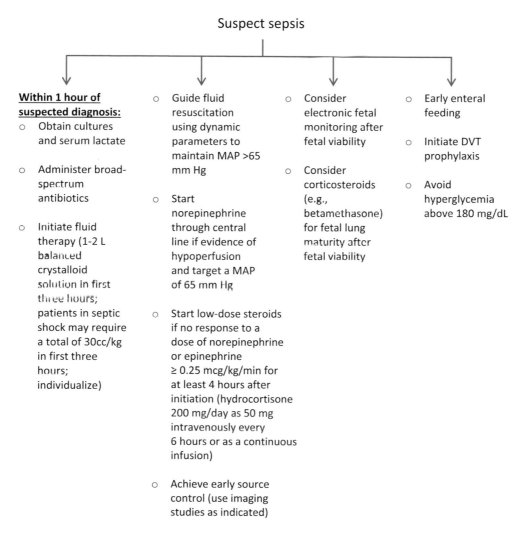

Suspect sepsis

**Within 1 hour of suspected diagnosis:**
o   Obtain cultures and serum lactate

o   Administer broad-spectrum antibiotics

o   Initiate fluid therapy (1-2 L balanced crystalloid solution in first three hours; patients in septic shock may require a total of 30cc/kg in first three hours; individualize)

o   Guide fluid resuscitation using dynamic parameters to maintain MAP >65 mm Hg

o   Start norepinephrine through central line if evidence of hypoperfusion and target a MAP of 65 mm Hg

o   Start low-dose steroids if no response to a dose of norepinephrine or epinephrine ≥ 0.25 mcg/kg/min for at least 4 hours after initiation (hydrocortisone 200 mg/day as 50 mg intravenously every 6 hours or as a continuous infusion)

o   Achieve early source control (use imaging studies as indicated)

o   Consider electronic fetal monitoring after fetal viability

o   Consider corticosteroids (e.g., betamethasone) for fetal lung maturity after fetal viability

o   Early enteral feeding

o   Initiate DVT prophylaxis

o   Avoid hyperglycemia above 180 mg/dL

**FIGURE 4.4**   Initial treatment of sepsis during pregnancy.

Adapted from Society for Maternal-Fetal Medicine.[40]

Table 4.12 reviews appropriate antibiotic selection for sepsis in pregnancy. Importantly, group A streptococcal infections during pregnancy or the postpartum period can rapidly progress to death within 2–8 hours of the initial presentation. Invasive group A streptococcal infections present most commonly in the postpartum period, though they can rarely present in the intrapartum period. Clinical signs can include disproportionate pain on exam and with abnormal vital signs. The Infectious Diseases Society of America recommends treatment of group A streptococcal infection with high-dose penicillin and clindamycin.

**TABLE 4.12**   Antibiotic Selection for Sepsis in Pregnancy[41]

| First-line agents | • Penicillin 3 million units IV every 4 hours, plus<br>• Gentamicin 1.5 mg/kg IV, then 1 mg/kg IV every 8 hours or 5 mg/kg every 24 hours, plus<br>• Clindamycin 900 mg IV every 8 hours |
|---|---|
| Alternative | • Vancomycin 15 mg/kg IV, then dose by pharmacy, plus<br>• Piperacillin-tazobactam 4.5 grams IV every 6 hours |
| Penicillin allergic | • Vancomycin 15 mg/kg IV, then dose by pharmacy, plus<br>• Meropenem 500 mg IV every 6 hours |

**KEY POINTS**

- Clinical signs and symptoms of sepsis include:
  - Body temperature changes (hypothermia and hyperthermia)
  - Tachycardia (heart rate >120)
  - Changes in WBC count (high or low WBC count)
  - Hypotension (systolic BP <90, diastolic BP <60 mean arterial pressure <60–65)
- Recognizing sepsis in a pregnant person can be challenging given that normal physiologic changes in pregnancy may mask symptoms and signs of sepsis
- Group A streptococcal infection is an important cause of postpartum sepsis and should be treated rapidly with high-dose penicillin and clindamycin

# 4.14  BAACC TO LIFE: EMERGENCY HYPERTENSION/ECLAMPSIA

Essential hypertension affects 6%–8% of all pregnancies in the U.S.[42] Pregnant patients affected by hypertension have increased risks of significant morbidity, including preeclampsia, eclampsia, pulmonary edema, and stroke.[40] Presenting symptoms of preeclampsia typically occur after 20 weeks gestation, and include headache, swelling, malaise, right upper quadrant abdominal pain, nausea, and vomiting. Presenting signs of preeclampsia include persistent systolic blood pressure elevations ≥140, and/or diastolic blood pressure elevations ≥90 in patients without preexisting hypertension, or worsening control of blood pressure in those with preexisting hypertension with or without proteinuria. Edema is a common finding in preeclampsia and results from fluid retention due to proteinuria and reduced intravascular oncotic pressure. Jaundice is rarely seen in preeclampsia. Laboratory findings include elevated hemoglobin and hematocrit due to hemoconcentration, low platelets, elevated liver enzymes, elevated serum creatinine, proteinuria, and hemolysis. The diagnosis of preeclampsia with severe features is based on both clinical and laboratory findings and is reviewed in Table 4.13.

Preeclampsia affects 6%–8% of all first-time pregnancies in the U.S.[43] The incidence is even higher in those with other comorbidities such as chronic hypertension, a history of preeclampsia in a prior pregnancy, obesity, multiple gestation, or underlying renal disease. Pregnant patients affected by hypertension and other comorbidities have increased risks of significant morbidity, including preeclampsia, eclampsia, pulmonary edema, and stroke.

Treat preeclampsia with severe features to prevent eclamptic seizures with a continuous IV infusion of magnesium sulfate and blood pressure control. A patient with persistent, severe systolic blood pressure ≥160 or persistent, severe diastolic blood

**TABLE 4.13**   Severe Features of Preeclampsia

| | |
|---|---|
| Acute renal insufficiency or failure (serum creatinine >1.1 mg/dL or doubling of baseline serum creatinine) | Pulmonary edema |
| Elevated liver enzymes (two times the upper limit), or right upper quadrant/epigastric pain | Systolic blood pressure ≥160 mm Hg or diastolic blood pressure ≥110 mm Hg |
| New-onset headache, vision changes, or mental status changes | Thrombocytopenia (platelet count <100,000) |

pressures ≥110 should be promptly treated within 15–30 minutes with antihypertensive therapy to avoid maternal stroke. Most protocols on the acute treatment of severe hypertension in pregnancy include the following first-line agents:

- Hydralazine (IV or IM)
- Labetalol (IV)
- Nifedipine, immediate release (oral)

Short-acting oral nifedipine is the treatment of choice in a conscious patient without IV access. Labetalol is contraindicated in patients with asthma.

The following presents treatment of generalized seizures. If eclamptic seizures occur, they are usually self-limited but should be treated aggressively and timed, if possible, from the onset of the first seizure. Start magnesium sulfate to prevent further seizures from occurring. In a patient without a seizure history, a seizure is most likely to be due to eclampsia, and intravenous access should be established to administer a 6-g bolus of magnesium sulfate over 15–20 minutes, followed by a a maintanence infusion of 2 g/hour. If the patient is already receiving a maintenance magnesium sulfate infusion of 2 g/hour and experiences another seizure, a second 2-g bolus of magnesium sulfate is given over 15–20 minutes followed by resuming the 2 g/hour infusion.

If another seizure occurs after a second bolus of magnesium, give an alternate therapy such as a benzodiazepine (IV lorazepam 2–4 mg or midazolam 2.5–5 mg). Magnesium sulfate and/or benzodiazepines can also be given intramuscularly or intraosseously in patients who present with eclamptic seizures and do not have IV access. The usual IM dose of magnesium is 10 g, divided into two 5-g doses, administered as two intramuscular injections, one into each gluteal muscle. The intraosseous dosing is the same as the IV dosing described earlier.

For refractory seizures lasting more than 5 minutes without return to baseline (status epilepticus), benzodiazepines should be immediately administered, airway secured, and neurology consulted emergently or a Code Stroke activated. In the prehospital setting, midazolam can be administered intramuscularly in the field at a dose of 10 mg IM for adults >40 kg. Airway should be secured and a fingerstick glucose obtained per usual emergency medical services protocols for convulsive status epilepticus. Eclamptic seizures are typically generalized; any focality of seizure semiology, such as forced gaze deviation, unilateral jerking, or twitching should prompt a Code Stroke activation and immediate brain imaging, as this may indicate a structural lesion such as an intracerebral hemorrhage.

In the out-of-hospital setting, pregnant people presenting with seizures should not be assumed to have eclampsia, as those with epilepsy may experience "breakthrough" seizures during pregnancy due to hormonally induced neurophysiologic changes (see Chapter 2). As soon as seizures are controlled and the patient is stabilized, OBLS recommends emergent brain imaging with noncontrast head CT to rule out intracranial hemorrhage or ischemic stroke.

The Council on Patient Safety in Women's Health Care's Alliance for Innovation on Maternal Health Program has developed a bundle on unit readiness, recognition and prevention, response, and reporting of severe hypertension in pregnancy.[44] Its hypertension bundle endorses facility-wide implementation and dissemination of protocols to assist with recognition and rapid treatment of severe-range hypertension in pregnancy (within 30 minutes from recognition) to reduce the risk of stroke and maternal mortality.[45]

---

**KEY POINTS**
- Pregnant patients affected by essential hypertension have increased risks of major morbidity including preeclampsia, eclampsia, and stroke.
- Presenting symptoms of preeclampsia include headache, swelling, malaise, and right upper quadrant abdominal pain after 20 weeks gestation.
- Presenting signs of preeclampsia include blood pressure elevations ≥140/90 in patients without preexisting hypertension or worsening control of blood pressure in those with preexisting hypertension and proteinuria after 20 weeks gestation.
- A pregnant person with persistent severe-range blood pressure ≥160/110 is at risk for stroke. Treat severe blood pressure with antihypertensive therapy within 15–30 minutes.
- The treatment of choice for prevention of eclamptic seizures in those affected with preeclampsia with severe features is intravenous infusion of magnesium sulfate.
- Short-acting oral nifedipine is a first-line agent for acute severe hypertension in a patient without IV access.
- Do not give labetalol to people with asthma.

# CHAPTER 4. PRACTICE QUESTIONS

1. In OBLS, which mnemonic is used to remember etiologies of MCA?
   A. SURVIVE at 5
   B. 5 to be ALIVE
   C. LUD for LIFE
   D. BAACC TO LIFE

2. Which of the following is the MOST common cause for maternal mortality worldwide?
   A. Hemorrhage
   B. Venous thromboembolism
   C. Cardiovascular diseases
   D. Hypertension

3. A pregnant person at 40 weeks gestation has preeclampsia with severe features with acute renal insufficiency and oliguria. While being induced and treated with IV magnesium sulfate for seizure prophylaxis, the patient becomes inattentive, has slowed responses to stimulation, and pulse is in the 40s. Which of the following is the BEST next step after calling the rapid response team and stopping the magnesium sulfate infusion?
   A. Give an IV bolus of lactated Ringer solution
   B. Begin chest compressions
   C. Administer calcium gluconate
   D. Re-bolus the magnesium sulfate

4. A pregnant person at 20 weeks is diagnosed in the field with a left tension pneumothorax. Emergency medical services providers are administering bag-mask ventilation with an $ETCO_2$ <10 mm Hg. What is the most appropriate next step?
   A. Needle decompression
   B. Chest tube placement in the field
   C. Pericardiocentesis
   D. Intubation and mechanical ventilation

5. A patient with extreme obesity who just delivered their first child 12 hours ago by cesarean delivery reports sudden onset shortness of breath and chest pain. On exam, the patient is writhing in bed, blood pressure is 70/40 mm Hg, and pulse is 140 beats per minute. An abdominal exam is benign. The patient becomes unconscious and pulseless. What is the most likely etiology for the cardiac arrest?
   A. Eclampsia
   B. Opioid overdose
   C. Intra-abdominal hemorrhage
   D. Massive pulmonary embolism

# CHAPTER 4. ANSWERS

1. **ANSWER: D.** OBLS uses the mnemonic BAACC TO LIFE to recall the potential etiologies of MCA.
2. **ANSWER: A.** Maternal hemorrhage is the number one cause of maternal morbidity and mortality worldwide. Postpartum hemorrhage is the most common cause of maternal hemorrhage, occurring in 4%–6% of all pregnancies, with greater than 50% of maternal deaths from this cause occurring within the first 24 hours of delivery. Postpartum hemorrhage is caused by uterine atony in approximately 70%–80% of cases.
3. **ANSWER: C.** Patients with preeclampsia with severe features who are receiving IV magnesium sulfate are at risk for magnesium toxicity. This risk is even greater with underlying renal insufficiency. Monitoring for magnesium toxicity can occur by clinical exam assessing for the loss of deep tendon reflexes and decreased respiratory rate, and/or by periodic monitoring of magnesium levels, especially in patients with underlying renal disease. Development of signs and/or symptoms of magnesium toxicity should have **prompt discontinuation of magnesium sulfate** while a STAT

serum magnesium level is obtained. **Calcium gluconate** should be administered if significant magnesium toxicity is suspected, as in this patient.

4. **ANSWER: A.** Early recognition of injuries such as tension pneumothorax can lead to more timely treatment and prevention of cardiac arrest. Tension pneumothorax or hemothorax is most caused due to a punctured lung, typically from trauma (such as from fractured rib, gunshot or stab injury, or following chest surgery). Decompress a tension pneumothorax or hemothorax on the field by inserting a large-bore (14- or 16-gauge) needle into the fourth intercostal space in the midaxillary line. Follow with more definitive treatment via chest tube when the patient arrives at the hospital.

5. **ANSWER: D.** Patients with pulmonary embolism will typically present with acute-onset shortness of breath, tachycardia, and chest pain. Initial evaluation should consist of an electrocardiogram and chest radiography. If clinical suspicion is high for pulmonary embolism, start therapeutic anticoagulation therapy empirically with heparin or low-molecular-weight heparin while pursuing further evaluation with either CT angiogram of the chest, or ventilation-perfusion scan.

# CHAPTER 4. REFERENCES

1. Petersen EE, Davis NL, Goodman D, et al. Vital signs: Pregnancy-related deaths, United States, 2011–2015, and strategies for prevention, 13 states, 2013–2017. *MMWR Morb Mortal Wkly Rep.* 2019;68:423–429. doi: 10.15585/mmwr.mm6818e1.
2. Obstetric Hemorrhage (+AIM). *Council on Patient Safety in Women's Health Care.* Website. https://saferbirth.org/wp-content/uploads/U2-FINAL_AIM_Bundle_ObstetricHemorrhage.pdf. Accessed September 13, 2019.
3. Committee on Practice Bulletins—Obstetrics. Practice Bulletin No. 183: Postpartum hemorrhage. *Obstet Gynecol.* 2017;13(4):e168–e186. doi: 10.1097/AOG.0000000000002351.
4. Mhyre JM, Riesner MN, Polley LS, Naughton NN. A series of anesthesia-related maternal deaths in Michigan, 1985–2003. *Anesthesiology.* 2007;10(6):1096–1104. doi: 10.1097/01.anes.0000267592.34626.6b.
5. Saade G, Hankins GVD, Clark SL. SMFM Clinical Guideline No. 9. Amniotic fluid embolism: Diagnosis and management. *Am J Obstet Gynecol.* 2016 August;215(2):B16–B24. doi: 10.1016/j.ajog.2016.03.012.
6. Shamshirsaz AA, Clark S. Amniotic fluid embolism. *Obstet Gynecol Clin North Am.* 2016. doi: 10.1016/j.ogc.2016.07.001.
7. Mathews T, Hamilton B. Mean age of mothers is on the rise: United States, 2000–2014. NCHS data brief. No. 232. *National Center for Health Statistics.* 2016 January.
8. Centers for Disease Control and Prevention. *Pregnancy mortality surveillance system.* Website. www.cdc.gov/reproductivehealth/maternal-mortality/pregnancy-mortality-surveillance-system.htm. Accessed September 17, 2019.
9. California Maternal Quality Care Collaborative (CMQCC). *Improving health care response to cardiovascular disease in pregnancy and postpartum.* Website. www.cmqcc.org/resources-toolkits/toolkits/improving-health-care-response-cardiovascular-disease-pregnancy-and2019.
10. Schaufelberger M. Cardiomyopathy and pregnancy. *Heart.* 2019;105:1543–1551. doi: 10.1136/heartjnl-2018-313476.
11. Pregnancy and Heart Disease. ACOG Practice Bulletin No. 212. American College of Obstetricians and Gynecologists. *Obstet Gynecol.* 2019;133(5):320–356. doi: 10.1097/AOG.0000000000003243.
12. van der Pol LM, Tromeur C, Bistervels I, et al. Pregnancy-adapted YEARS algorithm for diagnosis of suspected pulmonary embolism. *N Engl J Med.* 2019;380:1139–1149. doi: 10.1056/NEJMoa1813865.
13. ACOG Committee Opinion. Number 723. Guidelines for diagnostic imaging during pregnancy and lactation. *Obstet Gynecol.* 2017. doi: 10.1097/00006250-200510000-00052.
14. MacKay AP, Berg CJ, Atrash H. Pregnancy-related mortality from preeclampsia and eclampsia. *Obstet Gynecol.* 2001;97(4). doi: 10.1016/s0029-7844(00)01223-0.
15. Saver J. Time is brain-quantified. *Stroke.* 2006;37(1):263–266.
16. Goyal M, Menon BK, van Zwam WH, et al. Endovascular thrombectomy after large-vessel ischaemic stroke: A meta-analysis of individual patient data from five randomised trials. *Lancet.* 2016;387(10029):1723–1731.
17. Inamasu J, Nakagawa Y, Kuramae T, Nakatsukasa M, Miyatake S. Subarachnoid hemorrhage causing cardiopulmonary arrest: Resuscitation profiles and outcomes. *Neurol Med Chir (Tokyo).* 2011;51(9):619–623. doi: 10.2176/nmc.51.619.
18. Hasegawa J, Ikeda T, Sekizawa A, et al. Maternal death due to stroke associated with pregnancy-induced hypertension. *Circ J.* 2015;79(8):1835–1840. doi: 10.1253/circj.CJ-15-0297.
19. Hemphill JC, Greenberg SM, Anderson CS, et al. Guidelines for the management of spontaneous intracerebral hemorrhage: A guideline for healthcare professionals from the American Heart Association/American Stroke Association. *Stroke.* 2015;46:2032–2060.
20. Mendez-Figueroa H, Dahlke JD, Vrees R, Rouse DJ. Trauma in pregnancy: An updated systematic review. *Am J Obstet Gynecol.* 209. doi: 10.1016/j.ajog.2013.01.021.
21. Murphy NJ, Quinlan J. Trauma in pregnancy: Assessment, management, and prevention. *Am Fam Physician.* 2014;90(0):717–724.
22. Advanced Trauma Life Support. *American College of Surgeons.* Website. www.facs.org/quality-programs/trauma/atls. Updated 2020.
23. Lutgendorf MA. Intimate partner violence and women's health. *Obstet Gynecol.* 2019;134:470–480. doi: 10.1097/AOG.0000000000003326.

24. Campo M. *Domestic and family violence in pregnancy and early parenthood overview and emerging interventions.* Website. https://aifs.gov.au/sites/default/files/publication-documents/cfca-resource-dv-pregnancy_0.pdf. Updated 2020.

25. Garcia-Moreno C, Jansen H, Ellsberg M, Heise L, Watts CH. Prevalence of intimate partner violence: Findings from the WHO multi-country study on women's health and domestic violence. *Lancet.* 2006;368. doi: 10.1016/S0140-6736(06)69523-8.

26. Petrosky E, Blair JM, Betz CJ, Fowler KA, Jack SP, Lyons BH. Racial and ethnic differences in homicides of adult women and the role of intimate partner violence—United States, 2003–2014. *MMWR Morb Mortal Wkly Rep.* 2017. doi: 10.15585/mmwr.mm6628a1.

27. ACOG Committee Opinion 518. Intimate partner violence. *Obstet Gynecol.* 2012. doi: 10.1097/AOG.0b013e318249ff74.

28. Campbell J, Matoff-Stepp S, Velez ML, Cox HH, Laughon K. Pregnancy-associated deaths from homicide, suicide, and drug overdose: Review of research and the intersection with intimate partner violence. *J Womens Health (Larchmt).* 2021;30(2):236–244. doi: 10.1089/jwh.2020.8875. Epub 2020 Dec 8. PMID: 33295844; PMCID: PMC8020563.

29. Grigoriadis S, Wilton AS, Kurdyak PA, Rhodes AE, et al. Perinatal suicide in Ontario, Canada: A 15-year population-based study. *CMAJ.* 2017. doi: 10.1503/cmaj.170088.

30. Metz TD, Rovner P, Hoffman MC, Allshouse AA, Beckwith KM, Binswanger IA. Maternal deaths from suicide and overdose in Colorado, 2004–2012. *Obstet Gynecol.* 2016;128(6):1233–1240. doi: 10.1097/AOG.0000000000001695.

31. National Institute on Drug Abuse. *Substance use while pregnant and breastfeeding.* National Institutes of Health; U.S. Department of Health and Human Services. May 4, 2022. Website. https://nida.nih.gov/publications/research-reports/substance-use-in-women/substance-use-while-pregnant-breastfeeding. Updated 2023.

32. Bateman BT, Franklin JM, Bykov K, et al. Persistent opioid use following cesarean delivery: Patterns and predictors among opioid-naïve women. *Am J Obstet Gynecol.* 2016. doi: 10.1016/j.ajog.2016.03.016.

33. Wendell AD. Overview and epidemiology of substance abuse in pregnancy. *Clin Obstet Gynecol.* 2013;56(1):91–96. doi: 10.1097/GRF.0b013e31827feeb9.

34. National Institute on Drug Abuse (NIDA). *Sex and gender differences in substance use.* National Institutes of Health; U.S. Department of Health and Human Services. May 4, 2022. Website. https://nida.nih.gov/publications/research-reports/substance-use-in-women/sex-gender-differences-in-substance-use. Updated 2023.

35. Warnecke RB, Oh A, Breen N, Gehlert S, et al. Approaching health disparities from a population perspective: The National Institutes of Health Centers for Population Health and Health Disparities. *Am J of Public Health.* 2008;98(9):1608. doi: 10.2105/AJPH.2006.102525.

36. American Committee Opinion No. 723. Guidelines for diagnostic imaging during pregnancy and lactation. American College of Obstetricians and Gynecologists. *Obstet Gynecol* 2017;130:e210–6.

37. Bauer ME, Lorenz RP, Bauer ST, Rao K, Anderson FW. Maternal deaths due to sepsis in the state of Michigan, 1999–2006. *Obstet Gynecol.* 2015;12(4):747–752. doi: 10.1097/AOG.0000000000001028.

38. Albright CM, Has J, Rouse L, Hughes L. Internal validation of the sepsis in obstetrics score to identify risk of morbidity from sepsis in pregnancy. *Obstet Gynecol.* 2017 October;13(4):747–755. doi: 10.1097/AOG.0000000000002260.

39. Evans L, et al. Surviving sepsis campaign: International guidelines for management of sepsis and septic shock 2021. *Crit Care Med.* 49(11):p e1063–e1143. doi: 10.1097/CCM.0000000000005337.

40. *SMFM consult series #47: Sepsis during pregnancy and the puerperium.* Society for Maternal Fetal Medicine. Website. www.smfm.org/publications/271-smfm-consult-series-47-sepsis-during-pregnancy-and-the-puerperium. Accessed September 18, 2019.

41. Barton JR, Sibai B. Severe sepsis and septic shock in pregnancy. *Obstet Gynecol.* 2012 September;12(3):689–706. doi: 10.1097/AOG.0b013e318263a52d.

42. Seely E. Hypertension in pregnancy: A potential window into long-term cardiovascular risk in women. *J Clin Endocrinol Metab.* doi: 10.1210/jcem.84.6.5785.

43. Mayrink J, Souza RT, Feitosa FE, et al. Incidence and risk factors for preeclampsia in a cohort of healthy nulliparous pregnant women: A nested case-control study. *Sci Rep.* 2019. doi: 10.1038/s41598-019-46011-3.

44. Severe Hypertension in Pregnancy (+AIM). *Council on Patient Safety in Women's Health Care.* Website. https://saferbirth.org/psbs/severe-hypertension-in-pregnancy/. Updated 2020.

45. https://saferbirth.org/wp-content/uploads/U1-FINAL_AIM_Bundle_SHP2022.pdf

# Review of Cardiopulmonary Resuscitation Modifications for Pregnant Patients in Basic Life Support

**5**

## 5.1 INTRODUCTION

As previously highlighted, understanding the anatomy and physiology of pregnancy is essential for recognizing imminent MCA and allows for the proper application of the unique techniques needed to resuscitate pregnant people experiencing MCA. The next two chapters review the BLS and ACLS algorithms, or surveys, with an emphasis on modifications for MCA in pregnancy. BLS and ACLS algorithms should be readily available on code carts. Using algorithms standardizes care, optimizing the response to high-risk and complex situations, minimizing the need to memorize every step.

## 5.2 LEARNING OBJECTIVES

Learner will appropriately

- Review current BLS guidelines for the nonpregnant person.
- Describe the critical steps in MCA response that improve the efficacy of resuscitation in pregnant people.

## 5.3 REVIEW OF BASIC LIFE SUPPORT

The BLS survey for nonpregnant adults is summarized in Figure 5.1. EMS providers use BLS as a systematic, evidence-based approach to evaluate the unconscious or unstable patient and determine the next steps of action. Once an unresponsive patient is found to have no pulse or no breathing, the EMS provider(s) should activate the emergency response system, get an AED, and start high-quality chest compressions.

DOI: 10.1201/9781003299288-6

## Adult Basic Life Support Algorithm for Healthcare Providers

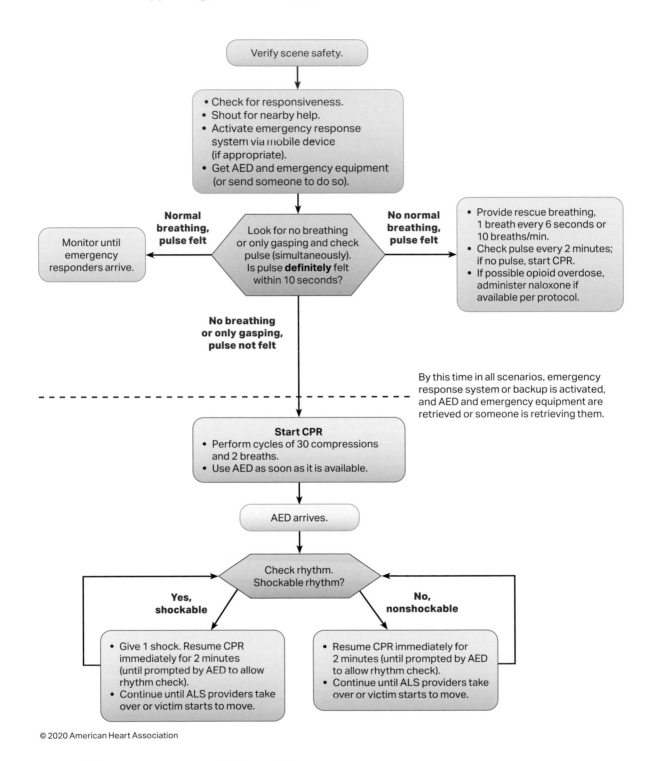

© 2020 American Heart Association

**FIGURE 5.1**    Basic life support treatment guidelines: Adults.

**KEY POINTS OF HIGH-QUALITY CARDIOPULMONARY RESUSCITATION**
- Effective chest compressions of 100–120/minute, with chest compression of 2 inches or one-third of chest depth with full recoil of the chest.
- Minimize interruptions in chest compressions. Pulse and rhythm checks should be <10 seconds and performed every 2 minutes.
- Switch CPR compressors at least every 2 minutes to avoid fatigue.
- Avoid over-ventilating a patient. Focus one breath every 5–6 seconds; alternatively, a 30:2 compression/respiratory ratio is acceptable. Prompt defibrillation of a shockable rhythm can be lifesaving and should be administered as soon as feasible.

## 5.4  BASIC LIFE SUPPORT CHANGES IN PREGNANCY

The start of the BLS survey is the same for pregnant and nonpregnant persons: activate help and immediately start high-quality chest compressions. Both actions are crucial to patient outcomes. It is critical to communicate that the arrest is in a **pregnant** patient when activating the emergency response system because at least three responders are needed to perform all basic modifications simultaneously.

## 5.5  CHEST COMPRESSIONS AND VENTILATION

Current recommendations for chest compressions on pregnant adults are to use the same hand placement on the chest as for nonpregnant adults. Place the heel of the hand in the middle of the sternum and place the other hand on top of this hand. The compression rate should be at least 100–120 per minute with a 30:2 compression to ventilation ratio,[1] or continuous compressions with ventilations every 5–6 seconds.[2] Compression depth should be at least 2 inches with full recoil of the chest.[3]

A pregnant patient's large, dense breasts may impede the ability to perform effective chest compressions as the fingers may rest atop the breast in an elevated position. This position may not allow for the proper force to be delivered with each chest compression. If this is the case, keep the heel of the hand on the sternum in the same place and slightly rotate the hand so the fingers point toward the patient's shoulder. This allows the hand to lay flat on the chest and allows maximum force to be applied to the sternum (Figure 5.2).

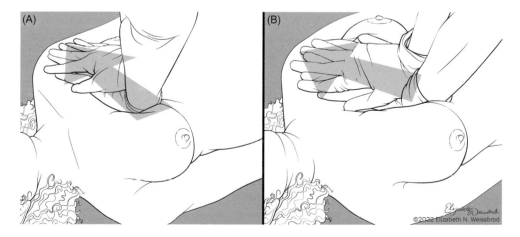

**FIGURE 5.2**  Proper hand placement for chest compressions on pregnant patients. (A) Proper hand placement on a pregnant patient. (B) If breast tissue is in the way, as can occur with large, pendulous breasts, slightly rotate the hand position toward the patient's shoulder to allow the proper delivery of downward force.

## 5.6 AUTOMATED CHEST COMPRESSION DEVICES

While automated chest compression devices (ACCDs) have not been studied in the pregnant population, it is reasonable to consider ACCD use for chest compressions. Using an ACCD can free up a team member to accomplish other tasks, such as LUD, obtaining IV access, and airway management during transport to the receiving hospital. If available, place the ACCD in a similar position to the recommended hand placement for effective compressions. Risks of use of an ACCD are like those in the nonpregnant patient. Therefore, do not place the ACCD over the abdomen or uterus as this could lead to ineffective chest compressions and injury to the pregnancy. Certain ACCDs encircle the lower chest and upper abdomen to deliver chest compressions. These types of devices should be avoided in pregnancy as there is a theoretical risk that they may cause liver lacerations, uterine rupture, and/or placental abruption.

## 5.7 DEFIBRILLATION

Defibrillation is a key component of resuscitation and should be administered without delay in a pregnant patient with a shockable rhythm. Deliver shocks via a manual defibrillator or an AED. Place pads either anterolateral or anteroposterior (Figure 5.3), depending on device manufacturer recommendations. If the patient has a suspected spinal cord injury, place the pads anterolateral to limit movement and potential further injury. In the anterolateral position, elevate and move medially any pendulous left breast tissue, and place the lateral pad **under** and just **lateral** to the left breast tissue. The pad should **not** lay on the breast tissue. Energy doses do not change during pregnancy; use the manufacturers' recommendations for specific devices.[3]

**Remove any fetal monitors prior to defibrillation**. Though not a significant safety concern if inadvertently left in place, removing fetal monitors focuses attention on maternal care and avoids the theoretical risk of arcing from the defibrillation pads to the fetal monitors.

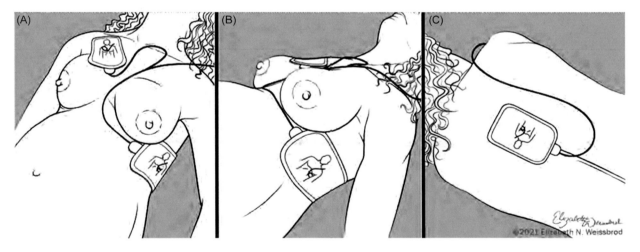

**FIGURE 5.3**  Proper automated external defibrillator pad placement. (A) Right anterior position. (B) Left anterolateral position. (C) Posterior position. **Note:** Posterior pad placement is not recommended in patients with suspected spinal cord injury, to limit movement that may cause further injury.

## 5.8 LEFT UTERINE DISPLACEMENT

The gravid uterus at term can decrease venous return to the maternal heart by 25%–30%. In the setting of MCA, the gravid uterus will also impede return of blood to the maternal heart during CPR. Thus, **LUD is a critical adjunct in performing high-quality CPR when the uterus is at the level of the umbilicus or higher**. If the pregnancy is clearly visible on abdominal exam, and the fundus (the top of the uterus) can be felt at or above the umbilicus, the uterus must be manually displaced upward and to the left to allow for improved blood return to the heart.

LUD may be accomplished in one of two ways:

1. Kneel on the **RIGHT** side of the patient, and **PUSH** the uterus leftward and slightly upward (Figure 5.4).

2. Kneel on the **LEFT** side of the patient, and using both hands, **PULL** the uterus leftward and slightly upward (Figure 5.5).*

**\* These steps are critical to ensure high-quality CPR in a pregnant person.**

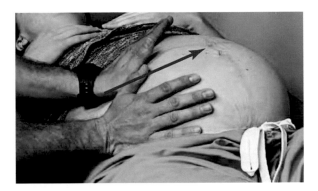

**FIGURE 5.4**  Proper left uterine displacement from maternal RIGHT side. Use hands to push the uterus up and over toward the maternal left side to lift the uterus off the great vessels.

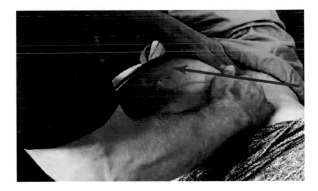

**FIGURE 5.5**  Proper left uterine displacement from the maternal LEFT side. Use the hands to pull the uterus up and over toward the maternal left side to lift the uterus off the great vessels.

**KEY POINTS**
- Ideally, at least **three** first responders perform the modifications of CPR in pregnancy: chest compressions, airway management, and LUD.
- For most pregnant patients, hand placement for chest compressions will not change. However, if a patient has large, dense breasts that are elevating the fingers, make sure the hand over the sternum lies flat on the chest by slightly rotating the hand more vertically on the chest and off of the breast tissue, keeping the heel of the hand perpendicular to the force of the chest compressions.
- Defibrillation pads can be placed anterolateral. Pads should **not** incorporate any breast tissue.
- High-quality CPR in a pregnant patient with the uterine fundus at or above the umbilicus requires early and continuous LUD to reduce compression of the great vessels and improve blood flow back to the heart.

## 5.9  BASIC LIFE SUPPORT IN THE REPRODUCTIVE-AGE FEMALE WITH UNKNOWN PREGNANCY STATUS

In general, a reproductive-age female in the United States is from age 12 years (average age of menarche) to age 51 years (average age of menopause).[4] Females 18–44 years of age comprise 35.6% of the overall population of the United States.[5] All medical personnel should be prepared to care for reproductive-age people who experience trauma or cardiac arrest. Those responding to MCA, especially to a patient in an unconscious state, should assess for pregnancy status early in the management. Confirming pregnancy at 20 weeks of gestation or greater, **or** if the uterus is at the level of the umbilicus or higher, necessitates that providers modify resuscitative care. If equipment and training allow, consider POC-US to evaluate pregnancy and assess gestational age.

## 5.10  VASCULAR ACCESS

In pregnancy, the expanding uterus compresses the aorta and inferior vena cava. Therefore, it is best to obtain IV access **above** the diaphragm. Placing the IV above the diaphragm allows for improved fluid resuscitation and drug administration, if indicated. However, in some circumstances, IV access can be difficult (such as some cases of preeclampsia with severe features or patients with long-standing diabetes or chronic kidney disease). An alternative to IV access is intraosseous (IO) access above the diaphragm in the proximal humerus. IO access into the humeral head is easy to obtain, is reliable, and offers the additional benefit of similar flow dynamics as that of a central line.[6] Complications of IO devices include discomfort and pain, difficulty penetrating the periosteum, trouble with aspiration of bone marrow, and bent or broken IO needles. A rare complication is compartment syndrome, seen in 0.6% of patients with IO access, which is caused by leaking at the needle's point of penetration into the cortex. Replace IO with a more long-term IV access after successful resuscitation.[6]

## 5.11  POINT-OF-CARE ULTRASOUND

If pregnancy status is unknown or difficult to discern (due to obesity or no family members or friends present to provide additional information), trained personnel should use a POC-US—when feasible—to perform an abdominal pelvic ultrasound to evaluate for pregnancy status. The POC-US should not interfere with chest compressions and should not be used to ascertain the fetal heart rate. Care should remain focused solely on effective maternal resuscitation. If pregnancy is identified with POC-US, the maternal fundus should be palpated within the abdomen. If the fundus is **palpable at or above the umbilicus**, LUD should be performed immediately. If the maternal fundus is **palpable below the umbilicus**, continue CPR as if the patient were not pregnant. If the fundus is **difficult to palpate**, trained personnel can use POC-US to measure the fetal femur length (FL) or biparietal diameter (BPD) to approximate gestational age. Refer to Chapter 7 for more details on how to effectively use and perform POC-US.

**KEY POINTS**
- Place IVs above the diaphragm on a pregnant patient.
- If IV access cannot be established, **IO access** above the diaphragm in the **proximal humerus** is the next best route of administration.
- POC-US is used to establish the presence or absence of pregnancy, **not** to establish fetal heartbeat. Stay focused on maternal care, thereby improving the patient's chances of survival.
- POC-US should not impede high-quality chest compressions.
- While POC-US can be performed during chest compressions, the image quality will likely be compromised but adequate for the purpose of determining gestational age and pregnancy status.
- Perform POC-US at any time during resuscitation. Pulse checks should last 10 seconds or less.

Regardless of the setting, providers who initiate BLS must be familiar with the important modifications of CPR in pregnant people who are at 20 weeks gestation or beyond, or when the uterine fundus can be palpated at or above the umbilicus. Applying the OBLS algorithm when pregnancy status is known or confirmed with the fundus palpable at or above the umbilicus will optimize maternal outcomes (Figures 5.6 and 5.7).

# OBSTETRIC LIFE SUPPORT

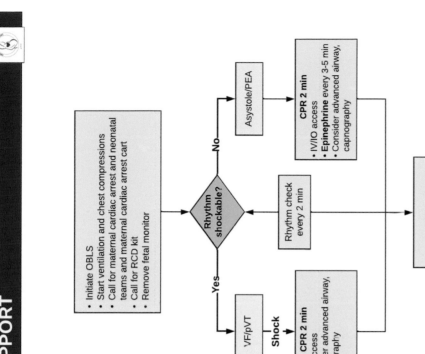

**Maternal cardiac arrest**
**No pulse, no response**

- Known pregnancy
- Fundus ≥ umbilicus
- In-hospital

- Initiate OBLS
- Start ventilation and chest compressions
- Call for maternal cardiac arrest and neonatal teams and maternal cardiac arrest cart
- Call for RCD kit
- Remove fetal monitor

**Rhythm shockable?**

**Yes** → **Shock** → VF/pVT → **CPR 2 min**
- IV/IO access
- Consider advanced airway, capnography

**No** → Asystole/PEA → **CPR 2 min**
- IV/IO access
- **Epinephrine** every 3-5 min
- Consider advanced airway, capnography

Rhythm check every 2 min

**Perform RCD 4 min** if no ROSC

Start post-arrest care if ROSC. Consider TTM

Start ECPR if no ROSC after delivery

Continuous high-quality chest compressions and LUD until delivery

**Abbreviations**

CPR - cardiopulmonary resuscitation
ECPR - extracorporeal cardiopulmonary resuscitation
IO - intraosseous
IV - intravenous
LUD - left uterine displacement
OBLS - Obstetric Life Support
PEA - pulseless electrical activity
pVT - ventricular tachycardia
RCD - resuscitative cesarean delivery
ROSC - return of spontaneous circulation
TTM - targeted temperature management
VF - ventricular fibrillation

| B | Bleeding |
| A | Anesthesia |
| A | Amniotic fluid embolism |
| C | Cardiovascular/cardiomyopathy |
| C | Clot/cerebrovascular |
| T | Trauma |
| O | Overdose (magnesium sulfate/opioids/other) |
| L | Lung injury/Acute respiratory distress syndrome |
| I | Ions (glucose/K+) |
| F | Fever (sepsis) |
| E | Emergency hypertension/eclampsia |

**FIGURE 5.6** Obstetric Life Support algorithm with modifications of cardiopulmonary resuscitation (known pregnancy >20 weeks).

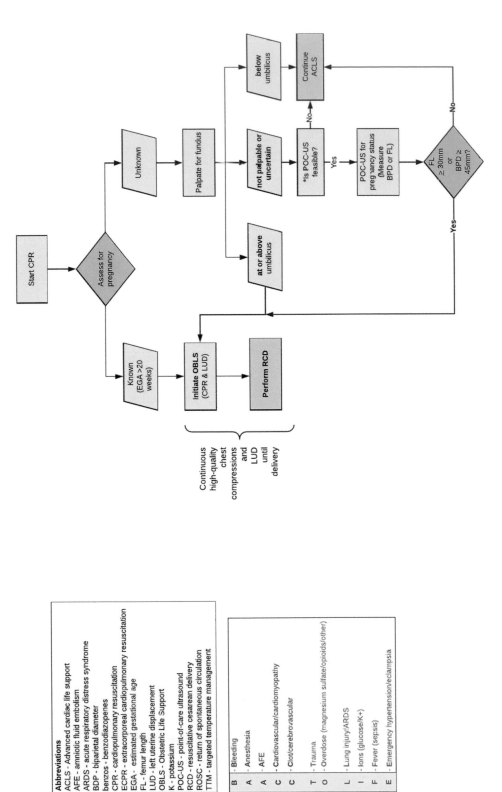

# OBSTETRIC LIFE SUPPORT

**Unconscious female, reproductive age.**
**No pulse, no or agonal breathing**
**OBLS should be done simultaneously with ongoing, high-quality CPR**

Start CPR

Assess for pregnancy

Known (EGA >20 weeks)

Unknown

Palpate for fundus

below umbilicus

at or above umbilicus

not palpable or uncertain

*Is POC-US feasible?

POC-US for pregnancy status (Measure BPD or FL)

FL ≥ 30mm or BPD ≥ 45mm?

Continue ACLS

Initiate OBLS (CPR & LUD)

Perform RCD

Continuous high-quality chest compressions and LUD until delivery

**Abbreviations**
ACLS - Advanced cardiac life support
AFE - amniotic fluid embolism
ARDS - acute respiratory distress syndrome
BDP - biparietal diameter
benzos - benzodiazopenes
CPR - cardiopulmonary resuscitation
ECPR - extracorporeal cardiopulmonary resuscitation
EGA - estimated gestational age
FL - femur length
LUD - left uterine displacement
OBLS - Obstetric Life Support
K - potassium
POC-US - point-of-care ultrasound
RCD - resuscitative cesarean delivery
ROSC - return of spontaneous circulation
TTM - targeted temperature management

B - Bleeding
A - Anesthesia
A - AFE
C - Cardiovascular/cardiomyopathy
C - Clot/cerebrovascular
T - Trauma
O - Overdose (magnesium sulfate/opioids/other)
L - Lung injury/ARDS
I - Ions (glucose/K+)
F - Fever (sepsis)
E - Emergency hypertension/eclampsia

**FIGURE 5.7**  Obstetric Life Support master algorithm (unknown pregnancy status).

**TABLE 5.1**  Key Assessments and Actions for Uterine Fundus Evaluation in Reproductive-Age People with Unknown Pregnancy Status and with Cardiac Arrest

| ASSESSMENT | ACTION |
|---|---|
| Fundus palpable at or above the umbilicus | • Pregnancy present, estimated to be at least 20 weeks gestation<br>• Assume that significant aortocaval compression is present, resulting in reduced effectiveness of chest compressions<br>• Perform **continuous LUD** in addition to high-quality CPR |
| Fundus palpable below the umbilicus | • Pregnancy present, assumed to be <20 weeks gestation<br>• Continue high-quality CPR without LUD |
| Fundus not palpable | • Pregnancy, or lack thereof, cannot be assumed<br>• Perform POC-US<br>• If pregnancy identified:<br>  • Obtain fetal FL and/or fetal BPD<br>  • Do not focus on fetal cardiac activity<br>  • POC-US should not impede or interrupt high-quality chest compressions and should not prolong pulse checks more than 10 seconds and should not prolong pulse check more than 10 seconds<br>• Apply LUD if >20 weeks by BPD (≥45 mm) or FL (≥30 mm), continue regular CPR if <20 weeks by BPD or FL (see Chapter 7 for more details)<br>• If pregnancy not identified, continue high-quality CPR without LUD |

**Case Vignette**

After collapsing, a 21-year-old patient at 38 weeks gestation is unconscious, and breathing is agonal. EMS providers do not find a pulse. One crew member begins chest compressions. Being told the patient is pregnant, the second crew member activates OBLS and requests additional personnel. They call for a second team and attach the defibrillator.

The team performs high-quality chest compressions, continuous LUD, and manages the patient's airway. Seeing the patient is in ventricular fibrillation, they deliver a shock. They resume chest compressions, intubate, and load for emergent transport to the closest emergency department with obstetrical services.

**REVIEW QUESTION**

Q. What are the modifications of BLS in pregnancy?

A. The modifications of BLS in pregnancy include LUD, calling for additional personnel, placing the AED pad to avoid breast tissue, and placing the IV above the diaphragm. These modifications improve blood flow back to the heart and the success of CPR on a pregnant patient.

# CHAPTER 5. PRACTICE QUESTIONS

1. Which of the following BEST describes the depth and speed of chest compressions during pregnancy?
   A. 1.5 inches deep, rate of 100–120/min
   B. 2 inches deep, rate of 100–120/min
   C. 1.5 inches deep, rate of 80–100/min
   D. 2 inches deep, rate of 80–100/min

2. What is the recommended minimum number of first responders to provide optimal maternal cardiac resuscitation?
   A. One
   B. Two
   C. Three
   D. Four

3. You placed the first AED pad on the sternum of a pregnant person at 35 weeks gestation with traumatic cardiac arrest and a suspected spinal cord injury from a fall. Which of the following is the BEST location for the second pad?
   A. Above the left breast
   B. Above the right breast

    C.  Underneath and lateral to the left breast

    D.  On the back

4. Your team is the first to respond to an MCA at 28 weeks gestation. Which of the following is the next BEST step after initiating BLS and calling for more help?
    A.  Endotracheal intubation
    B.  LUD
    C.  RCD
    D.  Wedging patient by 45 degrees

5. A person who is 30 weeks pregnant is in cardiac arrest. You begin CPR while your partner applies the AED. The AED states "shock advised." What should you do next?
    A.  Manually displace the uterus to the left and then defibrillate
    B.  Continue CPR while your partner intubates the patient
    C.  Position the patient on their left side and defibrillate
    D.  Deliver the shock and immediately resume CPR

# CHAPTER 5. ANSWERS

1. **ANSWER: B.** This is unchanged from high-quality chest compressions in a nonpregnant adult. Check carotid pulse for 5–10 seconds. If no pulse within 10 seconds, start CPR (30:2 or continuous compressions with ventilations every 5–6 seconds) beginning with chest compressions at the center of the chest (lower half of the sternum) hard and fast with at least 100–120 compressions per minute at a depth of at least 2 inches. Allow for complete recoil after each compression and minimize interruptions in compressions (10 seconds or less). Switch providers every 2 minutes to avoid fatigue.

2. **ANSWER: C.** The initial start of the BLS survey essentially remains the same for both pregnant and nonpregnant adults. Activating help and immediately starting high-quality chest compressions are crucial to the patient's outcome. Clearly communicate that the **pregnant** person is in arrest when activating the emergency response system; at least three responders are needed to perform all basic modifications to BLS simultaneously.

3. **ANSWER: C.** Pad placement can be either anterolateral or anteroposterior; however, place anterolaterally if the patient has a suspected spinal cord injury to limit movement and potential further injury of the patient. In the anterolateral position, the lateral pad should be placed **under** the left breast tissue.

4. **ANSWER: B.** Immediately perform LUD if the fundus is palpable at or above the umbilicus (which would be the case for a person at 28 weeks gestation). This will reduce aortocaval compression and promote high-quality CPR.

5. **ANSWER: D.** If the patient has no pulse, check for shockable rhythm with an AED as soon as it arrives and provide shocks as indicated. Follow each shock immediately with CPR, beginning with compressions. Shocks should not be delayed due to pregnant status.

# CHAPTER 5. REFERENCES

1. *Summary of high-quality CPR components for BLS providers.* Website. https://heartcprtrainingcenter.com/pdf/2020BLSSummary.pdf.
2. *Highlights of the 2020 focused updates to the American Heart Association guidelines for cardiopulmonary resuscitation and emergency cardiovascular care.* Website. https://cpr.heart.org/-/media/cpr-files/cpr-guidelines-files/highlights/hghlghts_2020_ecc_guidelines_english.pdf. Updated 2020.
3. Jeejeebhoy F W, R. Management of cardiac arrest in pregnancy. *Best Pract Res Clin Obstet Gynaecol.* 2014;28:607. doi: 10.1016/j.bpobgyn.2014.03.006.
4. Chumlea WC, Schubert CM, Roche AF, Kulin HE, Lee PA, Himes JH, Sun SS. Age at menarche and racial comparisons in US girls. *Pediatrics.* 2003;11(1):110–113. doi: 10.1542/peds.111.1.110.
5. U.S. Department of Health and Human Services, Health Resources and Services Administration, Maternal and Child Health Bureau. *Women's Health USA 2013.* Website. https://mchb.hrsa.gov/whusa13/population-characteristics/p/us-population.html. Updated 2013.
6. Fowler RL, Lippmann MJ. *Benefits vs. risks of intraosseous vascular access.* Website. https://psnet.ahrq.gov/web-mm/benefits-vs-risks-intraosseous-vascular-access. Updated 2019.

# Review of Cardiopulmonary Resuscitation Modifications for Pregnant Patients in Advanced Cardiac Life Support and Advanced Life Support

# 6

## 6.1 INTRODUCTION

As recommended by the AHA, the ACLS survey can be started either

1. after the BLS survey has been completed in an unconscious patient, or
2. immediately in the conscious but unstable patient.

While the BLS survey focuses primarily on high-quality CPR, the ACLS survey incorporates a differential diagnosis and applying advanced resuscitation techniques. The American Red Cross Advanced Life Support (ALS) also emphasizes an advanced survey and differential diagnosis to guide treatment.

## 6.2 LEARNING OBJECTIVES

Learner will appropriately

- Review current ACLS guidelines for the nonpregnant patient.
- Describe critical steps and actions of the ACLS survey, as applied to a pregnant patient.

## 6.3 REVIEW OF ADVANCED CARDIAC LIFE SUPPORT

ACLS follows the BLS survey and focuses on supporting a patient's circulation and ventilation (Figure 6.1). The ACLS survey follows the **ABCDE** approach, incorporating assessment of **A**irway, **B**reathing, **C**irculation, **D**isability, and **E**xposure (Figure 6.2). The ACLS survey also incorporates ECG rhythm interpretation and administration of medications to treat

DOI: 10.1201/9781003299288-7

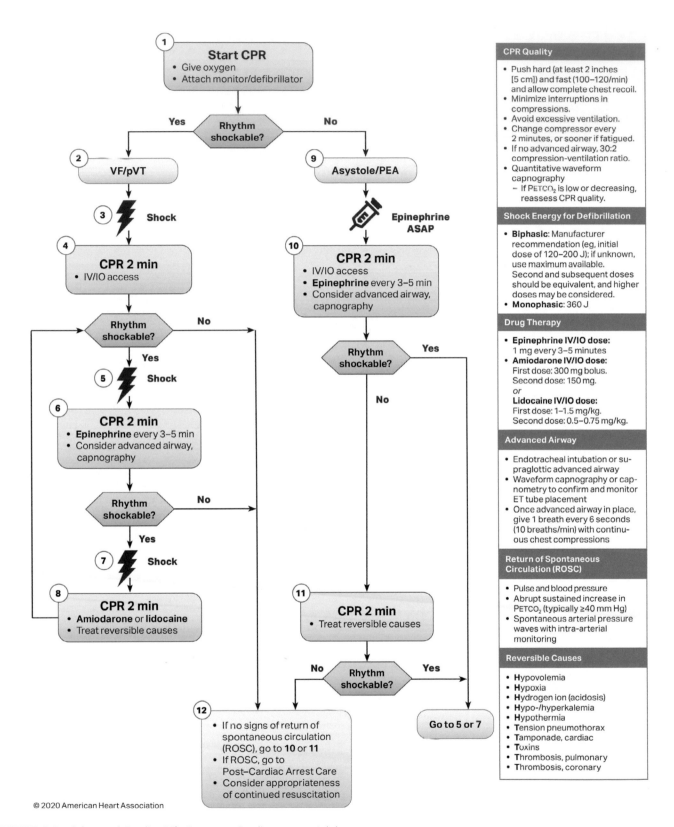

© 2020 American Heart Association

**FIGURE 6.1**   Advanced Cardiac Life Support. Cardiac arrest: Adult.

| Assess | Action as Appropriate |
|---|---|
| **Airway**<br><br>• *Is the airway patent?*<br>• *Is an advanced airway indicated?*<br>• *Is proper placement of airway device confirmed?*<br>• *Is tube secured and placement reconfirmed frequently?* | • **Maintain airway patency in unconscious patients** by use of the head tilt–chin lift, oropharyngeal airway, or nasopharyngeal airway<br>• **Use advanced airway management if needed** (eg, laryngeal mask airway, laryngeal tube, esophageal-tracheal tube, endotracheal tube)<br><br>*Healthcare providers must weigh the benefit of advanced airway placement against the adverse effects of interrupting chest compressions. If bag-mask ventilation is adequate, healthcare providers may defer insertion of an advanced airway until the patient does not respond to initial CPR and defibrillation or until spontaneous circulation returns. Advanced airway devices such as a laryngeal mask airway, laryngeal tube, or esophageal-tracheal tube can be placed while chest compressions continue.*<br><br>*If using advanced airway devices*<br>• **Confirm proper integration of CPR and ventilation**<br>• **Confirm proper placement of advanced airway devices** by<br>  – Physical examination<br>  – Quantitative waveform capnography<br>• **Secure the device to prevent dislodgment**<br>• **Monitor airway placement with continuous quantitative waveform capnography** |
| **Breathing**<br><br>• *Are ventilation and oxygenation adequate?*<br>• *Are quantitative waveform capnography and oxyhemoglobin saturation monitored?* | • **Give supplementary oxygen when indicated**<br>  – For cardiac arrest patients, administer 100% oxygen<br>  – For others, titrate oxygen administration to achieve oxygen saturation values of 94% or greater by pulse oximetry<br>• **Monitor the adequacy of ventilation and oxygenation** by<br>  – Clinical criteria (chest rise and cyanosis)<br>  – Quantitative waveform capnography<br>  – Oxygen saturation<br>• **Avoid excessive ventilation** |
| **Circulation**<br><br>• *Are chest compressions effective?*<br>• *What is the cardiac rhythm?*<br>• *Is defibrillation or cardioversion indicated?*<br>• *Has IV/IO access been established?*<br>• *Is ROSC present?*<br>• *Is the patient with a pulse unstable?*<br>• *Are medications needed for rhythm or blood pressure?*<br>• *Does the patient need volume (fluid) for resuscitation?* | • **Monitor CPR quality**<br>  – Quantitative waveform capnography (if $P_{ETCO_2}$ is less than 10 mm Hg, attempt to improve CPR quality)<br>  – Intra-arterial pressure (if relaxation phase [diastolic] pressure is less than 20 mm Hg, attempt to improve CPR quality)<br>• **Attach monitor/defibrillator for arrhythmias or cardiac arrest rhythms** (eg, ventricular fibrillation [VF], pulseless ventricular tachycardia [PVT], asystole, pulseless electrical activity [PEA])<br>• **Provide defibrillation/cardioversion**<br>• **Obtain IV/IO access**<br>• **Give appropriate drugs** to manage rhythm and blood pressure<br>• **Give IV/IO fluids if needed**<br>• **Check glucose and temperature**<br>• **Check perfusion issues** |
| **Disability** | • **Check for neurologic function**<br>• **Quickly assess for responsiveness, levels of consciousness, and pupil dilation**<br>• **AVPU: Alert, Voice, Painful, Unresponsive** |
| **Exposure** | • **Remove clothing to perform a physical examination, looking for obvious signs of trauma, bleeding, burns, unusual markings, or medical alert bracelets** |

$P_{ETCO_2}$ is the partial pressure of $CO_2$ in exhaled air at the end of the exhalation phase.

**FIGURE 6.2**  Advanced Cardiac Life Support. Primary assessment: Adult.

various cardiac dysrhythmias. Continuous high-quality CPR is critical. CPR should **not** be interrupted to place an advanced airway device. If bag-mask ventilation (BMV) is adequate, providers may defer insertion of an advanced airway until the patient fails to respond to initial CPR and defibrillation, or until spontaneous circulation occurs. In pregnancy, the pregnant patient's airway is more challenging due to pregnancy changes. Intubation attempts are best completed by experienced personnel.

Once an advanced airway is placed, correct airway placement should be confirmed with physical examination and continuous quantitative waveform capnography. The advanced airway should then be secured to prevent it being dislodged. The adequacy of ventilation and oxygenation should be monitored with chest rise and the presence or absence of cyanosis, quantitative waveform capnography (end-tidal $CO_2$ [$ETCO_2$]), and oxygen saturation. If quantitative waveform capnography shows an **$ETCO_2$ of <10 mm Hg**, attempts to improve CPR quality should be made.

Use **BAACC TO LIFE** to remember the differential diagnosis of MCA.

---

**KEY POINTS**

- **Do not** interrupt CPR to place an advanced airway device.
- If BMV is adequate, providers may defer the insertion of an advanced airway until the patient fails to respond to initial CPR and defibrillation or until spontaneous circulation returns.
- Confirm correct airway placement with physical exam and continuous quantitative waveform capnography.
- Monitor adequacy of ventilation and oxygenation with chest rise and presence or absence of cyanosis, $ETCO_2$, and oxygen saturation.
- If quantitative waveform capnography shows an $ETCO_2$ of <10 mm Hg, attempt to improve CPR quality.
- Use the mnemonic BAACC TO LIFE to remember differential diagnosis of causes of MCA.
- Administer 100% oxygen to patients in MCA.
- Ventilate at a rate of one breath every 5–6 seconds and avoid excessive ventilation.

---

# 6.4 INTERPRETATION OF CARDIAC RHYTHMS

The ACLS and ALS surveys build on BLS, incorporating cardiac rhythm interpretation and medications to treat various cardiac dysrhythmias. While OBLS does not review cardiac rhythms in depth, providers should be able to recognize key differences in treating the various rhythms found in cardiac arrest. Rhythms can be broken down into two basic groups: shockable and nonshockable rhythms. Shockable (or those that could respond to defibrillation) consist of ventricular fibrillation or pulseless ventricular tachycardia. Nonshockable rhythms are PEA and asystole. Each of these are further reviewed later.

---

# 6.5 SHOCKABLE RHYTHMS: VENTRICULAR FIBRILLATION AND PULSELESS VENTRICULAR TACHYCARDIA

Ventricular fibrillation (VF) (Figure 6.3) and pulseless ventricular tachycardia (VT; Figure 6.4) should be treated with high-quality CPR and biphasic defibrillation as soon as possible. Energy doses should be based on manufacturer's recommendations for their individual defibrillators, including fixed versus escalating energy doses. Please refer to Figure 6.1 for the recommended AHA algorithm for defibrillation.

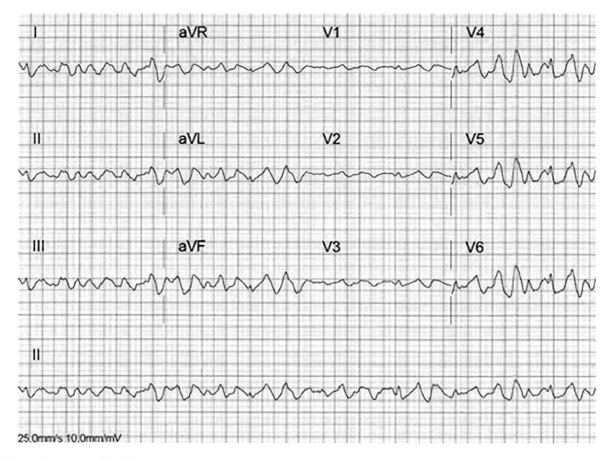

**FIGURE 6.3**   Ventricular fibrillation.

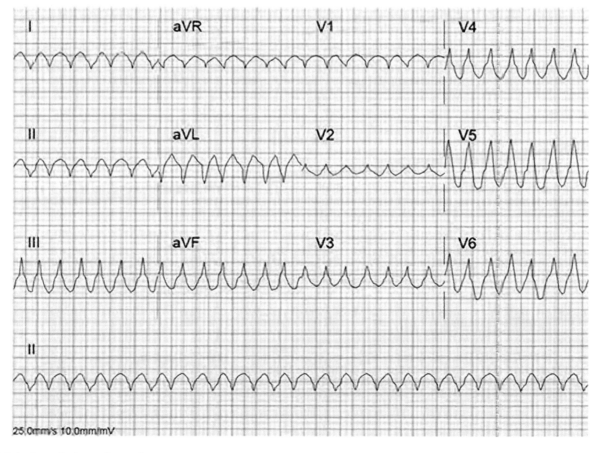

**FIGURE 6.4**   Ventricular tachycardia.

# 6.6 REFRACTORY VENTRICULAR FIBRILLATION AND VENTRICULAR TACHYCARDIA

Refractory VF/VT are dysrhythmias that persist despite one or more shocks. While medications such as epinephrine do not typically convert VF/VT, they do improve the restoration and continuation of a perfusing rhythm. While this aids in resuscitation, anti-arrhythmic drugs have not shown as much improvement in long-term survival as high-quality CPR has. In these cases, IV or IO access to administer medications should not be obtained at the expense of high-quality chest compressions. Table 6.1 lists the drugs and doses used in resuscitation and their indication by cardiac rhythm interpretation.

**TABLE 6.1**  Drugs Used in Basic Life Support and Advanced Life Support/Advanced Cardiac Life Support Surveys

| DRUG | DOSE | INDICATION |
| --- | --- | --- |
| Amiodarone | • First dose: 300 mg IV/IO push<br>• Second dose (if needed): 150 mg IV or IO push<br>• Max dose: 2.2 g IV over 24 hours | Cardiac arrest: VF/VT unresponsive to CPR, defibrillation, and epinephrine |
| Epinephrine | • 1 mg every 3–5 minutes IV or IO<br>• Follow dose with 20-mL bolus of IV fluid and elevate the extremity for 10–20 seconds | Cardiac arrest: VF, pulseless VT, asystole, PEA |
| Lidocaine | • Initial dose: 1–1.5 mg/kg IV/IO<br>• May give an additional 0.5–0.75 mg/kg IV push, repeat in 5–10 minutes; maximum 3 doses or total of 3 mg/kg | Alternative to amiodarone for VF/VT unresponsive to CPR, defibrillation, and epinephrine |

# 6.7 NONSHOCKABLE RHYTHMS: PULSELESS ELECTRICAL ACTIVITY AND ASYSTOLE

The patient experiencing PEA shows a rhythm on the monitor however exhibits no palpable pulse. In this case, this is **not** a shockable rhythm, therefore, high-quality CPR and IV or IO access are critical to managing the patient. Similarly, there is no shockable rhythm in asystole. As such, high-quality CPR and epinephrine are the priorities. It is not uncommon for PEA to result in asystole, but providers must ensure it is true asystole and not caused by loose or unconnected leads, a different rhythm (such as VF), or lack of power. Asystole is often the final rhythm prior to patient death for all cardiac dysrhythmias, including those that initially exhibited VF or VT. Figures 6.5 and 6.6 show examples of PEA and asystole. Please refer to Figure 6.1 for the AHA treatment algorithm.

**KEY POINTS**
- Electrocardiogram rhythm interpretation guides medication administration during a maternal code and does not differ from nonpregnant adults.
- Do **not** stop high-quality chest compressions to administer medications.
- IV/IO access above the diaphragm is critical to managing pregnant patients in cardiac arrest, especially if the initial rhythm is nonshockable, such as PEA or asystole.
- IO access in a pregnant patient is best placed above the diaphragm in the head of the humerus.
- Administer 1 mg of epinephrine every 3–5 minutes to optimize the survival of MCA patients in PEA.

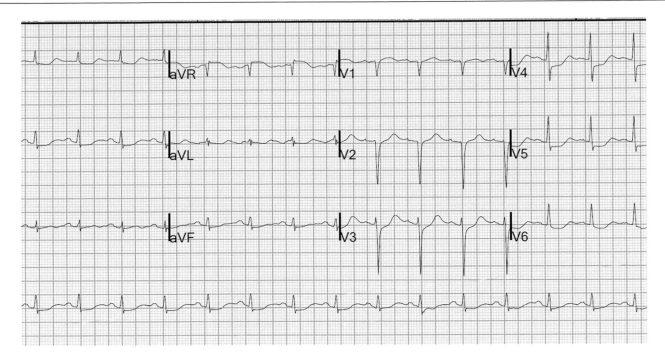

**FIGURE 6.5**   Pulseless electrical activity.

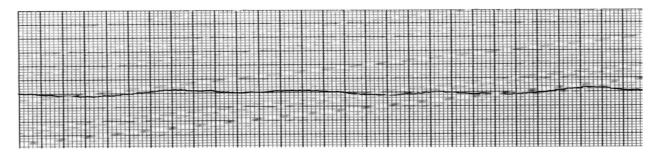

**FIGURE 6.6**   Asystole.

## 6.8 DIFFERENTIAL DIAGNOSIS

While many of the causes of cardiac arrest in a nonpregnant patient are similar in pregnancy, it is important to highlight pregnancy-specific causes of maternal cardiac arrest. The mnemonic **BAACC TO LIFE** is a reminder of the differential diagnosis for the most common etiologies of MCA (see Figure 4.1).

## 6.9 ADVANCED CARDIAC LIFE SUPPORT CHANGES IN PREGNANCY

There are several important changes and additions to ACLS that are critical to achieving ROSC during an MCA. Team orientation and communication are even more critical as many providers from different departments are required for effective ongoing resuscitation. In addition to continuous LUD during CPR, the resuscitation team must also prepare for immediate RCD, as well as the potential need for neonatal resuscitation. Preparation for a difficult airway must be considered, and all IV access must be above the diaphragm. Additionally, ECPR may be considered in cases of refractory cardiac arrest and is covered in more detail in Chapter 7.

# 6.10 OBSTETRIC LIFE SUPPORT COGNITIVE AID

The OBLS cognitive aid and **ALIVE AT FIVE** mnemonic are useful tools to quickly remember the necessary and important steps unique to caring for maternal patients in cardiac arrest (Figures 6.7 and 6.8). The **ALIVE AT FIVE** mnemonic is a simple way to remember the critical modifications and is easily taught to learners. The OBLS cognitive aids should be readily available (such as in EMS bags and on code carts) for use during a maternal code.

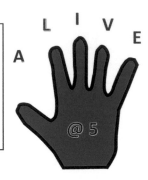

Activate OBLS

Left uterine displacement

IV placement above diaphragm/Intubate early

Ventilate/Verify equipment and personnel

Evacuate uterus by 5 minutes

**FIGURE 6.7**   ALIVE AT FIVE mnemonic.

# 6.11 AIRWAY MANAGEMENT: BASIC

High-quality CPR relies on effective chest compressions (**at least 2 inches in depth, rate of at least 100–120 compressions per minute, and with full chest recoil**) and continuous **LUD** in pregnancies >20 weeks gestation or when the uterus is at or above the umbilicus. If ventilation can be accomplished effectively with BMV with good chest rise, it is reasonable to continue with basic airway management until an experienced provider is available to secure an advanced airway. OBLS recommends ventilation with 100% $O_2$ at 15 L/min.

# 6.12 AIRWAY MANAGEMENT: ADVANCED

Pregnancy changes result in a difficult airway in pregnant people. Therefore, it is critical to assign advanced airway management to the most experienced provider and have advanced airway equipment readily available. The 2019 Focused Updates to the AHA Guidelines for Cardiopulmonary Resuscitation and Emergency Cardiovascular Care promote the use of BMV or an advanced airway strategy with supraglottic airway in the OH setting. Endotracheal intubation should only be used by EMS providers in settings of "high tracheal intubation rate of success or optimal training opportunities for endotracheal intubation."[1]

As the pregnant person's airway can present unique challenges, OBLS recommends continuing BMV if there is adequate chest rise in the OH setting, with the option of placing a supraglottic airway by a trained provider, if necessary. If an advanced airway is needed in the IH setting, an expert in airway management may choose either supraglottic airway or endotracheal intubation. In either setting, frequent experience or frequent retraining in endotracheal intubation is necessary to maintain skills, and "a program of on-going quality improvement to minimize complications and track overall supraglottic airway and endotracheal intubation success" is recommended for EMS providers.[2]

Consider a surgical airway such as percutaneous cricothyroidotomy if supraglottic airway and endotracheal intubation fail and BMV is inadequate.

As in nonpregnant patients, use continuous waveform capnography to evaluate and confirm proper endotracheal (ET) tube placement. $ETCO_2$ should be >10 mm Hg indicating effective chest compressions or ROSC. If proper ET tube placement is confirmed but $ETCO_2$ remains <10 mm Hg, providers should consider either ineffective chest compressions or causes such as massive pulmonary embolism, pericardial tamponade, tension pneumothorax, or exsanguination.

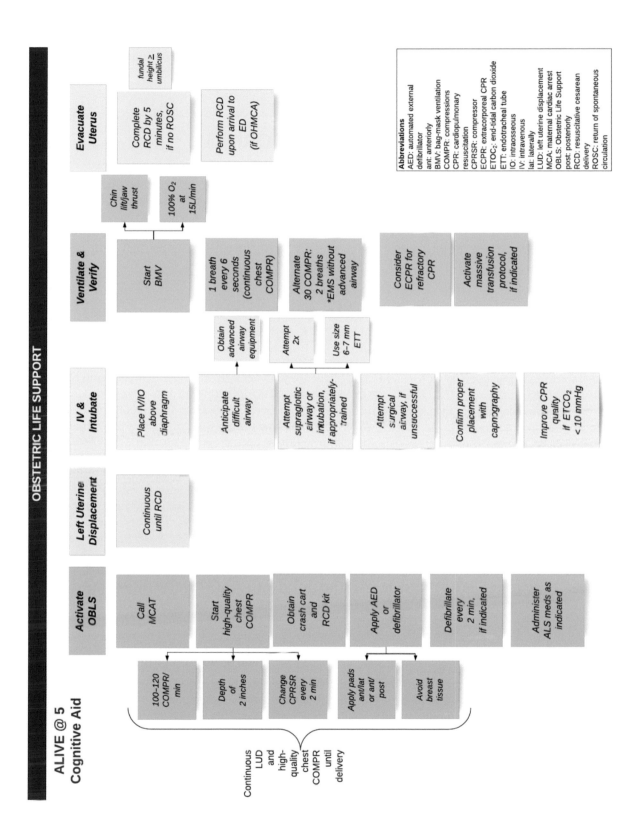

**FIGURE 6.8**  OBLS cognitive aid.

## 6.13  ANTI-ARRHYTHMIC DRUGS

Pregnancy does not alter the dose or route of medication administration during cardiac arrest. The pregnant patient should receive any indicated anti-arrhythmic medication at the same dose and timing as in nonpregnant patients. IV or IO access should be placed **above** the diaphragm to optimize fluid and medication administration.

## 6.14  FETAL MONITORING

Prioritizing maternal resuscitation is key to improving maternal survival. Therefore, focus attention on the mother during MCA. Do not place fetal monitors if pregnancy is confirmed, and remove any fetal monitors that may have been placed if MCA occurs. These actions help to keep the team focused on maternal resuscitation and facilitate easy access to the maternal abdomen if RCD is required. Removing fetal monitors also eliminates the theoretical risk of arcing should defibrillation be necessary. If ROSC occurs prior to RCD, fetal monitoring should be performed consistent with gestational age requirements. This is covered in more detail in Chapter 11.

## 6.15  RESUSCITATIVE CESAREAN DELIVERY

RCD is indicated for any pregnant person with a uterus at or above the umbilicus or ≥20 weeks gestation **and** has not achieved ROSC in the first 4 minutes of the arrest. RCD facilitates decompression of the inferior vena cava to improve blood flow back to the heart allowing for autotransfusion as the uterus contracts down after delivery. RCD should occur either at the site of arrest (if already hospitalized) or upon admission to the ED (if transported by EMS personnel). Studies show improved outcomes for both mother and fetus when RCD is performed as quickly as possible after MCA, even if outside the initial 4-minute parameter.[3–5]

Some studies recommend delivery within 4 minutes of arrest; however, under certain circumstances, (such as intrapartum, nonshockable rhythms), OBLS recommends immediately performing an RCD.[2] When MCA occurs OH, prepare for immediate RCD upon arrival at the ED. **Do not delay RCD** by moving the patient to the labor and delivery suite or an operating room. During transport, communicate with the hospital to activate the appropriate teams to perform RCD upon the patient's arrival.

Use a vertical midline skin incision to gain increased exposure. This incision allows for more exposure to control bleeding and explore the upper abdomen, especially in cases of trauma or uncertain etiology for MCA. Avoid Pfannenstiel skin incisions (long, horizontal abdominal incision made below the line of the pubic hair and above the mons) in MCA.

If an obstetrician is not immediately available, a general or trauma surgeon or emergency physician should perform the RCD. After entry into the abdomen with a vertical skin incision, make a vertical uterine incision and deliver the fetus. Hand the fetus to the waiting neonatal intensive care unit or pediatric team and remove the placenta. The uterine incision can then be packed with laparotomy sponges and clamped with Kelly or Pennington clamps; the incision can also be closed in a running locked fashion with delayed absorbable suture (such as 0-polyglactin or O-poliglecaprone). Similarly, the maternal abdomen can be packed with laparotomy sponges and the incision draped with a sterile towel until after the resuscitation is completed, at which time the uterus and abdomen can be closed. If ROSC is achieved, administer oxytocin and antibiotics (Ancef 2 g IV unless allergic). As oxytocin may precipitate rearrest, give it as an IV infusion, not an IV bolus.

In the setting of ROSC, operators should also prepare for bleeding from surgical sites by having additional suture, instruments, blood products, and/or massive transfusion protocol available. It may also be necessary to consider moving to an operating room once ROSC is achieved to complete the surgery and allow for improved visualization/surgical preparedness.

## 6.16  VAGINAL DELIVERY

Should MCA occur while the patient is in labor and the cervix is completely dilated, the delivering provider may consider an operative vaginal delivery with forceps instead of an RCD. An operative vaginal delivery in this scenario may be quicker than performing an RCD. Such decisions will be made by the delivering provider given the clinical scenario.

## 6.17 FACTORS THAT COULD DECREASE THE EFFECTIVENESS OF ADVANCED CARDIAC LIFE SUPPORT AND CARDIOPULMONARY RESUSCITATION IN PREGNANCY

High-quality CPR is directly correlated to improved maternal outcomes. However, several factors may negatively impact high-quality CPR in pregnant patients (see Table 6.2). Responders to MCA must be aware of and manage these factors to achieve high-quality CPR and improve maternal outcomes.

**TABLE 6.2**  Factors That Decrease the Effectiveness of Obstetric Life Support

| FACTOR | REDUCED EFFECTIVENESS IN PREGNANT PATIENTS DUE TO |
|---|---|
| Quality of CPR | • Dense/large breasts resulting in incorrect hand placement or shallow compressions<br>• Incorrect technique of rolling or wedging the pregnant patient to reduce aortocaval compression (historical teaching)<br>• Not performing LUD when indicated<br>• Not performing RCD when indicated |
| Inaction | • Too focused on fetal status, resulting in not performing or delaying RCD<br>• Fear that actions may adversely impact the pregnancy (such as withholding resuscitation medications)<br>• Fear of performing RCD due to limited or no real-life experience |
| Other | • Resuscitation team:<br>  • Does not know about or does not suspect pregnancy<br>  • Has poor communication<br>  • Lacks knowledge of modifications of CPR in pregnancy<br>• No communication with the command center about pregnancy in an OH arrest<br>• Crew transports patient to a hospital with inadequate resources to care for MCA |

## 6.18 MATERNAL CARDIAC ARREST TEAM

Hospitals, especially those providing maternal care, should designate a MCAT that is activated with a single call. A unified call to action will bring a designated response team with the proper personnel and resources to the patient's bedside. Decreasing the MCAT's response time is critical to improving maternal survival.

The MCAT can be broken into teams, as resources allow:

- Maternal team, consisting of OB (or surgery)
- Critical care or medicine
- Neonatal resuscitation team
- ECPR or extracorporeal membrane oxygenation (ECMO) team, if available

Table 6.3 outlines the composition of code teams and the members that make up each team. MCA code team leaders will require coordination between multiple leaders—for the adult resuscitation, obstetric modifications, neonatal resuscitation, and ECPR. Therefore, it is imperative that all team leads communicate effectively. Please refer to Chapter 12 for more details on effective communication among team members.

**TABLE 6.3**   Recommended Composition of a Maternal Cardiac Arrest Team

| Maternal Team | • OB<br>• Labor and delivery nurses<br>• Critical care or emergency physicians and nurses<br>• Respiratory therapy or equivalent<br>• Anesthesia (obstetric anesthesiologist if available), staff anesthesiologist, anesthesia assistant or Certified Registered Nurse Anesthetists (CRNAs)<br>• Consider trauma/general surgery, pharmacy representative, and internal medicine or family physician, if no critical care providers available |
|---|---|
| Neonatal Resuscitation Team | • Neonatal physician or pediatrician or family physician<br>• Neonatal or pediatric nurse<br>• Neonatal respiratory therapist or equivalent |
| ECPR Team | • Adult ECMO physician<br>• Adult ECMO specialist (nurse or respiratory therapist)<br>• Advanced technology specialist |
| Stroke Team | • Neurologist<br>• Neuro-intensive care unit RN |

**KEY POINTS**
- Consider an advanced airway strategy if BMV is not producing effective chest rise.
- EMS providers should remember "Stroke, STEMI, **Mama**, Trauma" and quickly transport a patient in MCA.
- If two attempts at supraglottic airway or intubation fail, and if BMV is inadequate, perform a surgical airway.
- Consider cricoid pressure during intubation on a case-by-case basis at the discretion of the laryngoscopist.
- Give pregnant patients all indicated anti-arrhythmic medications in the same dose and timing as in non-pregnant patients.
- Remove fetal monitors to maintain focus on maternal resuscitation.
- **Do not** delay RCD. Complete RCD by 5 minutes of arrest.
- Consider RCD for pregnant people with a uterus at or above the umbilicus or ≥20 weeks gestation **and** who has not achieved ROSC in the first 4 minutes of arrest.
- Perform RCD at arrest site (if IH) or upon admission to the ED (if OH).
- Performing an RCD during MCA improves cardiac output and may increase chances of successful ROSC.
- EMS providers focus on high-quality CPR, airway management, continuous LUD, and patient transport are vital to patient survival.
- In ideal circumstances, transport time of an MCA patient to the most appropriate facility is under 10 minutes.
- For OH MCA, the receiving facility should activate the MCA team so that the team is waiting in the ED with appropriate equipment and resources.

**Case Vignette**

A 21-year-old person at 38 weeks gestation calls 911 due to a severe headache and vaginal bleeding. The patient collapses shortly after EMS providers get an initial blood pressure reading of 210/120 mm Hg. The team starts BLS and notes that the patient looks "very pregnant" and has moderate vaginal bleeding. The crew leader radios the receiving hospital with an **OB Arrest Alert**, activating the MCAT.

Upon presentation to the ED, the patient is intubated and undergoes resuscitation for continued arrest. The EMS team reports giving two shocks for ventricular fibrillation without ROSC. While activating the massive blood transfusion protocol, the OB performs an RCD via a vertical midline incision.

Copious bloody amniotic fluid is noted on entry to the uterus, and the fetus and placenta are delivered together and handed off to the neonatologist. A placental abruption is diagnosed, and the team starts transfusing blood. The OB closes the uterus while high-quality CPR is continued. Severe preeclampsia is suspected as the root cause of the headache, blood pressure elevation, and abruption. After continued CPR and massive blood transfusion, the patient has ROSC.

## REVIEW QUESTION

Q. What are the modifications of ACLS in pregnancy?

A. The most critical modifications of ACLS in pregnancy are to keep the patient supine and apply continuous LUD during high-quality chest compressions. Start the IV above the diaphragm, be prepared for a difficult airway intubation, and do not withhold or change the dose of anti-arrhythmic drugs, if otherwise considered in a nonpregnant patient. Similarly, deliver a shock if the patient is in a shockable dysrhythmia.

If ROSC is not achieved within 4 minutes of resuscitation attempts, qualified providers (such as OB/GYN, general/trauma surgeon, or emergency physician) should perform RCD. Perform the RCD where the arrest occurred (if hospitalized) or in the ED upon presentation (if the arrest occurred OH). Alert the MCAT at the beginning of a maternal code to ensure adequate care for both the patient and fetus. Finally, in the event of refractory CPR, consider ECPR, where resources allow.

# CHAPTER 6. PRACTICE QUESTIONS

1. During resuscitation of an MCA patient with chest compressions, BMV, and LUD, the initial rhythm check demonstrates pulseless electrical activity. Which of the following is the BEST next step in management?
   A. Defibrillate and immediately resume high-quality chest compressions
   B. Stop chest compressions to allow placement of IV access
   C. Administer epinephrine 1 mg
   D. Administer amiodarone 300 mg

2. A pregnant person at 17 weeks gestation with a twin pregnancy arrives at the ED in cardiac arrest. When performing the primary survey, the ED provider palpates the fundus at 2 cm above the umbilicus. The patient does not have ROSC after 4 minutes of high-quality CPR and two shocks for ventricular fibrillation. What is the BEST next step in management?
   A. Perform an RCD
   B. Activate the massive transfusion protocol
   C. Perform point-of-care ultrasound to recheck gestational age
   D. Request a stat OB consult to confirm gestational age

3. Which of the following equipment needs are indispensable during a maternal cardiac arrest?
   A. 9-mm endotracheal tube
   B. Basic RCD kit
   C. Sutures and needle driver
   D. Uterine tamponade balloon

4. During a MCA, two attempts at intubation by the most experienced provider available have failed. What is the BEST next step in management?
   A. Reattempt intubation with cricoid pressure
   B. Place a supraglottic airway
   C. Continue BMV even if ETCO$_2$ <10 mm Hg
   D. Perform percutaneous cricothyroidotomy

5. Fetal monitors are in place during an MCA in the labor and delivery suite. You advise your technician to remove the monitors, but he challenges you that the fetal monitors will allow the team to ensure the fetus is okay during the resuscitation of the mother. Which response should you give him?
   A. Removing the monitors reduces target fixation away from resuscitation of the mother
   B. Fetal monitors reduce effectiveness of chest compressions and LUD
   C. The decision should be left to the discretion of the code leader
   D. Fetal monitoring can be done to indicate quality CPR in some circumstances

# CHAPTER 6. ANSWERS

1. **ANSWER: C.** The patient experiencing PEA shows a rhythm on the monitor but exhibits no palpable pulse. In this case, this is **not** a shockable rhythm; therefore, high-quality CPR and IV/IO access (for epinephrine 1 mg every 3–5 minutes) are critical steps to optimizing survival. The epinephrine dose is followed with a 20-mL bolus of IV fluid and elevated extremity for 10–20 seconds.
2. **ANSWER: A.** Consider RCD for any pregnant person with a uterus at or above the umbilicus and who has not achieved ROSC in the first 4 minutes of the arrest. RCD should occur either at the site of arrest if already hospitalized or upon admission to the ED if transported by EMS personnel. Studies have demonstrated improved outcomes for both mother and fetus if RCD can be performed as quickly as possible although in this case the fetuses are previable.
3. **ANSWER: B.** A basic RCD kit contains a scalpel, retractors, clamps (Kelly and Allis clamps), and umbilical cord clamps and should be available for the MCAT responding to MCA. Pregnant patients often require a **smaller** ET tube such as 6.0–7.0-mm. A 9.0-mm would be much too large. While suture and uterine balloon may ultimately be needed, these are not essential to perform RCD.
4. **ANSWER: B.** Pregnancy can result in a difficult airway. Therefore, it is critical to anticipate the difficult airway and assign advanced airway management to the most experienced provider. Ideally two attempts per technique are tried before switching to an alternative. It is appropriate to consider a slightly smaller ET tube (i.e., 6.0–7.0 mm inner diameter tube) to improve the likelihood of successful intubation. If two attempts at intubation have failed, a supraglottic airway is then recommended. If two attempts at supraglottic airway fail, and if BMV is inadequate, consider a surgical airway (such as percutaneous cricothyroidotomy).
5. **ANSWER: A.** Prioritize maternal resuscitation by focusing attention on the mother. Do not place fetal monitors if pregnancy is confirmed, and remove any fetal monitors that may have been placed. These actions help to focus on resuscitating the mother and facilitate easy access to the maternal abdomen if RCD is needed. Fetal monitors should be removed to reduce the theoretical risk of arcing in the event of defibrillation. If ROSC occurs prior to RCD, use fetal monitoring consistent with gestational age requirements.

# CHAPTER 6. REFERENCES

1. Jeejeebhoy F, Windrim R. Management of cardiac arrest in pregnancy. *Best Pract Res Clin Obstet Gynaecol*. 2014;28:607. doi: 10.1016/j.bpobgyn.2014.03.006.
2. Panchal AR, Berg KM, Cabanas JG, et al. 2019 American Heart Association focused update on systems of care: Dispatcher assisted cardiopulmonary resuscitation and cardiac arrest centers: An update to the American Heart Association guidelines for cardiopulmonary resuscitation. *Circ Arrhythm Electrophysiol*. 2019;140:895–903. doi: 10.1161/CIR.0000000000000733.
3. Katz V, Balderston K, DeFreest M. Perimortem cesarean delivery: Were our assumptions correct? *AJOG*. 2005;19(6):1916–1920; 1920–1921. doi: 10.1016/j.ajog.2005.02.038.
4. Rose C, Faksh A, Traynor K, Cabrera D, Arendt K, Brost B. Challenging the 4- to 5-minute rule: From perimortem cesarean to resuscitative hysterotomy. *Am J Obstet Gynecol*. 2015;21(5):653. doi: 10.1016/j.ajog.2015.07.019.
5. Link MS, Berkow LC, Kudenchuk PJ, et al. Part 7: Adult advanced cardiovascular life support: 2015 American Heart Association guidelines update for cardiopulmonary resuscitation and emergency cardiovascular care. *Circulation*. 2015;132(2):444–464. doi: 10.1161/CIR.0000000000000261.

# Special Procedures in Obstetric Life Support

# 7

## 7.1 INTRODUCTION

In addition to basic and advanced resuscitation CPR knowledge, OBLS requires familiarity with emerging techniques that may improve maternal survival and knowledge of when to apply modifications to the pregnant and postpartum population. This chapter details the indications for, and methods used to perform, RCD and POC-US during MCA. It also outlines the indications for ECPR during maternal resuscitation.

## 7.2 LEARNING OBJECTIVES

Learner will appropriately

- Summarize specific equipment and other resources needed to perform RCD.
- Describe appropriate timing of and criteria for RCD.
- Describe the benefits of RCD for pregnant patients in cardiac arrest.
- Describe the skills required to perform high-quality RCD.
- Describe the RCD procedure, including incision type used for different scenarios.
- Describe use of POC-US to verify pregnancy status in reproductive-age females with unknown pregnancy status.
- Describe use of POC-US to determine gestational age when indicated.
- Describe appropriate criteria for ECPR to treat MCA.

## 7.3 RESUSCITATIVE CESAREAN DELIVERY

Perimortem cesarean delivery is defined as the delivery of the fetus(es) during MCA or after maternal death. Recently, there has been a call to reconsider the nomenclature of this procedure to emphasize its resuscitative benefits. Experts have called for replacing the phrase "perimortem cesarean delivery", with a more accurate and positive term such as "resuscitative hysterotomy", or "resuscitative cesarean delivery". OBLS recommends the term **resuscitative cesarean delivery** because it accurately describes the procedure including the delivery of the fetus. Additionally, **cesarean delivery** is easily recognizable across medical teams. Although the term "hysterotomy" describes the surgical entry into the uterus, it does not include the delivery of the fetus and placenta.

Naming the procedure a RCD focuses the team to the main purpose and action of the procedure. It also may reduce communication errors during the maternal resuscitation, as the words resuscitative cesarean delivery are instantly recognizable to nonobstetric providers and staff who may be assisting in the resuscitation. Resuscitative vaginal delivery is a similarly accurate description where, in rare circumstances, expedited vaginal delivery and manual removal of the placenta can be performed more rapidly than RCD.

DOI: 10.1201/9781003299288-8

## 7.3.1 Indications for Resuscitative Cesarean Delivery

RCD is recommended for MCA when the uterus is at or above the umbilicus, regardless of fetal gestational age or fetal status, and at least one of the following criteria is met:

- No ROSC after two cycles of CPR
- Intermittent ROSC after two cycles of CPR
- Nonshockable rhythm
- For OH MCA: immediately upon arrival to the ED without ROSC

Delivery of the fetus early in MCA results in a greater than 50% probability of ROSC in the pregnant patient by improving maternal cardiac output through the reduction of aortocaval compression and the resultant autotransfusion of up to 500 milliliters of blood from the decompressed uterus.[1,2]

If the uterus is palpable at or above the umbilicus, preparations for delivery should be made with simultaneous initiation of maternal resuscitative efforts independent of fetal status. If the maternal arrest is not rapidly reversible, resuscitative delivery should be performed regardless of fetal viability or elapsed time since arrest.[2]

Experts have reported that rapid evacuation of uterine contents, even in the presence of intrauterine fetal death, will significantly improve maternal perfusion and outcomes during MCA.[2] Therefore, it is vital that the team does not focus on fetal status (such as single versus twin gestation or presence or absence of fetal cardiac activity). The decision to perform an RCD is based on the estimation of the relationship of the uterus to the umbilicus and the potential that the uterine size is causing compression of the major vessels and compromising CPR effectiveness.

Recent studies of patients with MCA found that only 11.2% presented with a shockable rhythm.[3] The high proportion of nonshockable rhythms in pregnancy highlights the need for adequate preparations for RCD during CPR with the immediate performance of RCD if the maternal cardiac rhythm is nonshockable. RCD should be performed when the uterus is at or above the umbilicus, irrespective of known gestational age or the presence of fetal cardiac activity. Timing of RCD for maternal survival, within 5 minutes of arrest (if IH) or at the time of admission to the ED, is critical to increasing maternal survival from MCA.

Though there is no upper time limit to perform an RCD, current data suggest that patients who have an RCD within 10 minutes of arrest have improved maternal and neonatal outcomes.[4] However, there are isolated case reports of survival after RCD was performed more than 10 minutes from witnessed arrest (and up to 40 minutes) that resulted in maternal survival.[4–7] As randomized trials in this area are not feasible, OBLS cannot clearly define a maximum time limit from arrest for benefit from RCD. Therefore, the team should not hesitate to perform an RCD for maternal benefit, especially in a person arriving at the hospital with an MCA, even if long periods have elapsed since the time of arrest with ongoing CPR. In this situation, OBLS recommends defining a late RCD as ≥30 minutes from the onset of maternal cardiac arrest. More information is needed to determine short- and long-term outcomes from late RCD. Currently, OBLS continues to recommend late RCD as consideration for ongoing maternal resuscitation.

---

**KEY POINTS**

- Performing an RCD relieves aortocaval compression and results in an autotransfusion of whole blood, which improves cardiac output and the chances of ROSC.
- Consider RCD for patients with MCA where the uterine fundus is at the umbilicus or higher.
- Ideally, RCD is performed within 5 minutes from arrest.

However, consider RCD as soon as feasible if CPR is ongoing and if any of the following indications are present, regardless of elapsed time:

- No ROSC after two cycles of CPR
- Intermittent ROSC after two cycles of CPR
- Nonshockable rhythm
- For out-of-hospital MCA: immediately upon arrival to the ED without ROSC

---

## 7.3.2 Preparations for Resuscitative Cesarean Delivery

Institutions that deliver obstetric care or have an ED that receives reproductive-age people should have planned and coordinated preparations for RCD **before** an MCA occurs. Institutions that deliver obstetric care should conduct simulation drills in MCA including areas where MCA is most likely to occur. These include the ED, labor and delivery (L&D), and ICUs. These drills will ensure adequate training and encourage a hospital culture of safety, so that all team members are prepared to respond when an actual event occurs.

For IH MCA, perform the RCD at the arrest location. Do not spend time transporting the patient to an operating room (OR) for an RCD. This delay in care results in decreased chances for both maternal and neonatal survival.[8] To ensure all necessary supplies and equipment are readily available at the bedside, an RCD kit should be available in all areas where MCA is likely to occur, such as the ED, L&D, and ICU. The OBLS-recommended basic RCD kit is outlined in Figure 7.1. If the arrest occurs at locations in the hospital where an RCD kit is not maintained, the MCAT and responding staff should know the location of the nearest RCD kit and bring it to the site of arrest in the hospital.

In addition to the RCD kit, an OB hemorrhage kit should also be brought to the maternal code. If ROSC is achieved following an RCD, there is a risk of postpartum hemorrhage from surgical bleeding or uterine atony. If amniotic fluid embolism (AFE) was the etiology of the MCA, there is a risk for significant bleeding from coagulopathy. Table 7.1 lists the recommended supplies for an OB hemorrhage kit. In addition to these medications, the use of TXA 1 g intravenously over 10 minutes is recommended after RCD (if acute thrombosis or pulmonary embolism is not suspected) to control bleeding from surgical sites and to assist with treatment in the acute phase of DIC.

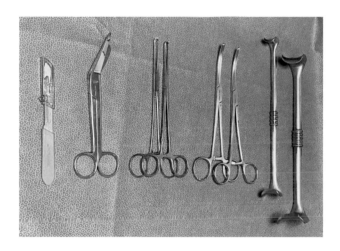

**FIGURE 7.1**   Instruments included in resuscitative cesarean delivery kit.

(From left to right → #10 blade scalpel, bandage scissors, Allis clamps, Kelly clamps, Richardson retractors.)

**TABLE 7.1**   RCD Kit: Recommended Supplies Immediately Available in All Locations Where MCA Is Likely to Occur (ED, L&D, ICU)

| SUPPLIES | EXAMPLE |
| --- | --- |
| Scalpel (#10 blade) | Disposable, #10 blade |
| Scissors | Bandage scissors, to extend incision |
| Retractors | Bladder blade, Richardson retractor |
| Clamps | Four Kelly, two Allis, umbilical cord clamp |
| Available to help close the abdomen after surgery* | |
| Forceps | One Russian forcep, one Bonnie or Ferris Smith forcep |
| Sutures, delayed absorbable | Three packs of O-polyglactin (Vicryl®) on CTX needle and 2–0 polyglactin on CT-1 needle |
| Needle driver | |
| Tamponade device | Uterine tamponade balloon |
| Laparotomy sponges | Two packs |
| Suture scissors | |

*In the event an OB/GYN or surgeon is not immediately available for closure, pack the uterus and abdomen with wet-to-dry laparotomy sponges until a more definitive closure can be performed.

**TABLE 7.2**  Obstetrics Hemorrhage Kit: Recommended Supplies

| | |
|---|---|
| Bakri balloon | Oxytocin* |
| Carboprost | Tranexamic acid |
| Methylergonovine | Urethral catheter |
| Misoprostol | Uterine banjo curette |

*Use care when administering undiluted IV oxytocin, as it can precipitate rearrest. Only use in settings where premix is available and IV infusion can be done safely, or administer intramuscularly. Refer to Table 4.3 for doses of these listed uterotonics.

**KEY POINTS**

- An RCD kit should be mobile and contain essential components such as a scalpel, bladder blade/retractor, clamps (Allis and Kelly), and umbilical cord clamps.
- An OB hemorrhage kit should accompany the RCD kit to manage bleeding that may occur after ROSC or as part of the underlying etiology of MCA such as AFE or obstetric hemorrhage.
- Perform RCD at the site of IH arrest. Do **not** transport the patient to the OR until after ROSC. For OH arrest, perform RCD upon arrival in the ED.*

*There may be some instances where an RCD-trained physician is in the field. In this specific situation, RCD may be considered in the field.

## 7.3.3 Technique for Resuscitative Cesarean Delivery

The technique for RCD is as follows:

1. Assemble supplies (ideally the RCD kit).
2. Announce, "I am going to perform a resuscitative cesarean delivery," to code team.
3. When ready, communicate with the rescuer performing LUD: "I am ready to cut, please stop LUD."
4. Rescuer stops LUD and checks back, "Stopping LUD." Rescuer backs away from the patient. Compressor continues high quality chest compressions during RCD.
5. Make a midline vertical skin incision with scalpel through the skin and subcutaneous tissue from just under the umbilicus to just above the pubic bone. (If present, follow the linea nigra, the dark vertical line that develops down the center of the abdomen during pregnancy.)
6. Use the scalpel to make an incision into the rectus fascia the same length as the skin incision.
7. Use your index fingers to hook under the rectus fascia and bluntly separate the rectus muscles pulling out laterally with both hands, simultaneously.
8. Once rectus muscles are separated, use a finger to bluntly pierce through the peritoneum and stretch it open laterally with both hands. (This may also be performed simultaneous with step 7.)
   If available, place retractor/bladder blade into abdomen to retract rectus fascia, muscles, subcutaneous tissue, and skin. If retractors are not available, use your hands. Another responder may be necessary to assist with this step, especially in the pregnant patient with obesity (Figure 7.2).
9. Make a vertical uterine incision approximately 5 cm in length with the scalpel (e.g., dotted white line in Figure 7.3). A low transverse incision may be considered by an experienced surgeon/OB as indicated.
10. Simultaneously hook your index fingers under the uterine muscle and bluntly extend the incision cephalad and caudad. A bandage scissors may be helpful with this step, especially with preterm deliveries. To use bandage scissors on the uterus, hook the fingers of the nondominant hand underneath the uterine wall in the direction you wish to cut. This protects the underlying fetus. Cut the muscle full thickness with the bandage scissors. Complete the same maneuver at the opposite aspect of the incision.
11. If the amniotic fluid sac is not ruptured, rupture using blunt (e.g., finger) or sharp (e.g., Allis clamp) dissection to enter the amniotic sac.

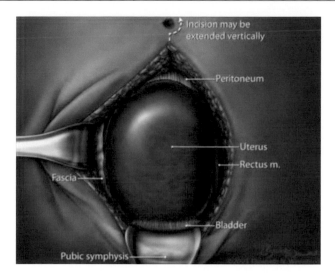

**FIGURE 7.2**   Uterine exposure with retractors (or hands) during resuscitative cesarean delivery.

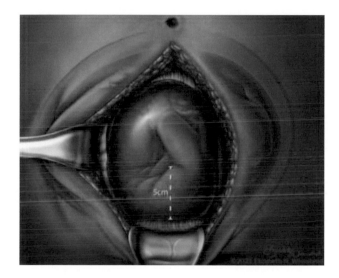

**FIGURE 7.3**   Vertical uterine incision to deliver the fetus during resuscitative cesarean delivery.

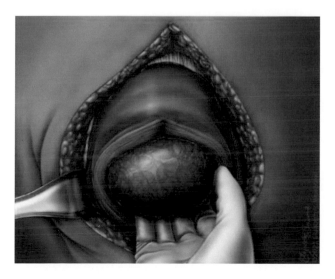

**FIGURE 7.4**   Deliver the fetus during resuscitative cesarean delivery.

12. Delivering the fetus.
    a. Fetus head down (cephalic): Insert the operator's hand into the uterine cavity and grasp the fetal head. Bring the fetal head up and out toward the uterine incision. If term or late preterm, use the nonoperating hand or an additional operator to apply fundal pressure to help deliver the head. Once the fetal head is delivered, encompass the head with both hands, and with gentle downward pressure on the head, continue fundal pressure until the anterior shoulder is delivered. Then apply gentle upward pressure to deliver the posterior shoulder. Once both shoulders are delivered, hook the fetal axilla bilaterally with your fingers to deliver the rest of the newborn (Figure 7.4).
    b. Fetus buttock down (breech): Insert the operator's hand into the uterine cavity and grasp the fetal buttock (or feet). Elevate the buttock (or feet) to the uterine incision, then apply gentle traction to the hips (or feet) to deliver the buttocks followed by the feet, then pull the fetal abdomen through the uterine incision to the level of the fetal shoulder blades (scapula). If the fetus is not in a back-up position, grab both fetal feet, and rotate them. Rotate the fetus to a side-lying position, and sweep the anterior arm across the fetal body and out. Rotate the fetus 180 degrees, and sweep the other arm. Rotate the fetus to a back-up position and hook the operator's index finger and third fingers on the fetal cheeks and flex the fetal head while applying fundal pressure to deliver the fetal head. Do not hook fingers into the fetal mouth and pull, as this may cause fetal injury.
    c. If the estimated gestational age is known to be viable (typically between 24 and 26 weeks), immediately clamp and cut the cord and hand the fetus to the awaiting neonatal team. Though delayed cord clamping is recommended at time of delivery, the lack of maternal (and consequently placental) circulation at time of RCD contraindicates this step. Therefore, when performing RCD, immediately clamp the cord when delivering the fetus.
    d. If a known nonviable gestation (typically <22–23 weeks), or the fetus has already been confirmed to be dead, deliver the fetus and placenta without stopping to clamp and cut the cord.
13. Deliver the placenta by manual extraction. Find a plane between the placenta and uterine wall and manually separate the entire placenta from the uterine wall. Once the placenta is delivered, sweep the uterine cavity to ensure no parts of membranes or placenta have been left behind.
14. Close the uterine incision.
    a. For delayed closure of the uterine incision: Pack the uterus with radiopaque laparotomy sponges tied together and clamp the uterine incision with Kelly or towel clamps. Record the number of sponges used to pack the uterus.
    b. For immediate uterine closure: Suture the uterus closed in a running, locked fashion with delayed absorbable suture (0-polyglactin or 0-poliglecaprone).
    c. The surgeon should not interfere with high-quality CPR when closing the uterus.
    d. Pack the abdomen until the patient is stable and can be taken to the OR or if exploration of the abdomen is anticipated (such as trauma or hemoperitoneum on entry). The surgeon should not interfere with high-quality CPR during abdominal closure.
15. If already in the OR, the surgeon may decide to proceed with an abdominal wall closure. This should not interfere with high-quality CPR.
16. If ROSC is achieved:
    a. Administer uterotonics as needed (see Table 7.2).
    b. Close the uterus and abdomen, if not already done.
    c. Administer antibiotics:
        i. Nonpenicillin allergic: cefazolin 2 g IV
        ii. Penicillin allergic: clindamycin 900 mg IV + gentamicin 1.5 mg/kg of actual body weight IV once available

## 7.3.4 Institutional Preparations for Resuscitative Cesarean Delivery

Every ED should be capable of performing an RCD. In general, both obstetricians and surgeons can perform this procedure. Given the variation in resources and staffing of hospitals, the healthcare community must be proactively prepared to respond to MCA. Therefore, OBLS recommends that medical professionals across all fields have a basic procedural competency in RCD. This training is especially crucial for hospitals that do not provide obstetric care or that do not have a general surgeon readily available:

1. Physicians must be credentialed and receive ongoing training in RCD.
2. Infrastructure must support the secondary consequences that may result from RCD or have the ability to transport the patient rapidly. Infrastructure includes the ability to transfuse IV antibiotics, initiate blood transfusion, secure a difficult airway, or perform the Neonatal Resuscitation Program, for example.

3. The receiving facility should be competent in managing maternal hemorrhage/DIC, including maternal ICU capability, and provide neonatal support, which may include resuscitation or palliative care.

## 7.4 OBLS IN A LOW-RESOURCE SETTING

During maternal cardiac arrest response in rural and remote locations, resource limitations may restrict providers' ability to implement the OBLS protocol. Therefore, following standard advanced life support protocols or further modifying the OBLS algorithms may become necessary in these circumstances. The following examples outline provider responses to maternal cardiac arrest in such cases:

- **Example 1.** A reproductive-age woman is in cardiac arrest. Unfortunately, ultrasound technology and a physician capable of performing an RCD are not available. In this case, responders should proceed with an advanced life support protocol until they achieve ROSC or make a determination of death.
- **Example 2.** A known pregnant patient is in cardiac arrest. Ultrasound technology is not available, but a physician credentialed to perform/capable of performing RCD is available. Here, responders must endeavor to assess the relationship of the fundus to the umbilicus. If the fundus is determined to be at or above the umbilicus, the team should consider performing an RCD. If the team cannot determine fundus location, they should default to an advanced life support protocol. Teams may choose to proceed with RCD as a final effort before making a determination of death if ROSC is not achieved.

  - 2A. Providers should continue OBLS if ECPR is indicated and not available.
  - 2B. Facilities should prioritize rapidly transporting the patient to a facility fully capable of caring for the patient. There is no standard guidance of when to stop CPR in a pregnant patient. Providers must consider multiple factors when considering when to stop CPR, including distance to the facility. Case reports of maternal cardiac arrest have demonstrated intact neurologic survival after 55 minutes of continued CPR.[7]

### KEY POINTS
- Providers trained in RCD should be familiar with the recommended skin and uterine incisions used during pregnancy and MCA. OBLS recommends a vertical midline abdominal and midline uterine incision.
- Emergency physicians and surgeons should be familiar with and trained in RCD, especially at those EDs without obstetric services.

## 7.5 POINT-OF-CARE ULTRASOUND

POC-US refers to the practice of using portable ultrasound equipment to guide diagnosis and treatment on site, whether in a hospital or in the field. POC-US is currently being incorporated into emergency protocols for the identification of

- Immediately reversible causes of cardiac arrest
- Clinical reclassification of pulseless electrical activity when there is identification of cardiac contractility activity without a palpable pulse
- Identification of the absence of cardiac contractility where further attempts at resuscitation may be futile

Despite the differences in maternal physiology from nonpregnant adults, there are multiple case reports highlighting the successful application of POC-US to assist in the management of MCA.[9–11] POC-US has been used for early diagnosis and treatment of pulmonary embolism, pneumothorax, and pericardial effusion for both IH and OH MCA. This section discusses the use of POC-US for a rapid identification of an intrauterine pregnancy and estimation of gestational age in the setting of MCA.

### 7.5.1 Point-of-Care Ultrasound for Rapid Identification of Pregnancy during Cardiac Arrest in Reproductive-Age Females

POC-US is a highly effective tool used to diagnose and guide treatment. It can be used to rapidly identify an intrauterine pregnancy, which then guides resuscitation management.[10–13]

The ease of use of POC-US at the site of MCA makes it an especially valuable tool in settings with limited diagnostic imaging capabilities, such as out-of-hospital and in limited-resource settings, where identification of pregnancy would otherwise be impossible. POC-US has the potential to improve MCA diagnosis and management. Knowing the patient is pregnant informs transportation to the most appropriate care location and mobilizes resources to perform RCD and ECPR (covered later in this chapter), potentially reducing significant care delays.

Currently, extended Focused Assessment of Sonography for Trauma (eFAST) protocols used in the setting of trauma do not incorporate an examination of the abdominopelvic area to detect pregnancy in reproductive-age people. However, at least one case demonstrated a timely diagnosis of intrauterine pregnancy during an eFAST exam in a reproductive-age female with gunshot wounds to the chest.[12] OBLS advocates incorporating a POC-US of the abdominopelvic area into eFAST protocols to evaluate reproductive-age people transported with trauma to allow for rapid identification of pregnancy (see Chapter 8).

### 7.5.2 Point-of-Care Ultrasound for Estimation of Gestational Age during Maternal Cardiac Arrest

There are specific circumstances where an estimation of gestational age by palpating the uterus in relation to the umbilicus is not possible, such as extreme obesity. In this situation, it may be necessary to use POC-US to quickly determine gestational age. FL and BPD measurements are the most accurate and easily reproducible.[14,16–19] Providers not familiar with this ultrasound technique should undergo limited, goal-directed ultrasound training to effectively perform quick and targeted POC-US to determine gestational age.[14]

POC-US can be performed anytime during CPR or pulse checks and should **not** interfere with CPR or prolong pauses in CPR. Pulse checks should continue to be less than 10 seconds.

POC-US requires, at minimum, a handheld ultrasound device and lubricant. To perform the ultrasound, place the wand below the patient's umbilicus and scan the abdomen and pelvis for the presence or absence of pregnancy. If pregnancy is found, a qualified provider can measure either a BPD of the fetal head and/or a femur length (Figures 7.5 and 7.6).

To measure a BPD, freeze the image of the widest part of the fetal head in the transaxial plane. An ideal plane includes the following landmarks: cavum septum pellucidum, thalamus, and choroid plexus (see Figure 7.5). Then, measure the BPD by placing the first caliper on the outer table of the skull and the second caliper on the inner table of the skull. On average, a BPD of 48 mm, or 4.8 cm, corresponds with 20 weeks gestation. OBLS recommends applying LUD on a pregnant patient with BPD of 45 mm to allow for a margin of error.

To obtain a FL, first identify the thigh and then measure the femur bone from blunt end to blunt end parallel to the shaft of the femur (see Figure 7.6). An average femur length at 20 weeks is 32 mm, or 3.2 cm. OBLS recommends applying LUD for a FL of 30 mm to account for a possible margin of error. For further correlation of ultrasound measurements and gestational age, refer to Figures 7.7 and 7.8, which show the average BPD and FL measurements throughout pregnancy, respectively.

A provider can acquire either FL or BPD (whichever is easiest) but does not need to do both.[17–19] Many portable ultrasound machines will have an obstetrical calculation mode that will provide an immediate estimation of gestational age based on individual biometric parameters, such as BPD and FL. In addition to LUD, OBLS recommends using a BPD ≥45 mm and FL ≥30 mm as measurements that correspond to a fundus at or above the umbilicus and performance of RCD in the setting of MCA.

POC-US should **not** interfere with high-quality CPR, postpone the start of chest compressions, or prolong pauses for pulse check.[8,20] Additionally, POC-US should not divert focus from maternal to fetal status (such as fixation on the presence or absence of fetal cardiac activity) or delay RCD. Additionally, POC-US for calculation of gestational age should not be performed if pregnancy status is confirmed, and the uterine fundus is palpable at or above the umbilicus.

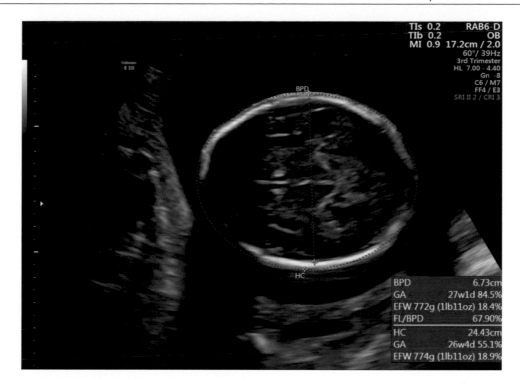

**FIGURE 7.5**   Ultrasound measurements of biparietal diameter.

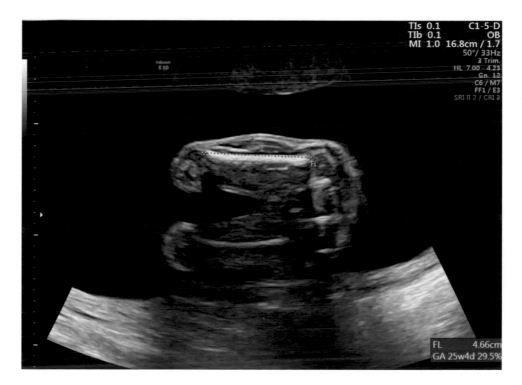

**FIGURE 7.6**   Ultrasound measurements of femur length.

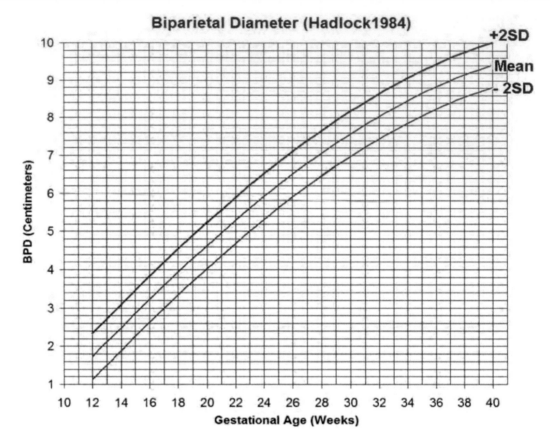

**FIGURE 7.7**    Average biparietal diameter by gestational age (weeks).

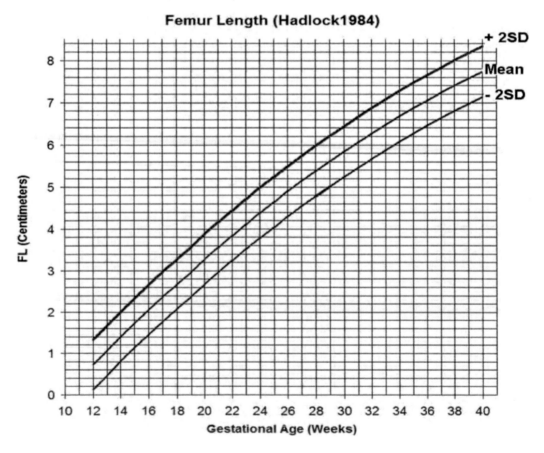

**FIGURE 7.8**    Average femur length (FL) measurements by gestational age (weeks).

# 7.6 OBESITY AND MATERNAL CARDIAC ARREST

Obesity is now an increasingly common and harmful pregnancy complication. According to the Centers for Disease Control and Prevention, 26% of pregnancies in the United States are impacted by obesity (defined as body mass index ≥30).[21] Therefore, further modifications to optimize effectiveness of CPR techniques must be considered in this population. Table 7.3 outlines the potential impact that obesity can have on CPR and the considerations that can be made for this patient population.

**TABLE 7.3**  Special Considerations for Patients with Morbid Obesity in Maternal Cardiac Arrest

|  | *POTENTIAL IMPACT ON CPR* | *RECOMMENDATIONS* |
|---|---|---|
| Airway management | More likely to encounter class 3 or 4 airway, especially in the latter half of pregnancy | Continue with bag-mask ventilation or supraglottic airway if sufficient, and allow most experienced laryngoscopist to attempt intubation |
| Breast tissue | May be more pendulous | Place left defibrillator pad underneath left breast tissue, or place pads anterior-posterior |
| Chest compressions | Chest compression depth: Compressor may tire more easily due to strength required to compress | Consider changing compressors after each minute |
| LUD | Person applying LUD may tire more easily due to amount of tissue they are displacing | Consider changing person performing LUD more frequently |
| Identification of pregnancy status and estimation of gestational age | If pregnancy status is unknown, it may be more difficult to identify by either assessment of uterine fundus or with ultrasound | Requires experienced personnel with ultrasound experience to identify or estimate gestational age<br>If resources allow, consider application of LUD until determination of pregnancy status can be made |
| RCD | A large overhanging pannus may make it difficult to make a low vertical incision from the umbilicus to just above the pubis symphysis | Recommend a high vertical incision above the umbilicus<br>Do not attempt to retract a large overlying pannus during CPR. This may interfere with chest compressions and result in maternal hypotension and respiratory compromise with ROSC. |

**KEY POINTS**
- Expand POC-US and eFAST exams to include examination of the abdomen and pelvis of reproductive-age females in the setting of unknown pregnancy status.
- Use POC-US when it is not feasible to determine gestational age by palpating the fundus, such as with some obese patients.
- If the uterine fundus cannot be confidently palpated in relation to the umbilicus during MCA response, use rapid bedside ultrasound to determine gestational age. RCD is recommended if a fetal femur length ≥30 mm or biparietal diameter ≥45 mm. Either measurement corresponds to a gestational age of ≥20 weeks or greater, and RCD should be performed.
- POC-US should **not** interrupt quality CPR or prolong brief pauses for pulse checks.
- POC-US should **not** be used to focus on the presence or absence of fetal cardiac activity.
- When available and with trained professionals, consider POC-US to evaluate for possible etiologies of and guide treatment during MCA.

# 7.7 EXTRACORPOREAL CARDIOPULMONARY RESUSCITATION

Despite high-quality CPR and prompt RCD, not all will achieve sustained ROSC. In these cases, ECPR is a potential additional beneficial intervention. ECPR is a method of CPR that passes the patient's blood through a machine to oxygenate the blood supply. A portable ECMO device is used to accompany standard CPR. ECPR is also known as emergency peripheral cardiopulmonary bypass or extracorporeal life support.[22]

ECPR has been used for many etiologies of MCA, including amniotic fluid embolism,[23,24] postpartum hemorrhage,[25] severe cardiomyopathy or cardiac disease,[26,27] sepsis,[28] and massive pulmonary embolism[29–33] in which CPR failed to result in sustained ROSC. When ECPR has been applied in the setting of MCA without ROSC, survival rates to discharge have been reported in as high as 77% for mothers and 67% for fetuses.[30] These rates compare favorably to the overall maternal survival rate to discharge of 40.7%.[3] As of 2020, there were 57 cases of ECPR used in MCA, with 50 survivors (87.7%).[34]

Although ECPR has been described at different gestational ages, it is generally applied after RCD in the second half of pregnancy. One case report of ECPR resulted in ROSC and survival with ongoing pregnancy in a patient at 10 weeks gestation following massive pulmonary embolism.[31]

The average time to application of ECPR for MCA varies, ranging between 18 and 100 minutes.[23,25,30] A recent case review of ECPR for MCA in five pregnant patients demonstrated a mean time to ECPR for MCA of 18 minutes, with the majority of patients receiving veno-arterial ECMO. Mean duration of circuit run was 32 hours with left ventricular function improving >10% within 3 days. Four of these five patients survived to discharge without neurologic sequelae. The authors noted that two of three patients who received ECPR for postpartum hemorrhage developed a hemorrhagic coagulopathy, a known complication of this procedure. The authors were uncertain if this was a complication of ECPR or a natural consequence of severe postpartum hemorrhage.[29]

Case reports have also highlighted the benefit of ECPR even after prolonged CPR efforts. One case of MCA described initiation of ECPR at 100 minutes after the start of CPR. The patient was discharged home on postoperative day 9 with normal cognitive function, with residual deficits of a persistent right foot drop and right flexion contracture of the upper limb post fasciotomy.[35] Another case report described a pregnant patient being transported to an ECMO-capable facility during CPR, with ECPR initiated upon arrival after 150 minutes, with a full cognitive recovery with residual deficits of mild right-hand motor weakness.[23] While ECPR appears very promising in the MCA population, there are limited data on the optimal techniques for applying ECPR during an MCA response.

The optimal perfusion strategy (site of cannulation, flow rate, and size or length of tubing) is uncertain. There is at least one case of survival following MCA with pediatric tubing used to initiate ECPR prior to transport to a hospital capable of continuing ECPR in an adult. The ideal site of ECPR cannulation during MCA is not known; some advocate for femoral artery cannulation to allow for ongoing CPR.[23] Additionally, the decision to use anticoagulation in prior case reports is highly variable; some patients received no anticoagulation while others received therapeutic anticoagulation. Experts suggest that the use of anticoagulation should be individualized in ECPR. In the setting of MCA, responders must also weigh the risk of thrombosis from the prothrombotic state of pregnancy and other prothrombotic conditions (e.g., autoimmune diseases, sepsis, etc.) against the risks of worsening bleeding, postpartum hemorrhage, bleeding from AFE, or a hemorrhagic cerebrovascular accident.[31] If anticoagulation is initiated as part of ECPR, protocols for monitoring of coagulation status are available.[31]

## 7.7.1 Criteria for Notification to Perform Extracorporeal Cardiopulmonary Resuscitation

Though there are no set criteria to recommend ECPR during MCA, OBLS advocates that when resources are available, any pregnant or postpartum person in cardiac arrest who is not responding to high-quality CPR or has undergone an RCD without ROSC should be considered a candidate for ECPR. Consider incorporating the ECPR team as part of the MCAT, if available at the institution. This ensures that the ECPR team is notified of the MCA as soon as possible and can begin preparations and increase availability to cannulate in the event of refractory CPR. If an ECPR team is not available, consider transporting the patient to an ECMO-capable facility. If not available, the code team must decide how long to continue resuscitation efforts in the setting of MCA refractory to CPR. The decision to discontinue CPR during an MCA is discussed in more detail in Chapter 11, in Section 11.14.

There are limited data to suggest that patients may be able to survive, with minimal neurologic injury, while undergoing high-quality CPR followed by initiation of ECPR as long as 100 minutes from the time of MCA.[32] In the setting of refractory MCA, the team should consider clinical factors, including the etiology of the MCA, time from arrest, $ETCO_2$, and underlying comorbidities, to decide if ECPR is reasonable. The team should promptly notify the ECPR team.

**KEY POINTS**

- ECPR is an emerging technique that has shown promise in pregnant and postpartum patients in cardiac arrest.
- The criteria for ECPR in MCA include refractory CPR (those without sustained ROSC after RCD).
- Determine the use of anticoagulation during ECPR on an individual basis and in consultation with the ECPR team.

## 7.7.2 Circulatory Determination of Death and Procurement of Organs during Extracorporeal Cardiopulmonary Resuscitation

If a pregnant person is not successfully resuscitated, ECPR has been used for the procurement of organs in circulatory determination of death.[36] While these data are currently limited to nonpregnant adults, the population of adults with MCA and refractory CPR are generally younger and in better health than the nonpregnant cardiac arrest population, making them ideal candidates for organ procurement. Moreover, organ donation may reduce feelings of sorrow related to death and provide comfort to families.[36,37]

Registry reporting and continued reevaluation of observational trials and case reports will play important roles in directing future applications of ECPR for MCA refractory to CPR and in refining the use of ECPR in this population. OBLS recommends verifying state regulations regarding organ and pregnancy status, as this may differ between states.

**KEY POINTS**

- ECPR has been shown to be effective for the procurement of organs in circulatory determination of death.
- People with refractory maternal cardiac arrest and circulatory determination of death are ideal candidates for organ procurement.
- Organ donation may reduce feelings of sorrow from the loss of a loved one and provide comfort to families.

# 7.8 TRANSPORT AND EMERGENCY MEDICAL STAFF PROVIDERS

EMS providers can apply OBLS techniques in Basic Life Support, Advanced Life Support, or Advanced Cardiac Life Support until the point of RCD. They can further improve outcomes by applying POC-US techniques, as described earlier in this chapter. While EMS providers are not expected to perform an RCD, they can improve the likelihood of successful RCD by performing high-quality CPR, airway management, manual LUD, and transporting the patient to the appropriate facility as quickly as possible. Appropriate facilities include those resourced with OB/GYN, general surgeons, or emergency medicine physicians who can perform RCD, neonatologists and/or pediatricians, and an ECPR team.

Current practice for many EMS teams is to "stay and play" for cardiac arrests, limiting hands-off time and improving CPR administration.[38] However, EMS teams are taught to quickly transport patients with suspected stroke, acute myocardial infarction, and trauma to the hospital to avail them of life-saving interventions. To remember which situations trigger rapid transport, EMS teams are taught the mnemonic "Stroke, STEMI, Trauma." MCA should also be a criterion for rapid transport to a hospital as an RCD may be a life-saving intervention in this situation. Therefore, OBLS recommends updating the mnemonic to "Stroke, STEMI, **Mama**, Trauma." EMS providers must inform the receiving hospital about the pregnancy status of the patient, so the MCAT can assemble and be prepared with the proper equipment in the ED. Ideally, transport time to the most appropriate facility is under 10 minutes.

### Case Vignette

A 40-year-old patient presents to the ED with severe chest pain and nausea. Before elaborating on prenatal care or gestational age, the patient becomes unresponsive. The ED team calls a code and activates the MCAT. They initiate high-quality CPR and determine the cardiac rhythm is ventricular fibrillation. The ED physician palpates for the uterine fundus but is unable to feel the fundus due to the body habitus.

The physician calls for an ultrasound machine, RCD kit, and a defibrillator. POC-US shows a BPD of 55 mm. The team applies automated external defibrillator pads and immediately defibrillates. They start LUD and debrief the just-arrived MCAT, who perform an RCD after two cycles of CPR. The neonate is handed to the neonatologist. ROSC is intermittently achieved following RCD, and the ECPR team is called to evaluate the patient.

## REVIEW QUESTIONS

**Q.** What are the possible etiologies of the patient's cardiac arrest?

**A.** Following BAACC TO LIFE™, the most common causes would include cardiovascular (such as acute myocardial infarction or cardiomyopathy), massive pulmonary embolism (or clot), or less common causes of chest pain such as cardiac tamponade (for instance, secondary to dissecting/ruptured aortic aneurysm, or trauma).

**Q.** What are the important modifications to CPR during a maternal cardiac arrest?

**A.** The important modifications to CPR during a maternal cardiac arrest are performing continuous LUD, activating the MCAT, and preparing for and performing RCD. These are in addition to ongoing, high-quality chest compressions. Additionally, use BAACC TO LIFE to consider the etiologies unique to pregnancy. These are important to guide treatment options and modalities.

# CHAPTER 7. PRACTICE QUESTIONS

1. A 25-year-old patient at 36 weeks gestation with a history of factor V Leiden deficiency has undergone an RCD due to respiratory collapse from suspected pulmonary embolism. Despite RCD and continued high-quality OBLS for 40 minutes, ROSC has not been achieved. What is your BEST next step in management?
   A. Perform POC-US to evaluate for pulmonary embolism
   B. Initiate ECPR for refractory cardiac arrest
   C. Continue high-quality OBLS
   D. Initiate ECPR for organ procurement

2. If an ultrasound must be performed to date a pregnancy, which fetal measurements will give the BEST estimation of gestational age?
   A. Femur length and biparietal diameter
   B. Abdominal circumference and femur length
   C. Humeral length and biparietal diameter
   D. Head circumference and biparietal diameter

3. A patient is experiencing cardiac arrest. An eFAST exam confirms twin pregnancy and at the first pulse check ultrasound dating corresponds with a 16-week gestation. Fundus is palpated at the umbilicus. What is the BEST next step in management?
   A. Administer shock if rhythm check demonstrates asystole
   B. Continue with Advanced Cardiac Life Support algorithm as you would with nonpregnant adult
   C. Perform left uterine displacement
   D. Perform RCD

4. A pregnant person at 17 weeks gestation with a twin pregnancy arrives at the ED in cardiac arrest. When performing the primary survey, the ED provider palpates the fundus at 2 cm above the umbilicus. The patient does not have ROSC after 4 minutes of high-quality CPR and two shocks for ventricular fibrillation. What is the BEST next step in management?
   A. Perform RCD
   B. Activate the massive transfusion protocol
   C. Perform POC-US to recheck gestational age
   D. Request a stat OB consult to confirm gestational age

5. The RCD kit has been brought to the emergency room. What are the BEST suggested components?
   A. Scalpel, clamps, suture
   B. Scalpel, urinary catheter, suture
   C. Clamps, scissors, electrocautery
   D. Scalpel, clamps, urinary catheter

# CHAPTER 7. ANSWERS

1. **ANSWER: B.** OBLS advocates that any pregnant or postpartum person in cardiac arrest who is not responding to high-quality CPR or has undergone an RCD without ROSC should be considered a candidate for ECPR. Imaging for pulmonary embolism with POC-US should not delay initiation of ECPR and, therefore, is not the best answer. Case reports show patients undergoing ECPR even after >30 minutes of CPR for MCA have a high rate of improvement and discharge to home. As such, considering ECPR for organ procurement is not indicated.

2. **ANSWER: A.** There are specific circumstances where an estimation of gestational age by palpating the uterus in relation to the umbilicus is not possible, such as extreme obesity. In this situation, it may be necessary to use POC-US for a quick determination of gestational age. The **use of FL and BPD measurements are the most accurate and reproducible**. A FL of 30 mm or greater or a BPD of 45 mm or greater corresponds to a gestational age of ≥20 weeks. Perform OBLS with LUD. RCD should be performed after two cycles of high-quality CPR.

3. **ANSWER: C.** If the uterine fundus cannot be confidently palpated in relation to the umbilicus during MCA response, determination of gestational age can be performed by rapid bedside ultrasound. Following, the OBLS algorithm is recommended if the fetal FL ≥30 mm **or** BPD ≥45 mm, as either corresponds to a gestational age of ≥20 weeks and approximates the uterine fundus being at or above the umbilicus. If the uterine fundus can be palpated at or above the umbilicus in a twin pregnancy or higher multiple order pregnancy, then the patient is a candidate for RCD regardless of gestational age <20 weeks.

4. **ANSWER: A.** RCD is recommended for all MCA where the uterus is at or above the umbilicus, regardless of fetal gestational age or fetal status, and when one of the following criteria is met: (1) no ROSC after two cycles of CPR; (2) intermittent ROSC after two cycles of CPR; (3) nonshockable rhythm; or (4) for OH MCA: immediately upon arrival to the ED without ROSC.

5. **ANSWER: A.** An RCD kit should be available in all areas where MCA is likely to occur, such as in the ED, L&D, and ICU. The most basic RCD kit consists of a scalpel, bladder blade/retractor, clamps (Allis and Kelly), and umbilical cord clamps. Other surgical supplies to bring to site of MCA include sutures, forceps, needle driver, uterine tamponade device, laparotomy sponges, and suture scissors, which are needed to control bleeding and when closing the uterus and maternal abdomen. Following RCD and ROSC, these patients may also be packed and moved to the OR to complete the surgery.

# CHAPTER 7. REFERENCES

1. Katz V, Balderston K, DeFreest M. Perimortem cesarean delivery: Were our assumptions correct? *AJOG*. 2005;19(6):1916–1920; 1920–1921. doi: 10.1016/j.ajog.2005.02.038.
2. Einav S, Kaufmana N, Sela HY. Maternal cardiac arrest and perimortem caesarean delivery: Evidence or expert-based? *Resuscitation*. 2012. doi: 10.1016/j.resuscitation.2012.05.005.
3. Rose C, Faksh A, Traynor K, Cabrera D, Arendt K, Brost B. Challenging the 4- to 5-minute rule: From perimortem cesarean to resuscitative hysterotomy. *Am J Obstet Gynecol*. 2015;21(5):653. doi: 10.1016/j.ajog.2015.07.019.
4. Zelop CM, Einav S, Mhyre JM, Lipman SS, et al. Characteristics and outcomes of maternal cardiac arrest: A descriptive analysis of get with the guidelines data. *Resuscitation*. 2018;132(212):17–20. doi: 10.1016/j.resuscitation.2018.08.029.
5. Pecher S, Williams E. Out-of-hospital cardiac arrest in pregnancy with good neurological outcome for mother and infant. *Int J Obstet Anesth*. 2017;29:81–84. doi: 10.1016/j.ijoa.2016.11.002.
6. Kazandi M, Mgoyi L, Gundem G, Hacivelioglu S, Yücebilgin S, Ozkinay E. Post-mortem caesarean section performed 30 minutes after maternal cardiopulmonary arrest. *Aust N Z J Obstet Gynaecol*. 2004;44. doi: 10.1111/j.1479-828X.2004.00215.x.
7. Anast N, Kwok J, Carvalho B, Lipman S, Flood P. Intact survival after obstetric hemorrhage and 55 minutes of cardiopulmonary resuscitation. *A & A Case Rep*. 2015 July 1;5:9–12. doi: 10.1213/XAA.0000000000000163.
8. Jeejeebhoy FM, Morrison L. Maternal cardiac arrest: A practical and comprehensive review. *Emerg Med Int*. 2013. doi: 10.1155/2013/274814.
9. Venkataramani R, Im M, Rao S. Breathless to pulseless: A classic use of bedside ultrasonography to the rescue. *Crit Care Med*. 2016;44(2):491. doi: 10.1097/01.ccm.0000510336.34856.a0.
10. Brun PM, Chenaitia H, Dejesus I, Bessereau J, Bonello L, Pierre B. Ultrasound to perimortem caesarean delivery in prehospital settings. *Injury*. 2013;44(1). doi: 10.1016/j.injury.2012.08.029.
11. Byhahn C, Tobias M, Bingolda TM, Zwissler B, Maier M, Walcher F. Prehospital ultrasound detects pericardial tamponade in a pregnant victim of stabbing assault. *Resuscitation*. 2008;76(1):146–148. doi: 10.1016/j.resuscitation.2007.07.020.
12. de Assis V, Shields AD, Johansson A, Shumbusho DI, York BM. Resuscitation of traumatic maternal cardiac arrest: A case report and summary of recommendations from Obstetric Life Support™. *Trauma Case Rep*. 2023;44:100800. doi: 10.1016/j.tcr.2023.100800. PMID: 36895863; PMCID: PMC9988540.

13. MacArthur B, Foley M, Gray K, Sisley A. Trauma in pregnancy: A comprehensive approach to the mother and fetus. *AJOG*. 2019;22(5). doi: 10.1016/j.ajog.2019.01.209.

14. Shah S, Teismann N, Zaia B, Vahidnia F, River G, Price D, Nagdev A. Accuracy of emergency physicians using ultrasound to determine gestational age in pregnant women. *Am J Emerg Med*. 2010;28.7:834–838. doi: 10.1016/j. ajem.2009.07.024.

15. Snijders R, Nicolaides K. Fetal biometry at 14 weeks gestation. *Ultrasound Obstet Gynecol*. 1994;4(1):34–48. doi: 10.1046/j.1469-0705.1994.04010034.x.

16. MacGregor SN, Sabbagha RE. Assessment of gestational age by ultrasound. *Glob Libr Women's Med*. 2008. doi: 10.3843/GLOWM.10206.

17. Hadlock FP, Deter RL, Harrist RB, Park SK. Estimating fetal age: Computer-assisted analysis of multiple fetal growth parameters. *Radiology*. 1984;15(2):497–501. doi: 10.1148/radiology.152.2.6739822.

18. Loughna P, Chitty L, Evans T, Chudleigh T. Fetal size and dating: Charts recommended for clinical obstetric practice. *Ultrasound*. 2009;17(3):161–167.

19. Schwarzler P, Bland JM, Holden D, Campbell S, Ville Y. Sex-specific antenatal reference growth charts for uncomplicated singleton pregnancies at 15–40 weeks of gestation. *Ultrasound Obstet Gynecol*. 2004;23:23–29. doi: 10.1002/uog.966.

20. Hernandez C, Shuler K, Hannan H, Sonyika C, Likourezos A, Marshall J. C.A.U.S.E.: Cardiac arrest ultrasound exam—A better approach to managing patients in primary non-arrhythmogenic cardiac arrest. *Resuscitation*. 2008;76(2). doi: 10.1016/j.resuscitation.2007.06.033.

21. Deputy NP, Dub B, Sharma AJ. Prevalence and trends in prepregnancy normal weight—48 states, New York City, and District of Columbia, 2011–2015. *MMWR Morb Mortal Wkly Rep*. 2018 June 1;66:2020.

22. Neumar RW, Shuster M, Callaway CW, et al. 2015 American Health Association guidelines update for cardiopulmonary resuscitation and emergency cardiovascular care. *Circulation*. 2015;132:S315–S367. doi: 10.1161/CIR.0000000000000252.

23. Fang Z, Van Diepen S, Royal Alexandra Hospital and University of Alberta Hospital Cardiac Arrest Teams. Successful inter-hospital transfer for extracorporeal membrane oxygenation after an amniotic fluid embolism induced cardiac arrest. *Can J Anaesth*. 2016. doi: 10.1007/s12630-015-0548-z.

24. Seong GM, Kim SW, Kang HS, Kang HW. Successful extracorporeal cardiopulmonary resuscitation in a postpartum patient with amniotic fluid embolism. *Thorac Dis*. 2018. doi: 10.21037/jtd.2018.03.06.

25. Huang KY, Li YP, Lin SY, Shih JC, Chen YS, Lee CN. Extracorporeal membrane oxygenation application in post-partum hemorrhage patients: Is post-partum hemorrhage contraindicated? *J Obstet Gynecol Res*. 2017. doi: 10.1111/jog.13426.

26. Kim HY, Jeon HJ, Yun JH, Lee JH, Lee GG, Woo SC. Anesthetic experience using extracorporeal membrane oxygenation for cesarean section in the patient with peripartum cardiomyopathy—A case report. *Korean J Anesthesiol*. 2014;66(5):392–397. doi: 10.4097/kjae.2014.66.5.392.

27. van Zwet CJ, Rist A, Haeussler A, Graves K, Zollinger A, Blumenthal S. Extracorporeal membrane oxygenation for treatment of acute inverted Takotsubo-like cardiomyopathy from hemorrhagic pheochromocytoma in late pregnancy. *A & A Case Rep*. 2016;7(9):196–199. doi: 10.1213/XAA.0000000000000383.

28. Imaeda T, Nakada T, Abe R, Tateishi Y, Oda S. Veno-arterial extracorporeal membrane oxygenation for *Streptococcus pyogenes* toxic shock syndrome in pregnancy. *J Artif Organs*. 2016;19:200. doi: 10.1007/s10047-015-0884-3.

29. Fernandes P, Allen P, Valdis M, Guo L. Successful use of extracorporeal membrane oxygenation for pulmonary embolism, prolonged cardiac arrest, post-partum: A cannulation dilemma. *Perfusion*. 2015;30(2). doi: 10.1177/0267659114555818.30.

30. McDonald C, Laurie J, Janssens S, Zazulak C, Kotze P, Shekar K. Successful provision of inter-hospital extracorporeal cardiopulmonary resuscitation for acute post-partum pulmonary embolism. *Int J Obstet Anesth*. 2017;30:65–68. doi: 10.1016/j. ijoa.2017.01.003.

31. Takacs ME, Damisch KE. Extracorporeal life support as salvage therapy for massive pulmonary embolus and cardiac arrest in pregnancy. *J Emerg Med*. 2018;55(1):121–124. doi: 10.1016/j.jemermed.2018.04.009.

32. Marty T, Hilton L, Spear K, Greyson K. Postcesarean pulmonary embolism, sustained cardiopulmonary resuscitation, embolectomy, and near-death experience. *Obstet Gynecol*. 2005. doi: 10.1097/01.AOG.0000164054.53501.96.

33. Bataillard A, Hebrard A, Gaide-Chevronnay L, Casez M, Dessertaine G, Durand M, Chavanon O, Albaladejo P. Extracorporeal life support for massive pulmonary embolism during pregnancy. *Perfusion*. 2016;31(2):169–171. doi: 10.1177/0267659115586578.

34. Naoum EE, Chalupka A, Haft J, MacEachern M, Vandeven CJM, Easter SR, Maile M, Bateman BT, Bauer ME. Extracorporeal life support in pregnancy: A systematic review. *J Am Heart Assoc*. 2020;9(13):e016072. doi: 10.1161/JAHA.119.016072. Epub 2020 Jun 24. PMID: 32578471; PMCID: PMC7670512.

35. Moore SA, Dietl CA, Coleman DM. Extracorporeal life support during pregnancy. *J Thorac Cardiovasc Surg*. 2016;15(4):1154. doi: 10.1016/j.jtcvs.2015.12.027.

36. Rojas-Pena A, Sall L, Gravel M, et al. Donation after circulatory determination of death: The University of Michigan experience with extracorporeal support. *Transplantation*. 2014;98(3):328–334. doi: 10.1097/TP.0000000000000070.

37. Tavakoli AH, Rasoulian M, Ghadrigolestani M. The comparison of depression and consent in families of brain dead patients in donor and non-donor groups. *Iran J Psychol Clin*. 2006;11:4138.

38. ACOG Committee Opinion No. 736. Optimizing postpartum care. American College of Obstetricians and Gynecologists. *Obstet Gynecol*. 2018;131:140–150.

# Traumatic Maternal Cardiac Arrest

# 8

## 8.1 INTRODUCTION

Trauma in pregnancy is the leading cause of nonobstetric or indirect maternal mortality and affects approximately 7% of all pregnancies. Intimate partner violence and motor vehicle crashes are the most common traumatic injuries. Because trauma has been cited as a leading cause of MCA, it is likely that both OH and in-hospital personnel will encounter trauma-related cardiac arrest in pregnant and postpartum patients.

Traumatic MCA requires coordination of multidisciplinary teams to optimize maternal and neonatal outcomes. It is critical to promptly identify pregnancy, estimate gestational age, and modify CPR. Any delays can be detrimental to maternal and neonatal outcomes.

This chapter discusses the approach to caring for a patient with traumatic MCA and outlines the diagnostic approach for all reproductive-age people (generally defined as 12–51 years of age) with traumatic cardiac arrest, focusing on the care of pregnant and postpartum people.

## 8.2 LEARNING OBJECTIVES

Learner will appropriately

- Review components of traumatic cardiac arrest algorithm for pregnancy.
- Describe the eFAST exam applied to reproductive-age females who experience traumatic cardiac arrest.
- Summarize the common obstetric morbidities associated with traumatic MCA.
- Describe the importance of incision type for a resuscitative cesarean delivery procedure in pregnant people who experience traumatic cardiac arrest.

## 8.3 TRAUMATIC CARDIAC ARREST REVIEW

Traumatic cardiac arrest is defined as cardiac arrest due to blunt or penetrating trauma. Identifying and treating reversible causes of traumatic cardiac arrest is key to survival (Table 8.1). Most traumatic cardiac arrest is due to hypovolemia leading to pulseless electrical activity.[1] As such, blood product replacement is critical for survival in the vast majority of cases of traumatic MCA.

Current courses on traumatic life support teach providers to assess for pregnancy status during the secondary survey but do not provide instructions on how to do this. In the case of MCA, maternal and neonatal survival are more likely when providers quickly recognize pregnancy (especially when the fundus is at or above the umbilicus) and apply LUD and RCD. Most current trauma algorithms focus on fetal status and outcome; however, during MCA it is vital to maintain maternal focus and implement crucial lifesaving modifications to CPR even if the fetus is nonviable or has died.

Traumatic MCA can result from placental abruption or uterine rupture with resultant concealed internal bleeding, with the loss of ≥1,500 mL of blood before hemodynamic changes are evident in pregnancy. The ability to compensate for significant hemorrhage is due to an increased maternal circulating volume that may hinder the early recognition of shock.

DOI: 10.1201/9781003299288-9

**TABLE 8.1**    Reversible Causes of Traumatic Maternal Cardiac Arrest

| CAUSE | TREATMENT | INTERVENTION |
| --- | --- | --- |
| Hypoxia | Oxygenate | Give high-flow oxygen |
| Tension pneumothorax | Decompress chest | Perform thoracostomy |
| Cardiac tamponade | Decompress tamponade | Perform pericardiocentesis |
| Hypovolemia* | Rapid infusion of blood and blood products; damage control resuscitation (including damage control surgery) | Large-bore IV access (central or peripheral) and transfusion of blood/blood products via a rapid infusion device |

* Common cause of traumatic cardiac arrest.

Providers must be aware of the potential for sudden maternal decompensation with hemorrhage from trauma that may result in hypovolemic shock and MCA. Rapid treatment of hypovolemic shock with massive transfusion, RCD, and operative laparotomy may be lifesaving in these scenarios.

# 8.4  APPROACH TO REPRODUCTIVE-AGE FEMALES WITH CARDIAC ARREST IN ASSOCIATION WITH TRAUMA

Current traumatic life support protocols for pregnancy are available and based on the assumption that EMS providers are already aware of the person's pregnancy status. However, as most traumatic MCA occurs OH, pregnancy status is likely unknown. EMS providers must have the skills to identify the pregnancy and modify resuscitative efforts accordingly.

Figure 8.1 outlines the OBLS-recommended approach to reproductive-age people in cardiac arrest due to trauma, the Traumatic Maternal Cardiac Arrest (T-MCA) algorithm. Providers who care for people of reproductive age who present with traumatic cardiac arrest should consider the possibility of pregnancy. If pregnancy is suspected, EMS providers can palpate the uterus and assess its relationship to the umbilicus. If the uterus is at or above the umbilicus, LUD should be immediately applied. Currently, most EMS units in the United States do not have handheld ultrasound equipment available and are not required to train in this skill. However, POC-US training is straightforward and could lead to earlier identification of a pregnancy in a reproductive-age person in cardiac arrest. In the field, knowledge of a pregnancy would allow the EMS team to transport the patient to the most appropriate location for continued care. Early estimation of gestational age (either by uterine fundal assessment or POC-US) could result in lifesaving modifications to CPR and allow for early mobilization of resources to perform an RCD, extracorporeal cardiopulmonary resuscitation, and potentially reduce significant delays of care and optimizing maternal outcomes.

**KEY POINTS**
- In the setting of trauma in pregnancy, it is most important to stabilize and resuscitate the patient.
- Hypovolemia is a likely cause of traumatic MCA.
- PEA is the most likely presenting rhythm in a traumatic MCA.
- Evaluating reproductive-age people (between 12 and 51 years of age) for pregnancy in the setting of traumatic cardiac arrest is critical to the success of resuscitative efforts.

Advanced traumatic life support (ATLS®) protocols are initiated when a reproductive-age female with traumatic cardiac arrest arrives to the emergency room. Currently, eFAST protocols used in the setting of trauma do not incorporate an examination of the abdominopelvic area to detect pregnancy in reproductive-age people. OBLS advocates that eFAST protocols begin to incorporate an examination of the female abdomen and pelvis to assess for pregnancy status in the primary survey. A "T" approach can be performed during the eFAST exam, scanning the upper abdomen and flanks in a horizontal fashion and then straight down the midline to the suprapubic region as shown in Figure 8.2. This approach would detect a pregnancy as well as

# OBSTETRIC LIFE SUPPORT

**Traumatic cardiac arrest in reproductive age female.
No pulse, no response**

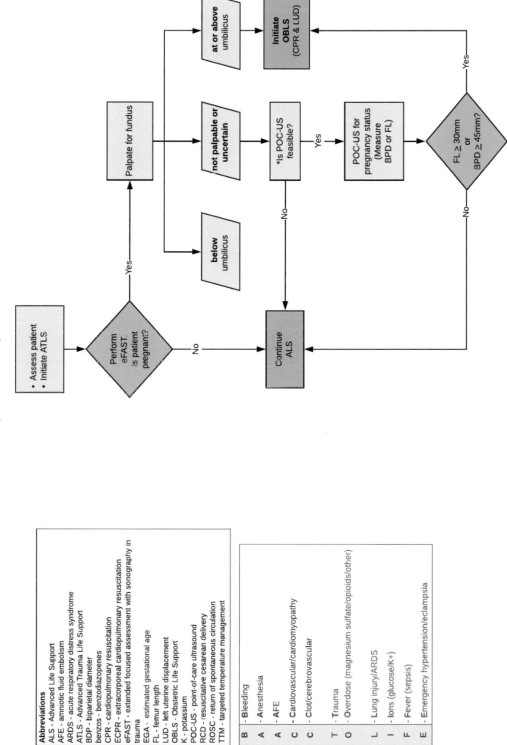

**Abbreviations**
ALS - Advanced Life Support
AFE - amniotic fluid embolism
ARDS - acute respiratory distress syndrome
ATLS - Advanced Trauma Life Support
BDP - biparietal diameter
benzos - benzodiazepenes
CPR - cardiopulmonary resuscitation
ECPR - extracorporeal cardiopulmonary resuscitation
eFAST - extended focused assessment with sonography in trauma
EGA - estimated gestational age
FL - femur length
LUD - left uterine displacement
OBLS - Obstetric Life Support
K - potassium
POC-US - point-of-care ultrasound
RCD - resuscitative cesarean delivery
ROSC - return of spontaneous circulation
TTM - targeted temperature management

B - Bleeding
A - Anesthesia
A - AFE
C - Cardiovascular/cardiomyopathy
C - Clot/cerebrovascular
T - Trauma
O - Overdose (magnesium sulfate/opioids/other)
L - Lung injury/ARDS
I - Ions (glucose/K+)
F - Fever (sepsis)
E - Emergency hypertension/eclampsia

**FIGURE 8.1**  Obstetric Life Support Traumatic Maternal Cardiac Arrest (T-MCA) algorithm.

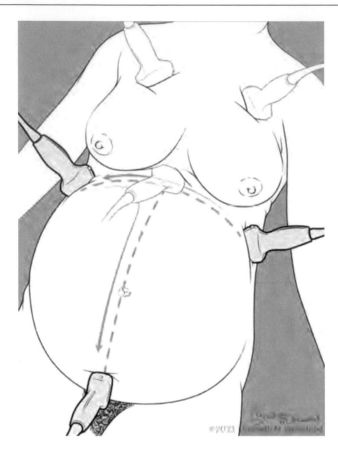

**FIGURE 8.2**   eFAST "T" scan.

provide evaluation of the bladder. Of note, fluid within the posterior cul-de-sac and paracolic gutters may be more difficult to detect with advancing gestational age due to the normal anatomic and physiologic changes of pregnancy. If an intrauterine pregnancy is confirmed, a quick assessment of the uterine fundus is recommended. If the uterus is at or above the umbilicus, OBLS is initiated. If below the umbilicus, continue ATLS® and ALS/ACLS.

As resources and training are available, POC-US can also be used in emergency protocols for identification of potentially reversible causes of cardiac arrest, such as identification of cardiac contractility without palpable pulse for clinical reclassification of PEA, and identification of the absence of cardiac contractility where further attempts at resuscitation may be futile.

In some circumstances such as extreme obesity, the application of POC-US for determination of gestational age may be necessary. The use of FL and BPD measurements are the most accurate and reproducible. Chapter 7 presents tables for FL and BPD throughout pregnancy. A FL of 30 mm or greater or a BPD of 45 mm or greater correspond to a gestational age of 20 weeks or greater, which generally corresponds to the uterus at the level of the umbilicus. A provider may acquire either FL or BPD, whichever is easiest or first visualized, but does not need to obtain both measurements.

POC-US in the setting of MCA should **not** interfere with proven and effective CPR techniques or prolong the initiation of chest compressions or pulse check pause in the setting of PEA. Additionally, POC-US should not divert focus away from the maternal status (e.g., presence or absence of fetal cardiac activity) or delay indicated RCD.

If the uterus is determined to be at or above the umbilicus, or the gestational age is known to be ≥20 weeks, an RCD is recommended to be started by 4 minutes of arrest. The preferred incision for an RCD is a vertical midline skin and uterine incision to allow for extension and exploration of the upper abdomen. See Chapter 7 for more details.

**KEY POINTS**
- The increased maternal circulating blood volume in pregnancy may mask changes in maternal vital signs and delay the recognition of hypovolemic shock from internal (concealed) hemorrhage due to uterine rupture or placental abruption associated with trauma in pregnancy. These cases may rapidly result in cardiac arrest if not recognized and treated early.

- In a reproductive-age female with traumatic MCA and unknown pregnancy status, include examination of abdominopelvic area during an eFAST exam to evaluate for pregnancy status.
- After confirming pregnancy with an eFAST, assess the uterine fundus in relation to umbilicus. If the uterine fundus cannot be palpated, gestational age can easily be assessed by measuring either fetal FL or BPD via POC-US.
- POC-US should only be performed during pulse checks, and should never interfere with high-quality CPR.

## Case Vignette

EMS providers treated an 18-year-old person with two gunshot wounds to the chest with high-quality CPR via automatic chest compression device. En route to the ED, they performed a right-sided needle decompression. At the ED, an eFAST exam revealed pericardial and intrathoracic fluid. The team performed an immediate resuscitative left anterolateral thoracotomy and right-sided tube thoracostomy. They noticed massive blood loss and identified and controlled a right atrial laceration. They cross-clamped the aorta, controlled right lung lacerations, and cannulated the right atrial appendage to aid with resuscitation.

During the secondary survey, an ultrasound exam revealed an intrauterine pregnancy, and the uterine fundus was noted to be a few centimeters above the umbilicus. The trauma surgeon initiated an RCD through a midline vertical skin incision 4 minutes after the patient's arrival to the ED. The on-call OB completed the RCD.

The neonatal intensive care unit (NICU) team resuscitated, intubated, and transferred the neonate to the NICU for further monitoring. To control ongoing uterine hemorrhage from intermittent return of spontaneous circulation, the uterine arteries were clamped bilaterally and the hysterotomy closed with 0-monocryl in a running fashion. Methylergonovine and oxytocin were administered, and surgical hemostasis from the uterus was achieved.

During ongoing intracardiac massage, multiple rounds of intracardiac epinephrine were administered and shocks delivered which resulted in intermittent organized cardiac rhythm. The atrial laceration was oversewn to attempt to gain control of bleeding in the chest. The patient was transferred to the operating room for the management of thoracic and pelvic wounds by cardiothoracic surgery and pelvic wounds by the gynecologic surgeon. Due to extensive wounds and blood loss, the patient was deemed not to be a candidate for veno-arterial bypass. Uteroovarian and uterine vessels remained clamped for hemostasis. Additional doses of oxytocin and methylergonovine resulted in minimal blood loss from the hysterotomy, or lower uterine segment.

In total, the patient received more than 20 units of blood products and the code continued for 60 minutes from arrival to the ED. At the 60-minute mark, there was no return of cardiac activity, no organized cardiac rhythm, no measurable PETCO$_2$, and no palpable pulse. The multidisciplinary team agreed that further attempts at resuscitation would be futile and stopped the resuscitation after 60 minutes.

## REVIEW QUESTIONS

**Q.** What are the steps to follow when assessing a reproductive-age person with traumatic cardiac arrest?

**A.** When assessing this patient population, responders should:
1. Evaluate for the presence of pregnancy. If the fundus is palpable, evaluate it in relation to the umbilicus. If the fundal height is **less** than the height of the umbilicus, continue the ATLS® and ALS/ACLS surveys. If fundus is **greater** than the umbilicus, initiate OBLS and ATLS®.
2. Evaluate the pelvis with an eFAST exam if pregnancy is suspected but the fundus is not palpable or if pregnancy status is unknown.
3. Measure the fetal BPD or FL to evaluate for an approximate fetal gestational age if pregnancy is confirmed.
4. Initiate OBLS with ATLS® if corresponding values are consistent with 20 weeks or greater.

**Q.** What are the important modifications to CPR during a MCA due to trauma?

**A.** Patients receiving CPR due to trauma are most likely in PEA (which is treated with high-quality CPR and epinephrine) due to hypovolemic shock. Patients in traumatic MCA should receive the same doses and timing of epinephrine in addition to high-quality CPR and LUD. They should also be considered for RCD if the fundus is at the level of or higher than the umbilicus, regardless of fetal gestational age or status.

Consider an OB hemorrhage kit and a massive transfusion protocol early in the treatment of traumatic MCA. These are important given that hypovolemia is a leading cause of traumatic MCA. An increased maternal circulating volume may mask the signs of hypovolemic shock, which can cause the patient to decline suddenly and rapidly.

**Q.** What type of skin incision is recommended for RCD in traumatic MCA?
**A.** OBLS recommends a vertical midline skin incision for RCD. The benefit of a vertical midline skin incision in the setting of trauma is that this incision can be easily extended to fully evaluate the abdominal cavity if indicated.

# CHAPTER 8. PRACTICE QUESTIONS

1. Which of the following is the MOST likely cause of traumatic cardiac arrest?
   A. Tension pneumothorax
   B. Cardiac tamponade
   C. Hypoxia
   D. Hypovolemia

2. What is the MOST likely presenting rhythm in a traumatic maternal cardiac arrest?
   A. PEA
   B. Asystole
   C. Ventricular tachycardia/ventricular fibrillation
   D. Bradycardia

3. According to the T-MCA algorithm, what exam should be added to all reproductive-age people in traumatic arrest to detect pregnancy?
   A. Palpation of the abdomen and pelvis during the primary survey
   B. Quick ultrasound of the abdomen and pelvis
   C. Perform deep peritoneal lavage
   D. Detection of fetal heart tones by handheld Doppler machine

4. According to the T-MCA algorithm, which of the following is the BEST next step in management if a pregnancy is confirmed during an eFAST protocol?
   A. Perform ultrasound to determine gestational age
   B. Palpate for uterine fundus and its relation to umbilicus
   C. Assess for fetal heart tones
   D. Evaluate the location of the placenta

5. If ultrasound must be performed to date a pregnancy, which fetal measurements will give the BEST estimation of gestational age?
   A. Femur length or biparietal diameter
   B. Abdominal circumference and femur length
   C. Humeral length and biparietal diameter
   D. Head circumference and biparietal diameter

# CHAPTER 8. ANSWERS

1. **ANSWER: D.** Traumatic cardiac arrest is defined as cardiac arrest due to blunt or penetrating trauma. Identifying and treating reversible causes of traumatic cardiac arrest is key to survival. Most traumatic cardiac arrest is due to hypovolemia. Other causes include hypoxia, tension pneumothorax, and cardiac tamponade.

2. **ANSWER: A.** Most traumatic cardiac arrest is due to hypovolemia leading to PEA. In such cases, blood product replacement is critical for survival.

3. **ANSWER: B.** OBLS advocates that eFAST protocols incorporate an examination of the female abdomen and pelvis to assess for pregnancy status in the primary survey. OBLS recommends a **T** approach to the eFAST exam, meaning the ultrasound wand is scanned in horizontal fashion across the bilateral upper quadrants of the abdomen and then down the midline. This would identify a pregnancy and provide evaluation of the bladder and posterior cul-de-sac.

4. **ANSWER: B.** If pregnancy is confirmed on eFAST protocol, an assessment of the uterine fundus is recommended. If the uterus is at or above the umbilicus, OBLS is simultaneously initiated. If below the umbilicus, follow ATLS or ALS/ACLS algorithms.

5. **ANSWER: A.** In some circumstances such as extreme obesity, the application of POC-US for quick determination of gestational age may be necessary. The use of FL and BPD measurements have been the most accurate and reproducible. A FL of 30 mm or greater and a BPD of 45 mm or greater corresponds to a gestational age of 20 weeks or greater, which generally corresponds to the uterus at the umbilicus. A provider can acquire either FL or BPD, whichever is first or easiest to obtain, but does not need to do both measurements.

# CHAPTER 8. REFERENCE

1. Davis NL, Hoyert DL, Goodman DA, et al. Contribution of maternal age and pregnancy checkbox on maternal mortality ratios in the United States 1978–2012. *Obstet Gynecol.* 2017;217:352.e1. doi: 10.1016/j.ajog.2017.04.042.

# Postpartum Cardiac Arrest

9

## 9.1 INTRODUCTION

Most anatomic and physiologic changes of pregnancy will persist for 8–12 weeks following delivery; therefore, a person's risk for significant morbidity and mortality during pregnancy extends into the postpartum period (up to 42 days postpartum). It is estimated that 22% of maternal deaths occur before delivery, 25% occur on the day of delivery and within 7 days postpartum, and 53% occur between 7 days and one year postpartum.[1,2] Continuous care is vital throughout the first year after delivery—some pregnancy-associated conditions can persist well into one year postpartum.

Unfortunately, only 40% of those who give birth in the U.S. attend a postpartum visit, contributing to increased risk for maternal morbidity and mortality.[2] To address this problem, in 2019 the American College of Obstetricians and Gynecologists recommended improving postpartum care in the "fourth trimester," including an early postpartum (within 1–3 weeks) and a late postpartum (up to 12 weeks) visit.[2]

## 9.2 LEARNING OBJECTIVES

Learner will appropriately

- Describe the common causes of postpartum cardiac arrest.
- Describe management strategies for the care of postpartum patients who are unstable or who have cardiac arrest.

## 9.3 CAUSES OF POSTPARTUM MATERNAL CARDIAC ARREST

In the U.S., the top three causes of postpartum MCA are hemorrhage, cardiovascular disease, and VTE/PE.[3–5] The most common causes of immediate (prehospital discharge) and delayed (post hospital discharge) MCA are listed in Table 9.1.

**TABLE 9.1**  Common Postpartum Causes of Maternal Cardiac Arrest

| Immediate MCA | • Cardiovascular disease/cardiomyopathy<br>• Infection<br>• Opioid overdose<br>• Preeclampsia/Eclampsia<br>• Postpartum hemorrhage<br>• Stroke<br>• VTE/PE |
|---|---|
| Delayed MCA | • Cardiovascular disease/Cardiomyopathy<br>• Infection (such as group A streptococcus)<br>• Opioid overdose<br>• Preeclampsia/Eclampsia<br>• Trauma (motor vehicle accident, suicide, homicide)<br>• Stroke<br>• VTE/PE |

DOI: 10.1201/9781003299288-10

# 9.4 MANAGEMENT OF POSTPARTUM CARDIAC ARREST BY CAUSE

Managing cardiac arrest in the postpartum patient is like that in the nonpregnant patient. Knowing the common causes of postpartum MCA allows the healthcare team to focus on the most likely etiology of arrest and promotes a focused evaluation during the assessment or primary and secondary surveys in the ED. There are unique signs, symptoms, and diagnostic considerations when caring for a postpartum patient in cardiac arrest that differ from care during pregnancy. The following section discusses some of the most common causes of MCA in the postpartum period and reviews treatment strategies for the unstable postpartum patient and the postpartum patient in cardiac arrest.

## 9.4.1 Postpartum Hemorrhage

PPH is the leading cause of maternal mortality.[6] PPH is a cumulative blood loss ≥1,000 mL or blood loss associated with signs or symptoms of hypovolemia during and within 24 hours of childbirth.[7] Significant vital sign changes do not typically occur until the patient has lost a substantial amount of blood, typically 25% or more of the total blood volume, around 1,500 mL. Therefore, it is imperative to recognize and treat PPH aggressively before the patient develops vital sign changes, hemodynamic instability, and hypovolemic cardiac arrest.

Primary causes of PPH (occurring in the first 24 hours after birth) include uterine atony, trauma, vaginal lacerations, postsurgical bleeding, retained products or placenta, abnormal placentation (placenta accreta spectrum disorder), acute coagulation deficit (such as disseminated intravascular coagulation or amniotic fluid embolism), and uterine injury from rupture or inversion. Secondary causes of PPH (>24 hours after birth and <12 weeks postpartum) include subinvolution of the placenta, infection, retained products or placenta, and inherited coagulation deficits (such as von Willebrand disease).

The goal of aggressive therapy is rapid recognition of bleeding to avoid maternal hypovolemia which may lead to significant morbidity and mortality. Aggressive fluid and blood replacement is recommended if MCA results from postpartum hemorrhage. See section 4.3 in Chapter 4 for a detailed discussion of maternal hemorrhage. The patient's risk for developing DIC is also increased, and massive transfusion protocols utilizing a fixed ratio of packed red blood cells to plasma to platelets (or whole blood, if available) may improve survival.

## 9.4.2 Preeclampsia/Eclampsia

Postpartum preeclampsia has a prevalence of 0.3%–27.5%. Signs and symptoms typically develop within the first 48–72 hours following birth. However, they can manifest any time in the first 6 weeks postpartum. Hypertensive disorders contribute to 10% of maternal deaths in the postpartum period.[8] Unfortunately, delays in diagnosis often occur unless patients had a previous diagnosis of hypertension in pregnancy or the immediate postpartum period. Therefore, practitioners must retain a high index of suspicion for preeclampsia in the postpartum period, especially in the setting of new-onset hypertension and/or a severe, unremitting headache.

The definition of severe hypertension in the postpartum period is the same as during pregnancy: systolic blood pressure ≥160, and/or diastolic blood pressure ≥110 mm Hg.[9] Implementation of hypertensive emergency bundles and checklists in ED and labor and delivery units improves response times for the administration of antihypertensive medications. Treat with anti-hypertensive medication as soon as possible within 30–60 minutes if there is sustained, elevated blood pressure (i.e., two measurements, 20 minutes apart).[9] In patients with chronic hypertension who develop superimposed preeclampsia with severe blood pressure, use caution when lowering blood pressure too quickly (e.g., avoid overtreatment), as a rapid decrease in blood pressure may result in stroke in the border zones of arterial territories of the brain ("watershed infarcts").[10] Table 9.2 reviews common treatment strategies for severe hypertension in the postpartum patient. Asthma is a relative contraindication for labetalol, as it can precipitate an asthmatic crisis.

Postpartum patients with hypertensive emergencies are at increased risk for multiple morbidities, including MCA, stroke, pulmonary edema, and encephalopathy due to cerebral edema. Half of the strokes that occur in the postpartum period, most often because of hypertensive emergency, occur within the first 2 weeks following delivery.[9] Stroke due to preeclampsia/eclampsia can be either hemorrhagic or ischemic. These patients require immediate brain imaging evaluation by a stroke team (e.g., Code Stoke). If preeclampsia or eclampsia results in a hemorrhagic stroke, blood pressure management is critical. Chapter 10 provides more details on stroke management. Patients with preeclampsia with severe features are also at increased risk for flash pulmonary edema, which can rapidly lead to respiratory failure. It is critical to have the most experienced laryngoscopist available for intubation of the difficult airway in the postpartum patient with preeclampsia, as laryngeal edema is common.

Multidisciplinary care for this patient with preeclampsia should include a maternal-fetal medicine specialist and/or obstetrician, a family medical provider, an anesthesiologist, and an intensivist. If the admitting hospital does not offer multidisciplinary critical care, the patient should be transported to a tertiary care center once stabilized. Additionally, during their pregnancy and, at a minimum, prior to discharge from the hospital, all postpartum patients should receive focused education on the signs and symptoms of hypertensive disorders and other postpartum emergencies and how and when to seek help with any concerns.

**TABLE 9.2**   Severe Hypertension Management in the Postpartum Patient

| DRUG | DOSE | TIME BETWEEN DRUG ADMINISTRATION | BP PARAMETERS |
|---|---|---|---|
| Hydralazine (IV) | 5 mg or 10 mg If requires more antihypertensive, switch to IV labetalol | Initial SBP ≥ 160 or DBP ≥110 for ≥15 minutes → repeat BP every 20 minutes until threshold met or switch to labetalol | Threshold: • SBP ≥160 • DBP ≥110 Below threshold: • SBP <160 • DBP <110 Once BP thresholds are achieved, repeat BP every 10 minutes × 1 hour → every 15 minutes × 1 hour → every 30 minutes × 1 hour → hourly × 4 hours |
| Labetalol (IV) | 20 mg → 40 mg → 80 mg If additional antihypertensive medication is required, switch to IV hydralazine | Initial SBP ≥ 160 or DBP ≥110 for ≥15 minutes → repeat BP every 10 minutes following labetalol until threshold met or switch to hydralazine | Threshold: • SBP ≥160 • DBP ≥110 Below threshold: • SBP <160 • DBP <110 Once BP thresholds are achieved, repeat BP every 10 minutes × 1 hour → every 15 minutes × 1 hour → every 30 minutes × 1 hour → hourly × 4 hours |
| Nifedipine— Immediate Release (oral) | 10 mg → 20 mg → 20 mg If additional antihypertensive medication is required, switch to 20 mg IV labetalol | Initial SBP ≥160 or DBP ≥110 for ≥15 minutes Repeat BP every 20 minutes following nifedipine until threshold met or switch to labetalol | Threshold: • SBP ≥160 • DBP ≥110 Below threshold: • SBP <160 • DBP <110 Once BP thresholds are achieved, repeat BP every 10 minutes × 1 hour → every 15 minutes × 1 hour → every 30 minutes × 1 hour → hourly × 4 hours |

Abbreviations: BP, blood pressure; DBP, diastolic blood pressure; SBP, systolic blood pressure.

**KEY POINTS**

- Aggressively manage severe-range blood pressure with antihypertensive medications such as labetalol, nifedipine, or hydralazine.
- Administer antihypertensive medications within 30–60 minutes of sustained severe-range pressures.
- Asthma is a relative contraindication to giving labetalol, which can precipitate an asthmatic crisis.
- Use available toolkits to improve response times to treatment of preeclampsia with severe features and eclampsia.

## 9.4.3 Cardiovascular Disease

Cardiovascular disease (CVD) affects 1%–4% of all pregnancies and is becoming more prevalent due to rising rates of acquired CVD.[11] A recent study from Illinois reported that 22% of maternal deaths resulted from cardiovascular causes, overwhelmingly due to acquired CVD.[12] In the postpartum period, the most common causes of maternal morbidity and mortality include cardiomyopathy, myocardial infarction (MI), arrhythmias, and aortic dissection.[11] There is significant room for improvement in maternal care in this area. Multiple studies show that more than 50% of maternal deaths due to CVDs could have been prevented.[13–15]

An indirect risk factor for acquired CVD in persons with the lived experience of racism is low socioeconomic status. Other risk factors include age, preexisting hypertension, and obesity. Even the presence of one of these risk factors should increase a clinician's suspicion for underlying maternal cardiovascular disease, and the increased risks of sequelae. CVD, and cardiomyopathy in particular, is the leading cause of late postpartum maternal mortality and can be seen as late as 1 year postpartum.[11]

Assess for red flags of CVD in any person in pregnancy or postpartum (Table 9.3). If present, expedite consultations with maternal-fetal medicine and primary care or cardiology (Figure 9.1).

Assessment of CVD in pregnant and postpartum people without preexisting CVD requires an awareness of the risk factors, abnormal vital signs, or physical exam findings that indicate the need for further evaluation (Figure 9.2). If a pregnant patient presents with chest pain or shortness of breath, a laboratory evaluation should include a B-type natriuretic peptide, cardiac enzymes, and electrocardiogram. Consider a D-dimer, understanding that this value remains elevated in the first 4–5 weeks postpartum. A chest radiograph and a cardiac echocardiogram should be considered and obtained based on their history and exam, especially if there is heightened concern for cardiomyopathy. If a pulmonary embolism or aortic dissection is suspected, a chest CT scan with IV contrast should be obtained for diagnostic purposes and not be withheld due to postpartum state or concerns about breastfeeding. CT pulmonary angiography is safe in pregnancy and postpartum, with minimal contrast excreted in the breast milk. These patients may continue to breastfeed without interruption after CT imaging.

Though atrial arrhythmias are common in pregnancy, they should be evaluated to ensure no underlying abnormal structural cardiac etiology is present. Ventricular arrhythmias are extremely rare in pregnancy (prevalence of 2 in 100,000 hospital admissions)[16] and the postpartum period and should also be thoroughly assessed.

The incidence of PPCM, also known as postpartum cardiomyopathy, is rising in the U.S. (incidence of 10.3 per 10,000 live births).[5] While many patients with PPCM ultimately regain full cardiac function, those patients with an initial ejection fraction of <30% on cardiac echocardiogram have lower rates of recovery, as well as increased morbidity and mortality. Alarmingly, approximately 13% of those who experience PPCM will also have a major adverse event associated with it.[17]

Acute coronary syndrome (ACS), though rare at 8 per 100,000 live births, is more often diagnosed in the postpartum period.[18] As with nonpregnant patients, pregnant patients with ACS benefit from expedited coronary reperfusion procedures as they are at risk for shock, arrhythmia, cardiac arrest and rearrest, recurrent infarctions, heart failure, and death.

Guidelines for initial treatment of chest pain are migrating from the cue **MONA**, which stands for **m**orphine, **o**xygen, **n**itroglycerin, and **a**spirin, to a more targeted approach, THROMBINS2, which stands for **t**hienopyridines, **h**eparin/enoxaparin, **r**enin-angiotensin system blockers, **o**xygen, **m**orphine, **b**eta-blocker, **i**ntervention, **n**itroglycerin, **s**tatin/**s**alicylate.[19] In the

**TABLE 9.3** Red Flags of Cardiovascular Disease in Pregnant or Postpartum People

| | |
|---|---|
| Oxygen saturations ≤94% with or without personal history of CVD | Resting HR ≥120 |
| Shortness of breath at rest | Resting systolic BP ≥160 mm Hg |
| Severe orthopnea—four or more pillows | Resting RR ≥30 |

Abbreviations: BP, blood pressure; CVD, cardiovascular disease; HR, heart rate; RR, respiratory rate.

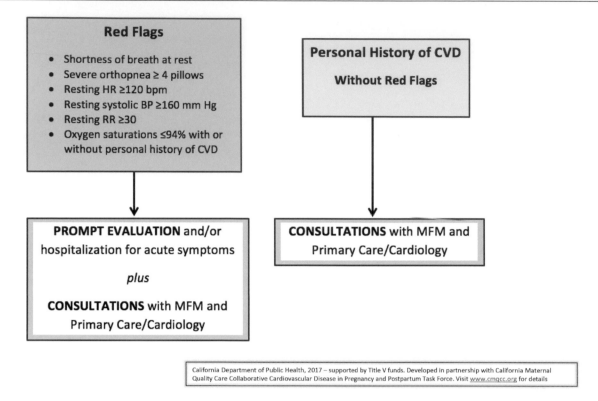

**FIGURE 9.1**    Cardiovascular disease assessment algorithm for pregnant and postpartum people.
Courtesy of the CMQCC.

out-of-hospital setting, consider giving pregnant patients with chest pain 324 mg chewable aspirin, titrated doses of morphine or fentanyl for pain control, oxygen supplementation if $O_2$ is <94%, and nitroglycerin if BP is elevated and there is no concern for inferior infarct. As with nonpregnant patients, ECG should be performed and transmitted as per protocol. Ideally, providers will transport pregnant patients with chest pain to a center capable of providing cardiac catheterization and obstetric and neonatal care, if indicated.

Once in the ED, it is reasonable to treat pregnant patients similarly to nonpregnant patients; however, Obstetric Life Support recommends multidisciplinary involvement to include maternal-fetal medicine/obstetrics, cardiology, and emergency medicine providers.

If the patient is undergoing ST-elevation myocardial infarction (STEMI), the catheterization laboratory (cardiac catheterization lab) is ready, and there are no emergent airway or hemodynamic issues, move the patient directly to the cardiac catheterization lab.

If the patient is undergoing STEMI, and the catheterization lab is **not** ready, repeat 12-lead ECG and administer bilevel positive airway pressure for acute pulmonary edema with severe distress or hypoxia (if awake and not hypotensive). Consider the following steps, including components of the mnemonic THROMBINS2[19]:

| | |
|---|---|
| **T**hienopyridines | • Administer clopidogrel 75 mg PO |
| **H**eparin | • Administer heparin 5,000 units IV |
| **R**enin-angiotensin system blockers | • Generally avoided during pregnancy, may use postpartum |
| **O**xygen | • Administer $O_2$, as indicated |
| **M**orphine | • Administer analgesics, as indicated |
| **B**eta-blockers | • Start within 24 hours if no evidence of heart failure, shock or heart block |
| **I**ntervention | • Shave groin if time permits for femoral artery access (although often use radial artery now) to prepare for cardiac catheterization |
| **N**itroglycerin | • Administer nitroglycerin, contraindicated in inferior MI (not a priority, no mortality benefit for MI) |
| **S**tatin/Salicylate | • Confirm administration of aspirin; statins are generally contraindicated if patient remains pregnant; okay to use postpartum |

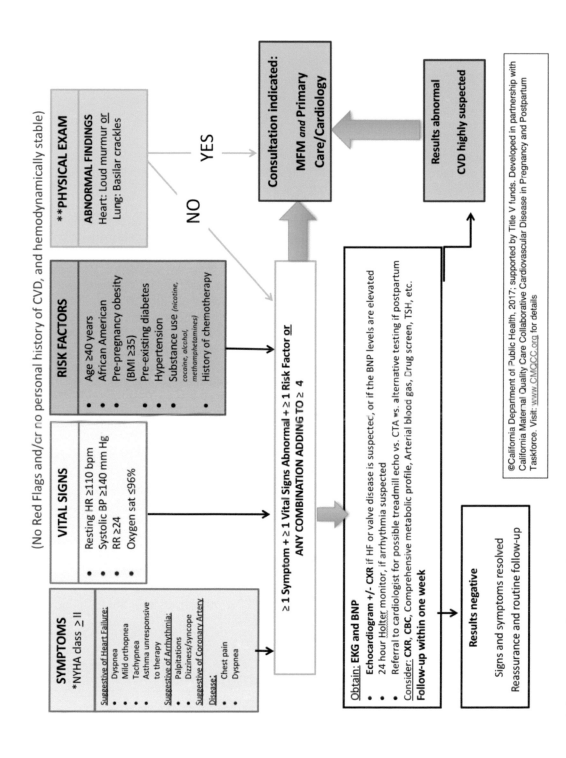

**FIGURE 9.2** Cardiovascular disease assessment in pregnant and postpartum people.
Courtesy of the CMQCC.

## 9.4.5 Spontaneous Coronary Artery Dissection

Spontaneous coronary artery dissection (SCAD), characterized by the spontaneous formation of an intramural hematoma of the coronary artery not associated with atherosclerosis or trauma, is now recognized as the most common cause of MI in pregnant and postpartum patients.[20] Despite advances in the understanding of pregnancy-associated SCAD (P-SCAD), it continues to be underrecognized, misdiagnosed, and mismanaged as atherosclerotic MI.[20]

Patients with P-SCAD are most likely to present in the third trimester or postpartum, with the majority occurring in the first 5 weeks postpartum.[20] The average age of patients with P-SCAD is 33–36 years. Associated demographic and comorbid conditions include age greater than 30 years, multiparity, a history of assisted reproductive technologies, and concurrent preeclampsia.[21] These patients present most commonly with the following:

- Chest pain
- Increased levels of cardiac enzymes with few or no cardiovascular risk factors
- STEMI
- Left ventricular ejection fraction <35%
- Involvement of more than one coronary vessel, and most commonly the left main and/or left anterior descending artery[20]

Once SCAD is suspected, a coronary angiography is performed as early as feasible, especially in the setting of STEMI.[20] If the patient is clinically stable on presentation and does not have high-risk anatomy (defined by left main or severe proximal two-vessel dissection), conservative therapy with inpatient monitoring for 3–5 days is recommended. If the patient is clinically stable with high-risk anatomy, consider a coronary artery bypass graft (CABG); however, conservative treatment may be a reasonable option but has not been well studied. It is important to recognize that percutaneous coronary intervention (PCI) for SCAD has been associated with lower technical success and a higher complication rate than PCI for atherosclerotic MI.[20] Therefore, PCI is reserved for patients with P-SCAD with active or ongoing ischemia or hemodynamic instability; alternatively, urgent CABG can be performed based on technical considerations and local expertise.[20]

Recurrence of P-SCAD may be reduced by initiating beta-blocker therapy, controlling blood pressure, and minimizing possible triggers such as extreme stress, extreme exertion, and future pregnancy. Manage patients with P-SCAD with a multidisciplinary pregnancy heart team in a level IV maternal care facility capable of managing cardiac emergencies, particularly if the patient remains pregnant following the P-SCAD event.[20,21] The mode and timing of delivery following P-SCAD are based on obstetrical indications, with neuraxial anesthesia being the preferred mode.

---

**KEY POINTS**

- In the U.S., cardiac disease is a leading cause of maternal morbidity and mortality in the postpartum period.
- Postpartum cardiomyopathy is the leading cause of late postpartum maternal mortality, occurring as late as 1 year postpartum.
- Evaluation of chest pain in the postpartum period should include cardiac enzymes, chest X-ray, ECG, and echocardiogram, as indicated.
- SCAD is the most common cause of MI in pregnant and postpartum patients.
- Red flags for cardiac disease in the postpartum period include orthopnea, shortness of breath at rest, and tachycardia, and should prompt an immediate cardiac workup.

---

## 9.4.6 Venous Thromboembolism/Pulmonary Embolism

Pregnancy greatly increases the risk of VTE by four- to five-fold as compared with nonpregnant people.[22] The risks are most significant in the initial weeks following delivery. VTE is a common cause of maternal mortality due to cardiac obstructive shock, and is responsible for 9.3% of all maternal deaths.[22] The two most important risk factors for VTE are a personal history of VTE and an existing thrombophilia (acquired or inherited). Other risk factors include cesarean delivery (especially if accompanied by complications such as obesity, infection, or hemorrhage), underlying cardiovascular disease, autoimmune diseases, and hypertensive disease such as preeclampsia.[22]

Any postpartum patient who reports acute-onset shortness of breath, chest pain, tachycardia, or decreased oxygen saturation should be evaluated for possible VTE or PE. These patients should be evaluated similarly to their nonpregnant counterparts and undergo ventilation-perfusion scan or CT angiography.[22,25] High suspicion or confirmation of VTE on imaging requires prompt anticoagulation therapy to prevent further clotting.

In addition, patients with a patent foramen ovale who develop VTE are at risk for arterial ischemic stroke due to "paradoxical embolism." Of note, one in four people has a patent foramen ovale,[23] and the prevalence is as high as 50% in people with a history of migraine with aura.[24] Postpartum people are also at higher risk for cerebral venous sinus thrombosis (CVST), which typically presents with progressive, severe headache that is worst in the supine position; left untreated, CVST may progress to cause cerebral edema, intracranial hemorrhage, and brain herniation.

Severe PE is associated with evidence of right heart strain. Signs of right heart strain on CT include right ventricular enlargement (right ventricle larger than the left ventricle), pulmonary trunk enlargement (pulmonary trunk larger than the aorta), and features of right heart failure (such as reflux of contrast into the inferior vena cava). Severe PE can be classified as **submassive** (defined as acute PE without systemic hypotension - SBP ≥90 mm Hg but with either right ventricular dysfunction or myocardial necrosis or **massive** (defined as acute PE with obstructive shock, SBP <90 mm Hg or cardiac arrest).

One systematic review looking at PE in pregnancy and the postpartum period found that 30% of PEs occurred in the postpartum period, 82% of PEs were considered massive, and over 20% of them resulted in MCA. Thrombolysis via either recombinant tissue plasminogen activator (59%) or streptokinase (14.5%) were used in over half of the cases, while almost 40% received either percutaneous thrombectomy or surgical thrombectomy. Of these, 11% required ECPR during their therapy, with a maternal survival (both pregnancy and postpartum) rate of 94% after therapy.[26] Of those postpartum-related events, almost half (46%) occurred within 24 hours of delivery, and over three-fourths were following a cesarean section.

Severe postpartum hemorrhage can result from thrombolytic therapy used to treat massive PE. A systematic review of pregnant and postpartum patients receiving thrombolysis for treatment of massive PE saw significant vaginal bleeding or postoperative bleeding in 18% and 58% of cases, respectively, with an overall bleeding complication rate of 28.4%.[26]

Similarly, postoperative bleeding is also a concern following surgical thrombectomy in the postpartum patient. While major bleeding is not as frequent following the treatment of massive PE with percutaneous fragmentation, additional treatment with either surgical thrombectomy or ECPR is frequently necessary. Only a limited number of cases of ECPR used in conjunction with anticoagulants (without thrombolytics) have been reported, but survival rates were favorable, and none of those patients had significant complications such as severe hemorrhage.[26]

---

**KEY POINTS**

- PE risk is highest in the early postpartum period, and it is one of the leading causes of maternal death during the postpartum period.
- Red flags such as acute shortness of breath, tachycardia, and oxygen desaturation should prompt an evaluation for PE with CT angiography or ventilation-perfusion scan.
- Massive PE is associated with right heart strain and hemodynamic instability. Aggressive treatment includes catheter-directed thrombolytics, embolectomy, and/or ECPR.
- Severe bleeding complications are common in pregnant and postpartum people undergoing treatment for massive PE and should be anticipated and treated aggressively.

## 9.4.7 Postpartum Stroke

The risk of maternal stroke is highest during the postpartum period, especially within the first 2 weeks after delivery.[27] A nationwide study found that the median time to readmission for stroke after delivery was 8 days.[28] Causes of postpartum stroke include CVST, arterial ischemia, and most commonly, intracerebral hemorrhage and/or subarachnoid hemorrhage.[29] While the overall incidence of maternal stroke is relatively rare at 30 per 100,000 deliveries,[30] some populations, such as those with hypertensive disorders, are at higher risk.[31] Risk factors for maternal postpartum stroke are reviewed in Table 9.4.

Reviews of maternal deaths due to stroke have found that up to 60% of these deaths could have been prevented by earlier recognition of warning signs and more aggressive treatment of hypertension.[32,33] Stroke can cause death directly by brain swelling and herniation or through neurogenic myocardial stunning causing cardiac arrest. Stroke can also result in maternal death indirectly due to common post-stroke complications such as VTE/PE, sepsis, and aspiration pneumonia.

Headache is quite common in the postpartum period, especially in people with a history of migraines or tension headaches. However, postpartum people presenting with a headache deserve a thorough evaluation, as headache can be a warning sign or a symptom of stroke. Carefully evaluate those who report postpartum headache for "red flag" headache features. These include

**TABLE 9.4**  Risk Factors for Postpartum Stroke[12]

| CESAREAN DELIVERY | LOWER SOCIOECONOMIC STATUS |
|---|---|
| Heart disease, including peripartum cardiomyopathy[34] | Longer delivery admission |
| History of migraines[35] | Lived experience of racism |
| Hypertensive disorders of pregnancy, including chronic hypertension, gestational hypertension, and preeclampsia/eclampsia | Older age |
| Infection during delivery admission[36] | Prothrombotic disorders (e.g., sickle cell disease, factor V Leiden) |

sudden or "thunderclap" onset, reaching maximum intensity within 60 seconds; severity ("worst headache of my life"); positionality (worse in supine position can indicate CVST); change in character of headache from usual migraines (e.g., pressure-like instead of throbbing); altered mental status; presence of any focal neurologic deficits, such as dizziness, vision changes, weakness/numbness, or speech difficulties; unrelieved by typical medications such as acetaminophen or ibuprofen; or elevated blood pressure.

These can be remembered by the mnemonic **SCAN ME**:

**S**udden/Severe/Seizure
**C**hange in position or quality
**A**ltered mental status
**N**eurologic deficits/Nausea and vomiting
**M**edications without relief
**E**levated blood pressure (hypertension) or temperature (fever)

Any of these should prompt a rapid neurologic evaluation and consideration of brain imaging. Any sudden neurologic change should prompt activation of the Code Stroke protocol. Postpartum stroke is discussed in more detail in Chapter 10.

**KEY POINTS**
- The risk of maternal stroke is highest during the postpartum period, especially in the first 2 weeks after delivery.
- People with hypertensive disorders of pregnancy are at the highest risk for postpartum stroke.
- Headache can be a warning sign for stroke. Carefully evaluate patients with headache for red flag features.

## 9.4.8 Trauma

Trauma affects approximately one in ten pregnant people and is a leading cause of maternal death.[37] The maternal mortality ratio is a health system indicator that refers to the number of pregnancy-related maternal deaths per 100,000 live births. The maternal mortality ratio includes direct pregnancy causes of maternal death (such as preeclampsia or CVD) and does not include indirect causes such as trauma (motor vehicle collisions, suicide, and homicide). Because of this, the number of maternal deaths is substantially underestimated. Violent or intentional trauma is inflicted on pregnant people more frequently than nonpregnant people (16% versus 10%, respectively) and is more likely to result in death during pregnancy. In Colorado, 30% of maternal deaths were due to suicide,[38] and in Illinois, trauma-related deaths accounted for more maternal deaths than hemorrhage, VTE, CVD, or infections.[12] Motor vehicle collisions accounted for three-fourths of the trauma cases in pregnant women.[39,40]

Given the high rates of trauma, suicide, and intimate partner violence in pregnancy, pregnant and postpartum people should be screened for intimate partner violence and postpartum depression. Universal screening may help to identify those at risk and protect them from violence before it occurs.[41] Additionally, pregnant and postpartum people should be counseled on seat belt use at prenatal and postpartum visits.

Pregnant or postpartum people presenting with trauma should undergo primary and secondary surveys. It is important to remember that normal pregnancy physiologic changes may persist in the early postpartum period. Point-of-care ultrasound with an extended Focused Assessment of Sonography for Trauma can help guide diagnostic and therapeutic treatments. A multidisciplinary approach to caring for postpartum trauma victims is paramount.

## 9.4.9 Infection

Sepsis is the second leading cause of maternal death. In the U.S., sepsis caused 13.9% of pregnancy-related deaths between 2016 and 2018[42] and is a common cause for delayed maternal mortality. Sepsis can occur from a variety of sources such as endometritis (infection of the uterus), postoperative complications, mastitis (infection of the breast), and urinary tract infection.

Perhaps one of the most insidious causes of sepsis is group A streptococcal (GAS) infection, historically referred to as puerperal sepsis. GAS infections typically present within 2–48 hours after delivery. Vaginal colonization of group A *Streptococcus* is extremely rare (0.03%) compared to group B *Streptococcus*, which impacts 10%–30% of pregnancies. Group A *Streptococcus* can be carried asymptomatically on the skin or throat in adults and children and is easily transmitted to postpartum patients.[43] Patients with GAS infections can rapidly deteriorate within 2–3 hours and die from GAS sepsis. Source control can be lifesaving, and many with GAS sepsis ultimately require surgical source control, such as hysterectomy.[43] A multidisciplinary approach to caring for a patient with GAS infection is crucial to optimize survival. Treatment for suspected GAS infections is with IV penicillin and clindamycin.

Treating sepsis requires prompt recognition and treatment of both sepsis and shock, as septic shock results in hemodynamic instability and increases the risk of maternal mortality. The Surviving Sepsis Campaign (SSC) recommends using the Hour-1 Bundle to reduce mortality rates (see Appendix C). The bundle encourages providers to start specific interventions in the first hour from sepsis recognition.[44] These include drawing blood cultures and a serum lactate and starting broad-spectrum antibiotics (see Table 4.12) and IV fluid resuscitation. In addition to obtaining a serum lactate, laboratory evaluation includes a complete blood count, comprehensive metabolic panel, and cultures (e.g., blood, urine, respiratory, and other sources such as endometrium). In the setting of hypotension refractory to IV fluid management, norepinephrine is considered the first-line vasopressor.[45]

> **KEY POINTS**
> - Infection/sepsis is the second most common cause of postpartum MCA.
> - Risk for infection is higher in postoperative patients.
> - Obstetric Life Support endorses using the SSC Hour-1 Sepsis bundle to improve maternal morbidity and mortality.
> - Treatment of sepsis includes early initiation of broad-spectrum antibiotics, intravenous fluid resuscitation, and source control, if indicated.

## 9.4.10 Opioid Overdose

Opioid-related overdose deaths have more than quadrupled over the past 15 years,[46] with, on average, 130 Americans dying a day from opioid overdoses.[47] The rates of prescription opioid-related overdose deaths are rising faster in women than in men, particularly women of reproductive age.[48] One-third of postpartum people have some form of narcotic at home for pain control, most commonly prescribed to treat postsurgical pain from cesarean delivery.[49] The Centers for Disease Control and Prevention report an overall cesarean delivery rate of 32% for the year 2017, with individual state rates ranging between 22% and 38%.[50]

Across the U.S., maternal deaths in the postpartum period due to opioid overdose are rising.[48] In the state of Texas, almost 20% of maternal deaths occurred as a result of drug overdose, with over half of fatal overdoses from opioids, all occurring in the postpartum period.[51] Over half of the maternal mortalities occurred as a result of drug combinations, with many occurring more than 2 months postpartum. Opioid overdose was also one of the few causes of maternal mortality,[52] where the Caucasian race was associated with the highest risk. The Alliance for Innovation on Maternal Health has a bundle with guidelines and tools that can be used to recognize and treat opioid/drug overdose with the goal of decreasing severe maternal morbidity and mortality.[52]

While treatment relies largely on prevention of opioid overdoses, if a postpartum person presents in cardiac arrest and an opioid overdose is the suspected etiology, give naloxone: 2 mg intranasally or 0.4 mg intramuscularly. Postpartum status should not change any drug administration that would otherwise be recommended in cardiac arrest. Continue high-quality CPR. Advanced Cardiac Life Support recommends administering a second dose of naloxone after 4 minutes if there is no response to the original dose.

> **KEY POINTS**
> - Opioid overdose is a significant cause of delayed maternal mortality in the United States.
> - If there is suspicion for opioid overdose, immediately administer naloxone: 2 mg intranasally or 0.4 mg intramuscularly.

**Case Vignette**

A 35-year-old person with obesity is 1-week postpartum after a low transverse cesarean section. Discharged home on postoperative day 3 after an uncomplicated hospital course, the patient notices left leg swelling and pain when walking. The obstetrician confirms a left lower extremity deep vein thrombosis via duplex Doppler ultrasound and starts the patient on therapeutic low-molecular-weight heparin.

Two days later, dispatched emergency medical services providers find the patient unresponsive and with a thready pulse. They start Basic Life Support and place an automated external defibrillator. During the pulse check, "no shock" is advised, and rhythm is concerning for pulseless electrical activity. The crew continues high-quality CPR and gives two rounds of epinephrine. Apparently, the patient was not taking the prescribed blood clot medication.

Emergency medical services providers transport the patient to the nearest facility with ECMO capability while continuing high-quality CPR. Upon arrival, the maternal code team and ECPR team are present and assume high-quality CPR and administer IV heparin due to suspected massive PE. Targeted point-of-care ultrasound revealed concern for massive PE and severe right heart strain.

They transport the patient to the operating room with ongoing CPR where the cardiothoracic surgeon performs a median sternotomy, and the ascending aorta and the right atrial appendage are cannulated to start cardiopulmonary bypass (CPB). An embolectomy is performed under mild hypothermia and CPB. Following surgery, an inferior vena caval filter is placed. The patient is weaned off CPB, and, after an uneventful recovery, is released from the hospital on day 10.

## REVIEW QUESTIONS

**Q.** What is the differential diagnosis for MCA occurring in the postpartum period?

**A.** The most common causes of MCA in the postpartum period include hemorrhage, CVD (including cardiomyopathy), infection/sepsis, opioid overdose, and VTE/PE.

This patient has risk factors for several of these etiologies. Given the lack of compliance with the anticoagulation therapy for DVT, massive PE is the most likely cause of MCA. Advanced maternal age and obesity are also risk factors for CVD. Additionally, the patient recently had surgery, a risk factor for opioid overdose and infection/sepsis.

**Q.** What are the treatment options for a postpartum patient suspected of having cardiac arrest from a massive PE?

**A.** Treatment options for massive PE may consist of anticoagulation such as IV heparin or thrombolytics, surgical evacuation via embolectomy, and/or ECMO therapy. Given this patient was already in cardiac arrest due to PE, it was prudent to proceed with surgical evacuation and consideration for ECMO.

Treatment modality will depend on the patient's stability and an institution's capabilities.

# CHAPTER 9. PRACTICE QUESTIONS

1. In the U.S., what is the leading cause of late postpartum maternal cardiovascular mortality and can be seen even as late as 1 year postpartum?
   A. Cardiomyopathy
   B. Acute MI
   C. Spontaneous coronary artery dissection
   D. Cardiac arrhythmia

2. Pregnancy-related deaths are most likely to occur at what point in pregnancy?
   A. Antepartum
   B. Intrapartum

C. Postpartum
D. Equally distributed throughout pregnancy

3. Which of the following signs or symptoms in the postpartum period would be a red flag for CVD?
A. Shortness of breath with exertion
B. Orthopnea: four or more pillows
C. Maternal pulse of 110
D. $O_2$ saturation 95%

4. A patient with extreme obesity just delivered their first child 12 hours ago by cesarean section. The nurse responds to reports of shortness of breath at rest and chest pain. On exam, the patient is writhing in bed, blood pressure is 70/40, $O_2$ saturations are 85%, and pulse is 140. Abdominal exam is not concerning for an acute abdomen. The patient becomes unconscious and pulseless. What is the most likely etiology for the cardiac arrest?
A. Preeclampsia/eclampsia
B. Opioid overdose
C. Intra-abdominal hemorrhage
D. Saddle/massive PE

5. Emergency medical services providers are called to the home of a 45-year-old who became unresponsive while breastfeeding. On examination, the patient has a pulse and is unresponsive. The crew learns that the patient had been struggling with the pain from a cesarean delivery for several months. What is the BEST next step?
A. Administer intranasal naloxone
B. Transport the patient to the nearest facility
C. Perform left uterine displacement
D. Perform immediate intubation

# CHAPTER 9. ANSWERS

1. **ANSWER: A.** CVD affects 1%–4% of all pregnancies and is becoming more prevalent due to rising rates of acquired CVD. In the postpartum period, the most common causes of maternal morbidity and mortality include cardiomyopathy/heart failure, myocardial infarction, arrhythmias, and aortic dissection. Importantly, cardiomyopathy is the leading cause of late postpartum maternal mortality and can be seen as late as 1 year postpartum.

2. **ANSWER: C.** The anatomic and physiologic changes of pregnancy will persist for 8–12 weeks following delivery; therefore, the risk for significant morbidity and mortality during pregnancy extends into the postpartum period. This is traditionally defined as after delivery to 42 days postpartum. It is estimated that 53% of maternal deaths occur between 7 days and 1 year postpartum. The remainder of maternal deaths are equally distributed prior to delivery (22%) and at delivery and within 7 days postpartum (25%).

3. **ANSWER: B.** Red flags for CVD in pregnant or postpartum patients includes shortness of breath at **rest**; severe orthopnea, four or more pillows; resting heart rate ≥120, resting systolic blood pressure ≥160 mm Hg; resting respiratory rate ≥30; and oxygen saturation ≤94%, with or without personal history of CVD.

4. **ANSWER: D.** A massive PE can cause cardiac arrest and should be suspected as an etiology for cardiac arrest in any postpartum patient. The postpartum state is a significant risk factor for VTE; additionally, patients who have had surgery, who are obese, who use tobacco products, who are immobilized, or who are using contraceptives containing estrogen are at increased risk for VTE. In the setting of massive PE (defined as systolic blood pressure <90, acute drop in blood pressure >40 mm Hg, or the need for inotropic support, or cardiac arrest), thrombolytic therapy or even thrombectomy should be considered.

5. **ANSWER: A.** Treat postpartum patients in cardiac arrest and suspected opioid overdose with naloxone either intranasally (2 mg) or intramuscularly (0.4 mg). Postpartum status should not change any drug administration that would otherwise be considered for a nonpregnant person in cardiac arrest. Focus remains on high-quality CPR and giving naloxone after 4 minutes if there is no response to the initial dose.

# CHAPTER 9. REFERENCES

1. Centers for Disease Control and Prevention. Four in 5 pregnancy-related deaths in the U.S. are preventable. Website. https://www.cdc.gov/media/releases/2022/p0919-pregnancy-related-deaths.html. Accessed March 18, 2023.
2. Optimizing Postpartum Care. ACOG Committee Opinion No. 736. American College of Obstetricians and Gynecologists. *Obstet Gynecol.* 2018;131:140–150.
3. Jeejeebhoy FM, Morrison L. Maternal cardiac arrest: A practical and comprehensive review. *Emerg Med Int.* 2013. doi: 10.1155/2013/274814.
4. *The World Health Report: 2005: Make every mother and child count.* World Health Organization. Website. www.who.int/whr/2005/en/.
5. Kikuchi J, Deering S. Cardiac arrest in pregnancy. *Semin Perinatol.* 2018;42(1):33–38. doi: 10.1053/j.semperi.2017.11.007.
6. GBD 2015 Disease and Injury Incidence and Prevalence, Collaborators. Global, regional, and national incidence, prevalence, and years lived with disability for 310 diseases and injuries, 1990–2015: A systematic analysis for the Global Burden of Disease Study 2015. *Lancet.* 2016;388(10053):1545–1602.
7. Committee on Practice Bulletins-Obstetrics. Practice Bulletin No. 183: Postpartum hemorrhage. *Obstet Gynecol.* 2017;13(4):e168–e186. doi: 10.1097/AOG.0000000000002351.
8. Ybarra N, Laperouse E. Postpartum preeclampsia. *J Obstet Gynecol Neonatal Nurs.* 2016. doi: 10.1016/j.jogn.2016.03.061.
9. ACOG Committee Opinion 767. Emergent therapy for acute-onset, severe hypertension during pregnancy and the postpartum period. *Obstet Gynecol.* 2019;133. doi: 10.1097/AOG.0000000000003075.
10. McNaughton CD, Self WH, Levy PD, Barrett TW. High-risk patients with hypertension: Clinical management options. *Clin Med Rev Vasc Health.* 2013;20(24). doi: 10.4137/CMRVH.S8109.
11. Pregnancy and Heart Disease. ACOG Practice Bulletin No. 212. American College of Obstetricians and Ggynecologists. *Obstet Gynecol.* 2019;133(5):320–356. doi: 10.1097/AOG.0000000000003243.
12. Briller J, Koch AR, Geller SE. Maternal cardiovascular mortality in Illinois, 2002–2011. *Obstet Gynecol.* 2017;12(5):819–826. doi: 10.1097/AOG.0000000000001981.
13. Hameed AB, Lawton ES, McCain CL, Morton CH, Mitchell C, Main EK, Foster E. Pregnancy-related cardiovascular deaths in California: Beyond peripartum cardiomyopathy. *Am J Obstet Gynecol.* 2015;21(3):379–379. doi: 10.1016/j.ajog.2015.05.008.
14. Kuklina E, Callaghan W. Chronic heart disease and severe obstetric morbidity among hospitalisations for pregnancy in the USA: 1995–2006. *BJOG.* 2011;11(3):345–352. doi: 10.1111/j.1471-0528.2010.02743.x.
15. Cantwell R, Clutton-Brock T, Cooper G, Dawson A, Drife J, Garrod D, et al. Saving Mothers' Lives: Reviewing maternal deaths to make motherhood safer: 2006–2008. The Eighth Report of the Confidential Enquiries into Maternal Deaths in the United Kingdom. *BJOG.* 2011;118:1–203. doi: 10.1111/j.1471-0528.2010.02847.x.
16. Li JM, Nguyen C, Joglar JA, Hamdan MH, Page RL. Frequency and outcome of arrhythmias complicating admission during pregnancy: Experience from a high-volume and ethnically-diverse obstetric service. *Clin Cardiol.* 2008;31:538–541.
17. Kolte D, Khera S, Aronow WS, et al. Temporal trends in incidence and outcomes of peripartum cardiomyopathy in the United States: A nationwide population-based study. *J Am Heart Assoc.* 2014;3(3):e001056. Published 2014 June 4. doi: 10.1161/JAHA.114.001056.
18. Smilowitz NR, Gupta N, Guo Y, Zhong J, Weinberg CR, Reynolds HR, Bangalore S. Acute myocardial infarction during pregnancy and the puerperium in the United States. *Mayo Clin Proc.* 2018. doi: 10.1016/j.mayocp.2018.04.019.
19. Cathlabdigest. *THROMBINS2 is the new MONA.* 2018 November 1. Website. www.cathlabdigest.com/content/THROMBINS2-New-MONA. Accessed February 12, 2021.
20. Hayes SN, Kim E, Saw J, Gulati R, Tweet M. Spontaneous coronary artery dissection: Current state of the science. A scientific statement from the American Heart Association. *Circulation.* 2018:8;137(19):e532–e557. doi: 10.1161/CIR.0000000000000564.
21. Tweet MS, Hayes SN, Codsi E, Gulati R, Rose CH, Best PJM. Spontaneous coronary artery dissection associated with pregnancy. *J Am Coll Cardiol.* 2017;70:426–435. doi: 10.1016/j.jacc.2017.05.055.
22. ACOG Practice Bulletin No. 196. Summary: Thromboembolism in pregnancy. *Obstet Gynecol.* 2018. doi: 10.1097/AOG.0000000000002706.
23. Hagen PT, Scholz DG, Edwards W. Incidence and size of patent foramen ovale during the first 10 decades of life: An autopsy study of 965 normal hearts. *Mayo Clin Proc.* 1984;59(1):17–20. doi: 10.1016/s0025-6196(12)60336-x.
24. Domitrz I, Mieszkowski J, Kaminska A. Relationship between migraine and patent foramen ovale: A study of 121 patients with migraine. *Headache.* 2007;47(9):1311–1318. doi: 10.1111/j.1526-4610.2006.00724.x.
25. van Mens TE, Scheres LJJ, de Jong PG, Leeflang MMG, Nijkeuter M, Middeldorp S. Imaging for the exclusion of pulmonary embolism in pregnancy. *Cochrane Database of Systematic Reviews.* 2017(1). doi: 10.1002/14651858.CD011053.pub2.
26. Martillotti G, Boehlen F, Robert-Ebadi H, Jastrow N, Righini M, Blondon M. Treatment options for severe pulmonary embolism during pregnancy and the postpartum period: A systematic review. *J Thromb Haemost.* 2017. doi: 10.1111/jth.13802.
27. Miller EC, Leffert L. Stroke in pregnancy: A focused update. *Anesth Analg.* 2020. doi: 10.1213/ANE.0000000000004203.
28. Too G, Wen T, Boehme AK. Timing and risk factors of postpartum stroke. *Obstet Gynecol.* 2018. doi: 10.1097/AOG.0000000000002372.
29. Zambrano MD, Miller EC. Maternal stroke: An update. *Curr Atheroscler Rep.* 2019. doi: 10.1007/s11883-019-0798-2.
30. Swartz RH, Cayley ML, Foley N, et al. The incidence of pregnancy-related stroke: A systematic review and meta-analysis. *Int J Stroke.* 2017;12(7):687–697. doi: 10.1177/1747493017723271.
31. Ladhani N, Swartz R, Foley Nea. Canadian Stroke Best Practice Consensus Statement: Acute stroke management during pregnancy. *Int J Stroke.* 2018. doi: 10.1177/1747493018786617.
32. Hasegawa J, Ikeda T, Sekizawa A, et al. Maternal death due to stroke associated with pregnancy-induced hypertension. *Circ J.* 2015;79(8):1835–1840. doi: 10.1253/circj.CJ-15-0297.

33. Katsuragi S, Tanaka H, Hasegawa J, et al. Analysis of preventability of stroke-related maternal death from the nationwide registration system of maternal deaths in Japan. *J Matern Fetal Neonatal Med.* 2018. doi: 10.1080/14767058.2017.1336222.

34. Lappin JM, Darke S, Duflou J, Kaye S, Farrell M. Fatal stroke in pregnancy and the puerperium. *Stroke.* 2018. doi: 10.1161/STROKEAHA.118.023274.

35. Wabnitz A, Bushnell C. Migraine, cardiovascular disease, and stroke during pregnancy: Systematic review of the literature. *Cephalalgia.* 2015. doi: 10.1177/0333102414554113.

36. Miller EC, Medina J, Friedman AM, Elkind MS, Boehme AK. Infection during delivery hospitalization is associated with increased risk of readmission for postpartum stroke. *Stroke.* 2019;50. doi: 10.1161/str.50.suppl-1.WMP86.

37. Mendez-Figueroa H, Dahlke JD, Vrees R, Rouse DJ. Trauma in pregnancy: An updated systematic review. *Am J Obstet Gynecol.* 209. doi: 10.1016/j.ajog.2013.01.021.

38. Garcia-Moreno C, Jansen H, Ellsberg M, Heise L, Watts CH. Prevalence of intimate partner violence: Findings from the WHO multi-country study on women's health and domestic violence. *Lancet.* 2006;368. doi: 10.1016/S0140-6736(06)69523-8.

39. Vivian-Taylor J, Roberts C, Chen J, Ford J. Motor vehicle accidents during pregnancy: A population-based study. *BJOG.* 2012. doi: 10.1111/j.1471-0528.2011.03226.x.

40. Weiss HB, Sauber-Schatz EK, Cook LJ. The epidemiology of pregnancy-associated emergency department injury visits and their impact on birth outcomes. *Accid Anal Prev.* 2008. doi: 10.1016/j.aap.2007.11.011.

41. Paterno MT, Draughon JE. Screening for intimate partner violence. *J Midwifery Womens Health.* 2015;61(3):370–375. doi: 10.1111/jmwh.12443.

42. Centers for Disease Control and Prevention. *Pregnancy Mortality Surveillance System.* 2022. Available at https://www.cdc.gov/reproductivehealth/maternal-mortality/pregnancy-mortality-surveillance-system.htm. Accessed March 12, 2023.

43. Sosa MEB. Streptococcal A infection: reemerging and virulent. *J Perinat Neonat Nurse.* 2009; 23:141–147. doi:10.1016/j.clp.2010.02.003.

44. Evans L, Rhodes A, Alhazzani W, et al. Surviving sepsis campaign: International guidelines for management of sepsis and septic shock 2021. *Intensive Care Med.* 2021;47:1181–247.

45. Avni T, Lador A, Lev S, Leibovici L, Paul M, Grossman A. Vasopressors for the treatment of septic shock: Systematic review and meta-analysis. *PLoS One.* 2015. doi: 10.1371/journal.pone.0129305.

46. Rudd RA, Seth P, David F, Scholl L. Increases in drug and opioid-involved overdose deaths—United States, 2010–2015. *MMWR Morb Mortal Wkly Rep.* 2016. doi: 10.15585/mmwr.mm655051e1.

47. America's Drug Overdose Epidemic: Data to Action. *Centers for Disease Control and Prevention.* Website. www.cdc.gov/injury/features/prescription-drug-overdose/index.html. Updated 2020. Accessed March 24, 2020.

48. Mack KA. Centers for Disease Control and Prevention (CDC): Drug-induced deaths—United States, 1999–2010. *MMWR Suppl.* 2013;62(03):161–163.

49. Bateman BT, Franklin JM, Bykov K, et al. Persistent opioid use following cesarean delivery: Patterns and predictors among opioid-naive women. *Obstet Gynecol.* 2016;71(3):353. doi: 10.1016/j.ajog.2016.03.016.

50. Cesarean Delivery Rate by State. *Centers for Disease Control and Prevention.* Website. www.cdc.gov/nchs/pressroom/sosmap/cesarean_births/cesareans.htm. Updated 2019. Accessed September 18, 2019.

51. Texas Department of Health and Human Services. Regional analysis of maternal and infant health in Texas. Public Health Region 9/10. *Maternal & Child Health Epidemiology.* 2018. Website: https://www.dshs.texas.gov/maternal-child-health/maternal-child-health-epidemiology-reports. Accessed March 12, 2023.

52. Alliance for Innovation on Maternal Health. *Care for pregnant and postpartum people with substance use disorder.* Website. https://saferbirth.org/psbs/care-for-pregnant-and-postpartum-people-with-substance-use-disorder/. Published 2021. Accessed 2023.

# Maternal Stroke and Acute Cerebrovascular Disease

# 10

## 10.1 INTRODUCTION

Maternal stroke is a significant cause of severe maternal morbidity and mortality. While the treatment of acute stroke in the nonpregnant population has been revolutionized in recent years through thrombolytics and mechanical thrombectomy, pregnant and postpartum people have historically been excluded from acute stroke clinical trials. Thus, there is a paucity of high-quality evidence to guide the management of maternal stroke. This chapter describes maternal stroke risk factors and subtypes, reviews the typical signs and symptoms of maternal stroke, and proposes an approach to the "OB Stroke Alert" to be used in the out-of-hospital, emergency triage, and inpatient settings. It also briefly reviews special considerations in post-stroke care for pregnant or postpartum people.

## 10.2 LEARNING OBJECTIVES

Learner will appropriately

- Define stroke, including stroke subtypes.
- Recognize the risk factors and presenting symptoms and signs of a maternal stroke.
- Use the **SCAN ME** mnemonic to recall "red flag" features of headache.
- Understand out-of-hospital protocols for maternal stroke.
- Describe acute stroke protocols in the emergency department and inpatient setting, including neuroimaging and activation of the Maternal Stroke Team (MAST).
- Describe the initial management of hyperacute ischemic stroke, including large vessel occlusion (LVO).
- Describe the initial management of cerebral venous thrombosis.
- Describe the initial management of intracerebral and subarachnoid hemorrhage.
- Describe the post-stroke care needs of pregnant and postpartum people.

### 10.2.1 Overview and General Principles of Maternal Stroke Care

Pregnant and postpartum people have approximately triple the risk of stroke than nonpregnant people of childbearing age.[1] Stroke is responsible for 7.7% of maternal deaths in the United States.[2] However, the impact of stroke on maternal mortality may be underestimated since hypertensive pregnancy disorders account for another 6.9% of maternal deaths, and intracerebral hemorrhage, a particularly deadly stroke subtype, is a significant cause of death in people with hypertensive disorders of pregnancy. Additionally, pregnancy-specific disorders such as gestational hypertension, preeclampsia, and HELLP (hemolysis, elevated liver enzymes, and low platelets) syndrome are associated with acute cerebrovascular disease, including posterior reversible encephalopathy syndrome, reversible cerebral vasoconstriction syndrome, and hypertensive intracerebral hemorrhage.[3] Changes in the maternal coagulation system put people at higher risk of thromboembolic events, including ischemic stroke, during pregnancy and postpartum.

Far from being a single disorder, "stroke" is a heterogeneous collection of acute cerebrovascular disorders. There are two broad categories and many subcategories of stroke (Table 10.1). The first is **ischemic stroke**, caused by interruption of blood supply to a specific area of brain, retina, or spinal cord. The second is **hemorrhagic stroke**, defined as non-traumatic bleeding into the subarachnoid space, ventricles, or brain parenchyma.[4]

DOI: 10.1201/9781003299288-11

**Approximately half of maternal strokes are hemorrhagic. In contrast, only 13% of strokes are hemorrhagic in the general population**. It is often impossible to differentiate these stroke types without brain imaging. It is critically important that clinicians recognize the warning signs and symptoms of maternal stroke to ensure rapid diagnosis and appropriate treatment (Table 10.1).

While acute stroke treatment differs drastically depending on stroke subtype, some general stroke management principles apply to all strokes. The most important of these is "time is brain." Each minute of interruption of blood supply in a large vessel arterial ischemic stroke results in the loss of 1.9 million neurons and 14 billion synapses.[5] Patients can quickly deteriorate and may require emergent neurosurgical interventions to prevent devastating or fatal brain injury. Several unique considerations to rapid diagnosis and treatment apply to pregnant or postpartum people. As such, it is critical that obstetricians are involved in this acute decision-making process.

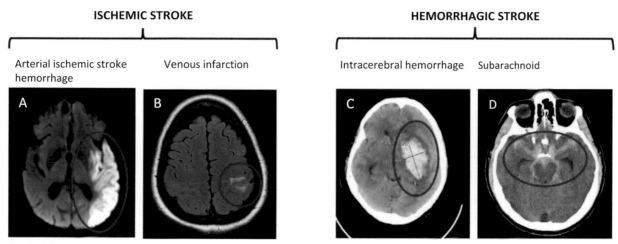

Stroke Subtypes
A. MRI showing acute arterial ischemic stroke in left middle cerebral artery territory.
B. MRI showing venous infarction from acute cerebral venous sinus thrombosis (not shown).
C. CT brain showing acute intracerebral hemorrhage in left basal ganglia
D. CT brain showing acute subarachnoid hemorrhage from a ruptured intracranial aneurysm.

**FIGURE 10.1**   Stroke types.

**TABLE 10.1**   Stroke Subtypes, Mechanisms, Symptoms/Signs, and Treatment Options

| STROKE SUBTYPE | COMMON MECHANISMS IN THE PREGNANT AND POSTPARTUM POPULATION | TYPICAL SIGNS AND SYMPTOMS* | TREATMENT OPTIONS |
|---|---|---|---|
| **Arterial ischemic stroke/Transient ischemic attack** | • Cardioembolism<br>• Cervical artery dissection<br>• Hypercoagulable state<br>• Paradoxical embolism (PFO)<br>• RCVS | • Focal neurologic deficits (e.g., facial droop, unilateral weakness, speech difficulty, vertigo, diplopia)<br>• Sudden-onset headache | • Anticoagulation<br>• Antiplatelet<br>• Decompressive hemicraniectomy (severe strokes)<br>• Intravenous thrombolysis (rtPA)<br>• Mechanical thrombectomy |
| **Venous infarction**[a] | • Cerebral venous sinus thrombosis<br>• Cortical vein thrombosis | • Altered mental status<br>• Blurred vision<br>• Gradual-onset headache<br>• Nausea/vomiting | • Anticoagulation<br>• Endovascular thrombolysis |
| **Intracerebral hemorrhage** | • Arteriovenous malformation rupture<br>• Cerebral venous thrombosis<br>• Coagulopathy<br>• Hypertensive hemorrhage with or without features of PRES | • Altered mental status<br>• Loss of consciousness<br>• Nausea/vomiting<br>• Posturing<br>• Seizures<br>• Sudden-onset headache | • Arterial embolization<br>• Blood pressure control<br>• Neurosurgical clot evacuation<br>• Ensure the reversal of coagulopathy |

*(Continued)*

**TABLE 10.1**    Stroke Subtypes, Mechanisms, Symptoms/Signs, and Treatment Options (Continued)

| STROKE SUBTYPE | COMMON MECHANISMS IN THE PREGNANT AND POSTPARTUM POPULATION | TYPICAL SIGNS AND SYMPTOMS* | TREATMENT OPTIONS |
|---|---|---|---|
| **Subarachnoid hemorrhage** | • Cerebral aneurysm rupture<br>• Cerebral venous thrombosis<br>• Coagulopathy<br>• RCVS | • Altered mental status<br>• Cardiac arrest<br>• Loss of consciousness<br>• Nausea/vomiting<br>• Posturing<br>• Seizures<br>• Sudden-onset headache | • Aneurysm coiling or clipping<br>• Blood pressure control<br>• Intraarterial calcium channel blocker infusion (RCVS)<br>• Reversal of coagulopathy |

Abbreviations: PFO, patent foramen ovale; PRES, posterior reversible encephalopathy syndrome; RCVS, reversible cerebral vasoconstriction syndrome; rtPA, recombinant tissue plasminogen activator.
ª (Cerebral ischemia secondary to congestion from venous thrombosis.)
* **Note**: This list of signs and symptoms is not comprehensive, and strokes of all types may present with variable symptoms depending on the part of the affected central nervous system. Any new focal neurologic deficit should prompt immediate activation of the Maternal Stroke Team.

## 10.2.2  Risk Factors

Figure 10.2 shows the risk factors for maternal stroke. Structural inequities encompass the structural forms of racism that have resulted in racial minorities bearing a disproportionate burden of morbidity and mortality.[6]

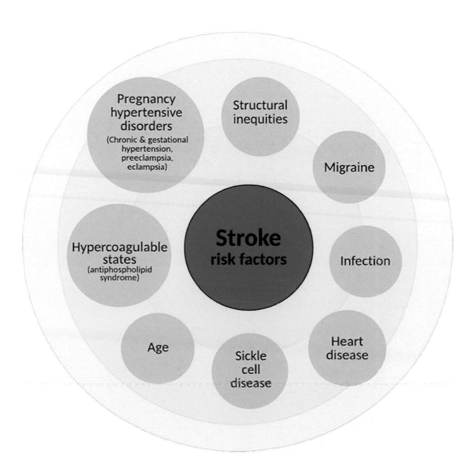

**FIGURE 10.2**    Stroke risk factors during pregnancy and postpartum.

# 10.3 TIMING

While stroke can occur at any time in pregnancy, most epidemiologic studies have found that the risk for maternal stroke is highest around delivery and in the first 2 weeks postpartum (Figure 10.3). Stroke risk can persist several months postpartum, and risk of some etiologies may persist even longer.

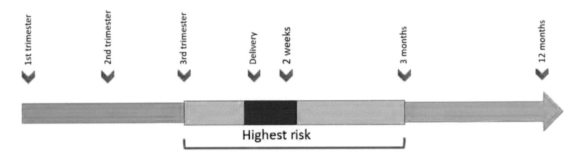

**FIGURE 10.3** Risk of stroke in pregnancy and postpartum.[7]

---

**KEY POINTS**

- Approximately half of maternal strokes are hemorrhagic.
- "Time is brain." Human nervous tissue is rapidly and irretrievably lost as stroke progresses.
- The highest risk period for maternal stroke is around the time of delivery and postpartum.

---

# 10.4 RECOGNIZING WARNING SIGNS AND SYMPTOMS OF MATERNAL STROKE

While useful to identify stroke symptoms, the BE-FAST mnemonic[8] (Balance, Eyes, Face, Arm, Speech, Time to call the emergency medical service) does not include those common in maternal stroke, such as headache or confusion. Carefully evaluate any pregnant or postpartum patient presenting with a headache for "red flag" features that could indicate a cerebrovascular cause. Recall these features with the **SCAN ME** mnemonic (Figure 10.4).

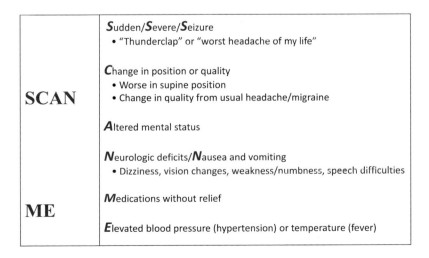

**FIGURE 10.4** SCAN ME: Red flag features of headache.

Any of these features should prompt immediate further neurologic evaluation and, in most cases, brain imaging. Obstetric Life Support recommends involving a neurologist if any red flag features of headache are present in a pregnant or postpartum person.

**KEY POINTS**
- Use the **SCAN ME** mnemonic to remember high-risk features of headache.
- Involve a neurologist if any red flag features of headache are present in a pregnant or postpartum person.

# 10.5 OUT-OF-HOSPITAL EVALUATION AND TRANSPORT OF MATERNAL STROKE

In cases of possible maternal stroke, the primary goals of an EMS provider are to do the following:

1. **STABILIZE** ABCs
2. **IDENTIFY** if patient is pregnant or postpartum, and any possible stroke symptoms
3. **HISTORY** obtain basic obstetric and neurologic history
4. **TRIAGE** patient to the appropriate receiving facility using the "OB Stroke Alert"
5. **NOTIFY** the MAST before arrival

## 10.5.1 ABCs

Assess and support airway, breathing, and circulation as for any patient and as described elsewhere in this manual. Check fingerstick blood glucose and administer glucose as indicated.

## 10.5.2 Identify Possible Stroke

Signs and symptoms of stroke are numerous and overlap across the stroke subtypes of acute ischemic stroke (AIS), ICH, and SAH. EMS providers should assess for facial droop, arm drift, and slurred speech—findings consistent with stroke (Table 10.2 and Figure 10.5). If clinical evidence of a stroke is present, EMS providers should activate the OB Stroke Alert and transport the patient immediately.

In addition to the standard Cincinnati Prehospital Stroke Scale (Figure 10.5), the VAN scale, which stands for Vision, Aphasia, Neglect, can help to identify large strokes that may benefit from thrombectomy[9,10] (Table 10.2). Patients who screen positive on the VAN scale should be transported to a thrombectomy-capable stroke center, if possible.

### 10.5.2.1 Important Note

- Posterior circulation strokes can be difficult to recognize using standard stroke screening tools. Be alert for signs such as **severe headache, nausea and vomiting, confusion, gait instability, or vision changes** which can be signs of posterior circulation stroke.
- When in doubt, activate the alert!

**TABLE 10.2**  Signs and Symptoms of Intracranial Hemorrhage and Subarachnoid Hemorrhage

BE ALERT for the following signs and symptoms:
- Severe headache
- Loss of consciousness
- Confusion or disorientation
- Seizure

**ASSESS** for:

1. **Facial droop.** Ask patient to smile. If one side of the face does not move as well as the other, this is abnormal.
2. **Arm drift.** Ask the patient to close their eyes and extend both arms in front of them for 10 seconds. If one arm cannot extend or drifts downward within 10 seconds, this is abnormal.

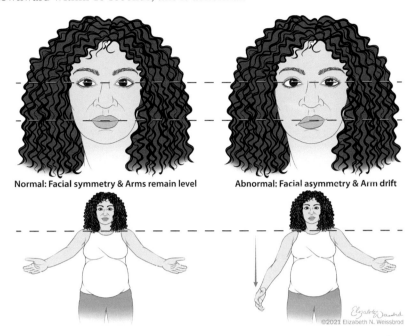

Normal: Facial symmetry & Arms remain level          Abnormal: Facial asymmetry & Arm drift

©2021 Elizabeth N. Weissbrod

3. **Speech disturbance.** Ask patient to repeat "The bird flew in the blue sky." If patient slurs words, uses the wrong words, or cannot speak, this is abnormal.

**FIGURE 10.5**   Screening for stroke: Cincinnati Prehospital Stroke Scale.[11]

**TABLE 10.3**   VAN (Vision, Aphasia, Neglect) Screening Tool for Large Vessel Occlusion

| | |
|---|---|
| **How weak is the patient?** Raise both arms up. | ☐ Mild (minor drift) |
| | ☐ Moderate (severe drift, touches or nearly touches) |
| | ☐ Severe (flaccid or no antigravity) |
| | ☐ No weakness → patient is VAN negative |
| Exceptions: In confused or comatose patients with dizziness, focal findings, or no reason for their altered mental status; basilar artery thrombus must be considered. | |
| **Visual disturbance** | ☐ Field cut (four quadrants) |
| | ☐ Double vision |
| | ☐ Blind, new onset |
| | ☐ None |
| **Aphasia** | ☐ Expressive (inability to speak or paraphasic errors; do not count slurring of words) |
| | ☐ Receptive (not understanding or following commands) |
| | ☐ Mixed |
| | ☐ None |
| **Neglect** | ☐ Forced gaze or inability to track to one side |
| | ☐ Unable to feel both sides at the same time, or unable to identify own arm |
| | ☐ Ignoring one side |
| | ☐ None |
| Patients must have weakness PLUS one or all of the V, A, or N to be VAN positive. | |

## 10.5.3  Seizure

Seizures during pregnancy or postpartum can be symptoms of stroke, particularly in the case of hemorrhagic stroke. Other common causes of seizures include the exacerbation of an underlying seizure disorder (epilepsy) or eclampsia, particularly when accompanied by systemic hypertension. As described in Chapter 4, eclamptic seizures are typically generalized; any focality such as forced gaze deviation or unilateral jerking or twitching, may indicate an underlying structural brain injury or lesion. A seizure in a pregnant or postpartum patient may be due to hormonal changes or noncompliance with anticonvulsant medications in a patient with a seizure history or eclampsia in a patient without a seizure history. See Table 10.4 for acute management of convulsive seizures.

**TABLE 10.4**  Acute Treatment of Maternal Seizure

| SEIZURE HISTORY | TREATMENT |
| --- | --- |
| Seizure in patient with no or unknown seizure history: possible eclampsia | First seizure: Magnesium sulfate IV/IO 6 g over 15–20 minutes, then start 2 g/hr infusion<br>*Alternative: Magnesium sulfate 5 mg IM into each gluteal muscle (prepare as a minimum of two injections, but preferably four due to volume)<br>Second seizure: Magnesium sulfate IV/IO 2 g over 15–20 minutes, then resume 2 g/hr infusion and consider brain imaging |
| Third seizure or seizurel lasting longer than 5 minutes or seizure in patient with known seizure history | IV/IO lorazepam 2–4 mg or IV/IO midazolam 2.5–5 mg<br>*Alternative: IM midazolam 10 mg for adults >40 kg |

Abbreviations: IM, intramuscularly; IO, intraosseous; IV, intravenous.
*Magnesium sulfate can be given IM or IO in patients presenting with seizures who do not have IV access.

## 10.5.4  Obtain a Basic Obstetric and Neurologic History

Identifying several key historical features can assist with triage and be helpful for receiving teams, especially if the patient's neurologic status declines en route to a receiving facility (Table 10.5).

**TABLE 10.5**  Important Elements of Patient History

- "Last known well," most recent time the patient was seen at her baseline level of consciousness and neurologic status, before symptom onset—the more specific, the better. If a patient wakes up with symptoms, the "last known well" or normal baseline may be the night before
- Gestational age or time since delivery
- Presence of pregnancy or birth complications (hypertension, blood clots, infections)
- Any history of neurologic conditions (stroke or seizure)
- Current medications—if possible, bring the bottles or list

## 10.5.5  Patient Transport

Pregnant or postpartum people (up to 1 year following delivery) who report or are found to have any of the previously listed signs or symptoms have a possible maternal neurologic emergency and should be transported as quickly as possible to the closest appropriate facility. When feasible, it is optimal to transport to a facility that provides both comprehensive stroke care and obstetric services.

If no such facility is available, transport patients to the nearest stroke-ready center in accordance with standard stroke guidelines. Regardless of the facility, patients should be taken to the adult ED and not to labor and delivery triage. The ED provides easier access to imaging facilities. EMS providers should alert the MAST at the receiving facility before transporting the patient.

**KEY POINTS**

- Stabilize the ABCs.
- Pharmacologically terminate seizures.
- EMS providers should share initial signs and symptoms of stroke and key elements of the patient history with the receiving MAST.
- If possible, transport patients with a suspected maternal neurologic emergency to a facility that provides both comprehensive stroke care and obstetric services.

# 10.6  OBSTETRIC STROKE PROTOCOL

Following are the primary goals of the MAST (Figure 10.6):

- Stabilize the ABCs.
- Evaluate for possible stroke with imaging.
- Obtain/confirm further history, as indicated.

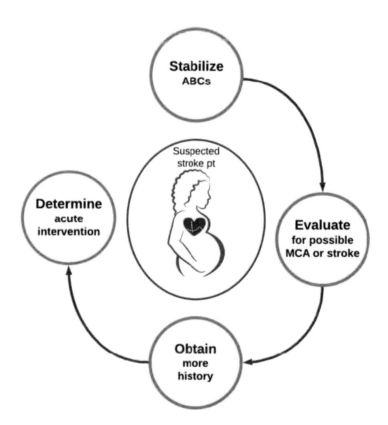

**FIGURE 10.6**  MAST responsibilities.

- Determine whether the patient is a candidate for acute intervention (tPA, thrombectomy, surgical evacuation of hemorrhage).
- Admit the patient to the proper inpatient team for further management with input from the MAST.

## 10.7  MATERNAL STROKE TEAM COMPOSITION

Hospitals should designate a MAST that is activated with a single call. A unified call to action will bring an established response team with the proper personnel and resources to the patient's bedside. Decreasing the MAST's response time is critical to improving maternal survival. MAST personnel are divided into two teams: core and contingency, as available:

- *Core*: personnel primarily managing the hyperacute stroke code
- *Contingency*: personnel ready for involvement, as indicated

Figure 10.7 and Table 10.6 outline the MAST teams and members. All team members must communicate effectively. See Chapter 11 for more details on effective communication among team members.

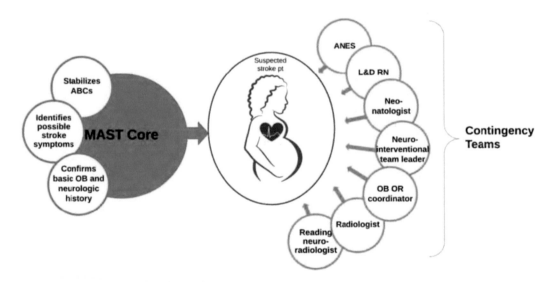

**FIGURE 10.7**   MAST core team responsibilities and contingency teams.

**TABLE 10.6**   Recommended Composition of a Maternal Stroke Team

| Core | • ED or primary team physician (team leader) |
| --- | --- |
| | • Inpatient pharmacist |
| | • Neurologist |
| | • Obstetrician and/or maternal-fetal medicine specialist |
| | • Nursing support |
| | • For inpatient stroke codes only: Rapid Response team |
| Contingency | • Anesthesiologist (ANES) |
| | • Labor and delivery charge nurse (RN) |
| | • Neonatologist |
| | • Neuro critical care intensivist |
| | • Neuro-interventional team leader |
| | • OB OR coordinator |
| | • Radiology technician and supervisors |
| | • Reading neuroradiologist |

# 10.8 STROKE CODE

First, activate the MAST and perform ABCs. Then obtain labs and establish IV access with an 18-gauge IV. All interventions are time sensitive, so it is imperative that the team and imaging are activated emergently to allow for all possible options. Interventions include rtPA or mechanical thrombectomy for AIS, surgical decompression for ICH, and extraventricular drain placement and hyperosmolar therapies for ICH and SAH.

## 10.8.1 Exam

The responding neurologist should perform a targeted neurologic exam, including a National Institutes of Health Stroke Scale (NIHSS). A remote neurologist can perform this task via telehealth technology, if necessary.

## 10.8.2 Imaging

Brain imaging is critical to making decisions about acute interventions during a stroke code. In general, **noncontrast CT head is the initial modality of choice** as it can rule out ICH, a necessary step in determining candidacy for tPA.[12,13] If resources allow, a rapid magnetic resonance imaging (MRI) can be obtained instead, though this is a lengthier procedure and often not readily available.[13] Do **not** delay the acquisition of a brain image by waiting for MRI. After getting an image and choosing whether to administer tPA, a CT angiography (CTA) or magnetic resonance angiogram (MRA) is warranted in most cases to assess for LVO or stenosis. This may be deferred at the discretion of the neurologist.

In general, the American College of Obstetricians and Gynecologists and the Society for Maternal-Fetal Medicine recommend that practitioners do **not** withhold potentially lifesaving imaging due to pregnancy. One caveat to this is MRI/A/venography (V) with gadolinium contrast. The use of gadolinium is not recommended during stroke imaging. The safety of gadolinium exposure of the fetus during the pregnancy has not been proven, and the use of gadolinium is unlikely to contribute more information than CTA during a stroke evaluation. For those patients undergoing imaging, wedge pregnant patients to the left during supine imaging to facilitate left uterine displacement after 20 weeks.[13] Table 10.8 describes the utility and speed of acquisition of different brain imaging modalities. See Figure 10.8.

**TABLE 10.7**  Initial Labs

| | |
|---|---|
| • Complete blood count (CBC) | • Point-of-care glucose |
| • Comprehensive metabolic panel (CMP) | • Type and screen |
| • aPTT | • Prenatal labs, as indicated |
| • Prothrombin time/international normalized ratio (PT/INR) | |

**TABLE 10.8**  Brain Imaging Types, Utilities, Rapidity, Availability

| TYPE | UTILITY | RAPIDITY AND AVAILABILITY |
|---|---|---|
| CT head without contrast | • Detects ICH<br>• May detect large AIS<br>• Detects mass effect/midline shift | • Rapid and easily available |
| MRI brain without contrast | • Detects AIS<br>• Detects ICH<br>• Detects mass effect/midline shift<br>• Detects edema | • Less rapid, not always available |
| CTA head and neck | • Detects LVO, aneurysm, and RCVS | • Rapid, usually available |
| MRA head and neck (without contrast) | | • Less rapid, not always available |
| CTV head | • Detects CVST | • Rapid, and usually available |
| MRV brain (without contrast) | | • Less rapid, not always available |

Abbreviations: AIS, acute ischemic stroke; CVST, cerebral venous sinus thrombosis; CT, computed, tomography; CTA, CT angiography; CTV, CT cerebral venography; ICH, intracerebral hemorrhage; LVO, large vessel occlusion; MRA, magnetic resonance angiography; MRI, magnetic resonance imaging; MRV: magnetic resonance venography; RCVS, reversible cerebral vasoconstriction syndrome.

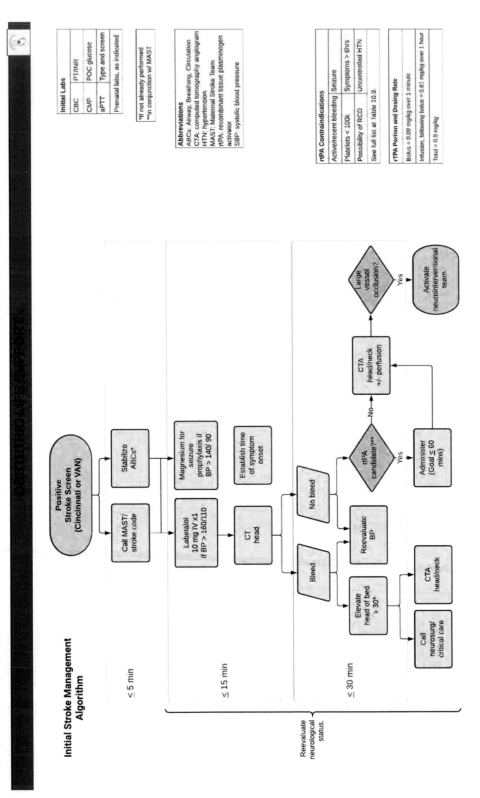

**FIGURE 10.8**   Initial Stroke Management algorithm.

## 10.8.3 Immediate Interventions for Acute Ischemic Stroke

If the initial exam and imaging suggest AIS, the patient may be a candidate for immediate reperfusion therapies, including rtPA and thrombectomy.

### 10.8.3.1 rtPA

rtPA can be administered within 4.5 hours of stroke onset or at the point at which the patient was last neurologically asymptomatic in the absence of certain exclusion criteria, see Table 10.9.

rtPA is thought not to reach or cause any direct molecular effects to the fetus—the rtPA molecule is too large to cross the placenta.[14] However, rtPA may increase the risk of maternal bleeding events, particularly in the case of imminent vaginal or surgical delivery or in the immediate postpartum period. It is not known whether rtPA increases the risk of placental abruption.[13] Notably, pregnancy, vaginal bleeding, early postpartum period, and recent lumbar dural puncture are all listed as relative but not absolute contraindications (Table 10.9).[12] **Communication between the neurologist, obstetrician/maternal-fetal medicine, and patient regarding risks and benefits is crucial.** This is particularly true in the case of fetal distress or maternal cardiac arrest that may otherwise require delivery. Clinicians should weigh the degree of suspicion for AIS, severity of neurologic deficits, risk of bleeding from rtPA, and risks to the fetus of delayed delivery in the context of the patient's wishes and values, while prioritizing the health and well-being of the patient.

rtPA is U.S. Food and Drug Administration–approved for use in patients ≥18 years of age. Therefore, practitioners may offer rtPA to pregnant or postpartum patients <18 years of age, clearly communicating that its use is off-label.

Blood pressure >185/110 is an absolute contraindication to tPA.[12] Therefore, administer IV antihypertensives as outlined in Table 9.2 before bolus infusion of rtPA.

Table 10.10 outlines rtPA dosing.[12]

**TABLE 10.9**   rtPA Contraindications (see AHA/ASA Guidelines for complete list of contraindications)[12]

| ABSOLUTE CONTRAINDICATIONS | RELATIVE CONTRAINDICATIONS |
|---|---|
| BP >185/110 mm Hg | Pregnancy |
| Mild (NIHSS ≤5) nondisabling stroke | Recent or active vaginal bleeding |
| Extensive regions of clear hypoattenuation on CTH | Early postpartum period (< 14 days after delivery) |
| Intracranial hemorrhage or head trauma | Lumbar dural puncture in the preceding 7 days |
| AIS, severe head trauma, or intracranial/spinal surgery during prior 3 months | 3–4.5 hours from last neurologic baseline and NIHSS >25 |
| History of intracranial hemorrhage | 3–4.5 hours from last neurologic baseline and prior stroke and diabetes |
| Signs and symptoms of SAH | Seizure at time of stroke onset |
| Structural gastrointestinal (GI) malignancy or recent GI bleed in the prior 21 days | Glucose levels < 50 or > 400 that are subsequently normalized |
| Platelets <100,000/mcL, INR >1.7, aPTT >40s, PT >15s* | Warfarin use and INR ≤1.7 or PT <15s |

*(Continued)*

**TABLE 10.9**    rtPA Contraindications (see AHA/ASA Guidelines for complete list of contraindications)[12] (Continued)

| ABSOLUTE CONTRAINDICATIONS | RELATIVE CONTRAINDICATIONS |
|---|---|
| Full treatment dose of low-molecular-weight heparin (LMWH) within prior 24 hours | Potential bleeding diathesis or coagulopathy |
| Dose of direct thrombin or factor Xa inhibitors within prior 48 hours | Arterial puncture of noncompressible blood vessel in the prior 7 days |
| Symptoms consistent with infective endocarditis | Major trauma not involving the head or major surgery within the prior 14 days |
| Known or suspected aortic arch dissection | Prior GI/genitourinary bleeding |
| Intra-axial intracranial neoplasm | Extracranial cervical or intracranial arterial dissection |
| Patient in maternal cardiac arrest who may be a candidate for resuscitative cesarean delivery | Unruptured intracranial aneurysm |
| | MI in the prior 3 months |
| | Acute pericarditis |
| | Systemic malignancy |
| | Hemorrhagic ophthalmic conditions |

Abbreviations: AIS, acute ischemic stroke; aPTT, activated partial thromboplastin time; GI, gastrointestinal; INR, international normalized ratio; MI, myocardial infarction; PT, prothrombin time; PTT, partial thromboplastin time; SAH, subarachnoid hemorrhage.

\*   In patients without a history of thrombocytopenia, treatment with tPA can be initiated before the availability of platelet count but should be discontinued if platelet count is <100,000/mm³. In patients without recent use of oral anticoagulants or heparin, treatment with tPA can be initiated before availability of coagulation test results. Discontinue tPA if INR is >1.7 or PT is abnormally elevated by local laboratory standards.

**TABLE 10.10**    rtPA Dosing[12]

| PORTION | DOSING AND RATE |
|---|---|
| Bolus | 0.09 mg/kg over 1 minute |
| Infusion, following bolus | 0.81 mg/kg over 1 hour |
| Total | 0.9 mg/kg |

## 10.8.3.2 Mechanical Thrombectomy

Endovascular mechanical thrombectomy can remove a clot from a large proximal vessel in the brain (LVO). Promptly perform CTA or MRA of the head and neck to detect an LVO, as mechanical thrombectomy is possible up to 6 hours after last known well, or 24 hours in select cases.[12] If appropriate, the rtPA bolus may be given before obtaining cerebrovascular imaging. If the patient has a LVO, the MAST should immediately consult the neurointerventional team (neurosurgery and/or interventional neuroradiology) to assess candidacy for thrombectomy. Given the severity of disability from a large vessel occlusion, do not withhold thrombectomy in cases of fetal distress.[13] In this situation, the neurologist, obstetrician, and neurointerventionalist should discuss the possibility of **concurrent delivery and thrombectomy** in the context of the patient's wishes and values.

**KEY POINTS**
- Administer rtPA within 4.5 hours of symptom onset or last known well in acute ischemic stroke in pregnant and postpartum patients in the absence of certain exclusion criteria. rtPA may increase risk of obstetric bleeding, and both pregnancy and the early postpartum period (<14 days) are relative exclusion criteria for rtPA.
- Perform mechanical thrombectomy in pregnant and postpartum patients within 6 hours of symptom onset or last known well, or within 24 hours in select cases, in the instance of a proximal large vessel occlusion in the brain.
- In cases of fetal distress, prioritize the health and well-being of the patient in the context of their wishes and values. Carefully weigh the risks, benefits, and relative timing of delivery and acute interventions.

## 10.9  INTRACRANIAL HEMORRHAGE

The management of ICH is quite different from that of AIS. Morbidity and mortality from ICH are often due to mass effect in the brain, causing elevated intracranial pressure (ICP), acute obstructive hydrocephalus, and in some cases, brain herniation. Primary goals in the acute management of ICH are to prevent expansion of the bleed and to manage elevated ICP. Early assessment for signs of elevated ICP is crucial (Table 10.12). Urgent cerebrovascular imaging (CTA or MRA) is warranted in all cases.[13] If vascular imaging reveals an aneurysm or vascular malformation, the neurosurgical consult should make recommendations on timing and method of securing the malformation. For a pregnant patient with impending maternal decompensation or evidence of fetal distress, this may involve concurrent delivery of the fetus.[15]

## 10.10  SUBARACHNOID HEMORRHAGE

SAH can occur secondary to rupture of a cerebral aneurysm or vascular malformation, CVST, reversible cerebral vaso-constriction syndrome, dissection, or trauma. Immediate morbidity and mortality are due to expansion of the bleed and to cerebral edema causing elevated ICP. The MAST should manage ICP and consult neurosurgery. For SAH, the blood pressure goal is SBP <140 given the possibility of an unsecured aneurysm and the risk of rebleed. If vascular imaging reveals an aneurysm or vascular malformation, the neurosurgical consultant should recommend the timing and method of securing the malformation. Patients with a SAH should generally be started on levetiracetam (500 mg by mouth, twice a day) for seizure prophylaxis given the risk of rebleed in the context of seizure and unsecured aneurysm.[15]

## 10.11  REVERSAL OF COAGULOPATHY IN INTRACRANIAL HEMORRHAGE AND SUBARACHNOID HEMORRHAGE

In most cases of ICH and SAH, coagulopathy (thrombocytopenia or treatment with heparinoids) should be reversed promptly.[16] In the case of a minor bleed and high suspicion for sinus venous thrombosis as the underlying cause, deferral of correction may be warranted. Confirm dosing regimens with a pharmacist and/or hematologist, as indicated.

**TABLE 10.11**    Reversal of Coagulopathy in Intracranial Hemorrhage and Subarachnoid Hemorrhage[16]

| CONDITION | TREATMENT |
|---|---|
| Platelets <100,000 | Platelet transfusion |
| Current therapy with heparin infusion or with subcutaneous heparin and significantly prolonged partial thromboplastin time (PTT) | Protamine sulfate 1 mg per 100 units of heparin (maximum single dose 50 mg) |
| Current therapy with low-molecular-weight heparin (off-label) | ≤8 hours from last dose: protamine sulfate 1 mg per 1 mg of enoxaparin (maximum single dose 50 mg) 8–12 hours from last dose: protamine sulfate 0.5 mg per 1 mg of enoxaparin (maximum single dose 50 mg) |
| Current therapy with vitamin K antagonist | Prothrombin complex concentrates (PCC) or fresh frozen plasma (FFP) and 5–10 mg IV vitamin K |
| Current therapy with antiplatelet | No treatment for reversal is recommended; discuss with neurosurgery if operative management is planned |

## 10.12 ELEVATED INTRACRANIAL PRESSURE IN INTRACRANIAL HEMORRHAGE AND SUBARACHNOID HEMORRHAGE

Elevated ICP may result from mass effect of blood, cerebral edema, and/or hydrocephalus. Table 10.12 reviews the signs of elevated ICP. Interventions for elevated ICP range from noninvasive (elevate the head of bed) to surgical (decompressive hemicraniectomy, surgical clot evacuation, and extraventricular drain placement). Table 10.13 lists immediate measures to begin for elevated ICP.

**TABLE 10.12**   Signs of Elevated ICP[17]

- Decreased attention and/or alertness
- Significant mass effect or midline shift on brain imaging
- Asymmetry in pupil size or reactivity to light
- Motor posturing

**TABLE 10.13**   Acute Interventions for Elevated ICP[17,18]

| PATIENTS | MONITOR GLASGOW COMA SCALE | ELEVATE HEAD OF BED 30° | HYPEROSMOLAR THERAPY | VITAL SIGNS |
|---|---|---|---|---|
| Embolic stroke | Yes | Yes | **No** | As per unit protocol |
| Signs or symptoms of ICP | Yes | Yes | • Mannitol 20% IV bolus 1 g/kg (maximum 100 g); use in-line 0.22 micron filter and infuse at maximum rate (999 mL/hr) or<br>• 3% NaCl 250 mL IV over 30 minutes (can be administered peripherally) or<br>• 23.4% NaCl 30 mL IV via central line only over 20 minutes | • Monitor for hypotension; replace urine output with IV fluids to maintain euvolemia<br>• Monitor for hypotension and pulmonary edema |

## 10.13 DELIVERY IN INTRACRANIAL HEMORRHAGE AND SUBARACHNOID HEMORRHAGE

Whether or not surgical intervention is planned, fetal delivery in ICH/SAH warrants certain special considerations due to the potential for worsening bleed, increasing ICP, and herniation with labor and dural puncture.[13]

- **Consider cesarean delivery** if poor mental status, elevated ICP (which Valsalva may worsen), or known/suspected underlying vascular lesion (including ruptured and unsecured aneurysm).
- **Consider vaginal delivery and/or forceps or vacuum extraction** if none of the previous considerations are present.
- **Discuss safety of spinal/epidural anesthesia with neurology and OB anesthesia given potentially increased risk of herniation with dural puncture** if there is significant mass effect on brain imaging.

It is imperative that the mode of delivery planning involve shared decision-making and multidisciplinary involvement with OB, neurology, and anesthesia.

**KEY POINTS**

- Causes of early morbidity and mortality in intracranial hemorrhage and subarachnoid hemorrhage are bleed expansion and herniation from elevated intracranial pressure.
- Treatments for elevated ICP include elevating the head of the bed, hyperosmolar therapies, and potentially neurosurgical decompression.
- Urgent vessel imaging is warranted in all cases of ICH or SAH.
- Start patients with SAH on prophylactic levetiracetam to prevent seizure.
- Delivery in ICH and SAH requires careful planning given the risks of worsening bleed, increasing ICP, and herniation with labor and dural puncture.

# 10.14 POST-STROKE CARE

The stroke code is only the first phase of stroke management. After stabilizing the patient, performing initial diagnostic procedures, and carrying out acute interventions, the MAST must admit the patient to the correct inpatient service, where providers can closely monitor the patient and complete the diagnostic evaluation. All patients should be treated to maintain normothermia, normoglycemia, and normonatremia. A course of antenatal corticosteroids for fetal lung maturation should be considered and is not contraindicated after stroke. For postpartum patients, offer patients breastfeeding support including the assistance of an occupational therapist and lactation consultants.

## 10.14.1 Patient Admission

In most cases, pregnant and postpartum patients with suspected or confirmed AIS, ICH, or SAH should be admitted to neurologic—not obstetric—services. This allows specially trained nurses to monitor and identify the neurologic changes that signal complications such as new or worsening hemorrhage, recurrent stroke, rising ICP, or seizure. The OB consult service should follow the patient during admission and should coordinate delivery, postpartum care, or fetal monitoring as needed.

Certain conditions warrant admission to an ICU. While neuro-ICU admission is ideal, this is not available at many hospitals. Patients admitted to a medical or surgical ICU should be followed by OB and neurology consult services. In the case of inpatient stroke, transfer from a non-neurology to a neurology unit or ICU service is often warranted.

## 10.14.2 Blood Pressure Management

Blood pressure management is crucial to prevent further neurologic injury after a neurovascular event. Blood pressure goals for various conditions and interventions are listed in Table 10.14, and acute BP management should be achieved as described in Table 9.2.

The International Society for the Study of Hypertension in Pregnancy (ISSHP) considers stroke and new-onset hypertension to be diagnostic of preeclampsia.[19] Lower blood pressure targets are therefore reasonable in all pregnant and postpartum patients with stroke.

**TABLE 10.14**  Blood Pressure Goals in Maternal Neurovascular Conditions

| CONDITION | BP GOAL |
|---|---|
| AIS, no tPA or thrombectomy | SBP ≤160, DBP ≤110 |
| AIS, tPA ± thrombectomy | SBP ≤160, DBP ≤105[12] or stricter per neurosurgery/ neurointerventional radiology based on degree of reperfusion achieved |
| AIS, thrombectomy, no tPA | SBP ≤160, DBP ≤105[12] or stricter per neurosurgery/neurointerventional radiology based on degree of reperfusion achieved |
| ICH | Initial SBP ≤160, DBP ≤110 followed by gradual reduction to SBP ≤140,[13] DBP ≤90 |
| SAH | SBP ≤140[18] |

Note: Blood pressure recommendation must be individualized, and factors such as baseline blood pressure and placental perfusion should be taken into account.

Abbreviations: AIS, acute ischemic stroke; DBP, diastolic blood pressure; ICH, intracerebral hemorrhage; SAH, subarachnoid hemorrhage; SBP, systolic blood pressure; tPA, tissue plasminogen activator.

## 10.14.3  Seizure Prophylaxis, Evaluation, and Treatment

Seizure can occur as a result of ICH and, less commonly, AIS. It is also a diagnostic feature of eclampsia, which can underlie both ICH and AIS. Refer to Table 10.3 for guidance on initial acute management of generalized seizures in the pregnant or postpartum patient.

Current American Stroke Association (ASA)/AHA guidelines recommend against empiric prophylactic antiepileptic medications in ICH in nonpregnant patients. Instead, patients with mental status changes deemed disproportionate to degree of ICH should be monitored on electroencephalogram and treated only if found to have seizures.[16] This approach is reasonable to pursue in pregnant patients as well. Magnesium sulfate for seizure prophylaxis is reasonable for any patient with stroke and SBP ≥140 and/or DBP ≥110. If seizures are identified with electroencephalogram, administer appropriate anti-seizure medications with the guidance of the neurology, neurosurgery, or neurocritical care team. In select cases, prophylactic anti-seizure medications (e.g., levetiracetam) may be recommended, particularly if neurosurgical procedures are planned. An individualized approach is favored based on the recommendations of the treating neurologist or neurosurgeon.

## 10.14.4  Venous Thromboembolism Prophylaxis

Patients with ICH, SAH, and AIS are at elevated risk of venous thromboembolism during hospitalization. Prophylactic measures should adhere to AHA/ASA guidelines to balance the risk of this complication with the risk of worsening ICH and hemorrhagic conversion of AIS (Appendix G).

## 10.14.5  Post-rtPA Care

Patients who receive rtPA require special monitoring and treatment for at least 24 hours after treatment to ensure early detection of hemorrhagic complications, particularly ICH. Table 10.15 lists the recommended care for patients who have received treatment with rtPA.

**TABLE 10.15**   Post-rtPA Care

- Perform frequent neuro and vitals checks per hospital policy
- Maintain BP <180/105 for at least 24 hours following rtPA[12]
- Avoid antiplatelet[12] and pharmacologic VTE prophylaxis for at least 24 hours following rtPA
- Repeat CT head or MRI 24 hours after tPA to assess for ICH, or immediately for any change in neurologic exam

## 10.14.6  Further Evaluation

The neurologic primary team or consult service may pursue additional diagnostic studies to elucidate stroke risk. While a description of the indications for such tests is beyond the scope of this manual, Table 10.16 provides a list of potential studies.

**TABLE 10.16**   Nonurgent Diagnostic Tests Following Maternal Neurovascular Event

- MRI brain without contrast
- Venous cerebral vessel imaging, if not already performed (CTV, MRV)
- Electrocardiogram
- Transthoracic echocardiogram ± bubble study; transesophageal echocardiogram
- Transcranial Dopplers
- Four-extremity venous Dopplers
- Hypercoagulable workup
- Urine toxicology screen

# 10.15  CEREBRAL VENOUS SINUS THROMBOSIS

CVST is a cause of both ischemic and hemorrhagic stroke for which pregnant and postpartum people are at increased risk, especially in the context of preeclampsia/eclampsia. Based on clinical presentation and initial imaging, further diagnostic testing for CVST may be warranted. Treatment for CVST is anticoagulation, even in the case of ICH, since worsening venous hypertension can worsen parenchymal bleeding. In very severe cases, patients may need endovascular thrombolysis or thrombectomy. AHA/ASA guidelines recommend treatment with LMWH over unfractionated heparin in pregnant people and continuation of LMWH or vitamin K antagonist with INR goal 2.0–3.0 for at least 6 weeks postpartum.[20] Some patients may require longer treatment.

## KEY POINTS

- Admit patients with a maternal neurologic emergency to a neurology service and/or ICU. The appropriate consultant teams should follow throughout admission.
- Inpatient stroke codes should proceed similarly to those in the ED. Following a stroke code, transfer those patients admitted to a non-neurology service to a neurology service or ICU.
- Adherence to blood pressure targets is essential to prevent secondary brain injury.
- Appropriate venous thromboembolism prophylaxis is critical to prevent this complication of stroke.
- Further diagnostic procedures may be warranted to determine the cause of stroke. If venous imaging reveals a cerebral venous sinus thrombosis, treatment with LMWH is indicated, even in ICH.

### Case Vignette

EMS providers brought a 32-year-old G1P0 at 37 weeks gestation to the ED. The patient had developed an acute inability to speak or move their right side. Last neurologic baseline 2 hours before hospital arrival. Blood pressure is 200/120, and vitals are otherwise normal. On neurologic exam, the patient is alert and attentive but has minimal and effortful speech output, answering one of two questions correctly and correctly performing one of two tasks. The team notes forced left gaze deviation, a right facial droop, right arm and leg drift to the bed within 5 seconds, and impaired sensation on the right side of body. NIHSS is 15.

### TESTS AND DATA

CT head shows no ICH. CTA shows a left middle cerebral artery occlusion. Blood glucose is 175 mg/dL. Platelets and coagulation factors are within normal limits. Fetal monitoring reveals persistent spontaneous decelerations in heart rate.

### TREATMENT DISCUSSION

The patient meets the criteria for rtPA except for elevated blood pressure and is a candidate for thrombectomy. Her deficits severely disable her. Fetal vital sign instability is an indication for emergent delivery. The team discusses the risks and benefits of rtPA and thrombectomy with the patient's partner and healthcare proxy because of the severity of aphasia. Their partner says the patient would not want to parent with this degree of disability and strongly desires the pregnancy. Because of the risks to the fetus of delayed delivery and the cesarean section risks after rtPA, the team and proxy choose not to use rtPA and proceed with thrombectomy and cesarean section.

### TREATMENT AND OUTCOME

The patient undergoes successful endovascular clot retrieval and reperfusion of the left middle cerebral artery, and immediate cesarean section. Admitted to the neurologic ICU, the patient is given magnesium prophylaxis for preeclampsia, and blood pressure is maintained (<160/110). Later, the patient is discharged to an acute inpatient rehabilitation facility. Three months later, they have mild speech difficulty, are walking as they were before giving birth, and can hold their child without assistance.

# CHAPTER 10. PRACTICE QUESTIONS

1. Which period has the highest risk of maternal stroke?
   A. The risk is equally distributed throughout pregnancy
   B. Antepartum
   C. Intrapartum/early postpartum
   D. Late postpartum

2. What is the SCAN ME mnemonic used to remember?
   A. Types of brain imaging and their indications
   B. Concerning features of headache
   C. Exam maneuvers in a potential maternal stroke
   D. Steps to perform in a maternal stroke code

3. Which of the following should a practitioner initially order in a maternal stroke code?
   A. CT head with contrast
   B. CT head without contrast
   C. MRI brain with contrast
   D. MRI brain without contrast

4. Which of the following is an absolute contraindication to rtPA administration?
   A. Recent or active vaginal bleeding
   B. Early postpartum period (<14 days after delivery)
   C. BP >185/110 mm Hg
   D. Lumbar dural puncture in the preceding 7 days

5. Treatments for elevated ICP include:
   A. Trendelenburg
   B. Furosemide
   C. Hyposmolar therapies
   D. Neurosurgical decompression

6. What is the MOST appropriate admitting service for the case vignette?
   A. Neurologic ICU
   B. Labor and delivery
   C. Regular neurology floor bed
   D. Medical ICU

# CHAPTER 10. ANSWERS

1. **ANSWER: C.** Most epidemiologic studies have found that the risk for maternal stroke is highest around delivery and postpartum, particularly in the first 2 weeks after delivery.
2. **ANSWER: B.** The **SCAN ME** mnemonic is useful to identify concerning features of headache that may indicate a neurovascular cause. SCAN ME stands for Sudden/Severe/Seizure, Change in position or quality, Altered mental status, Neurologic deficits/Nausea and vomiting, Medications without relief, and Elevated blood pressure or temperature.
3. **ANSWER: B.** A CT head without contrast is fast and effective at ruling out a bleed in the brain, which is a prerequisite for rtPA administration. MRI brain without contrast is more sensitive than CT at detecting AIS and may be obtained first in certain circumstances.
4. **ANSWER: C.** BP >185/110 is an absolute contraindication to rtPA administration; the other answer choices are relative contraindications.[11]
5. **ANSWER: D.** Treatments for elevated ICP include hyperosmolar therapies, elevating head of bed, and neurosurgical decompression. While hyperosmolar therapies have a diuretic effect, primary diuretics like furosemide are not effective in reducing intracranial pressure.

6. **Answer: A.** Neurologic ICU is the most appropriate. This patient requires close monitoring for hypertension and changes in neurologic exam that could indicate complications of rtPA.

# CHAPTER 10. REFERENCES

1. Swartz RH, Cayley ML, Foley N, et al. The incidence of pregnancy-related stroke: A systematic review and meta-analysis. *Int J Stroke.* 2017;12(7):687–697. doi: 10.1177/1747493017723271.

2. Centers for Disease Control and Prevention. *Pregnancy Mortality Surveillance System.* Website. www.cdc.gov/reproductivehealth/maternal-mortality/pregnancy-mortality-surveillance-system.htm?CDC_AA_refVal=https%3A%2F%2Fwww.cdc.gov%2Freproductivehealth%2Fmaternalinfanthealth%2Fpregnancy-mortality-surveillance-system.htm. Published February 4, 2020. Accessed October 17, 2020.

3. Roeder HJ, Lopez JR, Miller EC. Ischemic stroke and cerebral venous sinus thrombosis in pregnancy. *Handb Clin Neurol.* 2020;172:3–31. doi: 10.1016/B978-0-444-64240-0.00001-5. PMID: 32768092; PMCID: PMC7528571.

4. Sacco RL, Kasner SE, Broderick JP, et al. An updated definition of stroke for the 21st century: A statement for healthcare professionals from the American Heart Association/American Stroke Association. *Stroke.* 2013;44(7):2064–2089. doi: 10.1161/STR.0b013e318296aeca.

5. Saver JL. Time is brain-quantified. *Stroke.* 2006 January;37(1):263–266. doi: 10.1161/01.STR.0000196957.55928.ab. Epub 2005 December 8. PMID: 16339467.

6. National Academies of Sciences, Engineering, and Medicine. 2017. *Communities in action: Pathways to health equity.* National Academies Press. doi: 10.17226/24624. Too G, Wen T, Boehme AK, et al. Timing and risk factors of postpartum stroke. *Obstet Gynecol.* 2018;131(1):70–78. doi: 10.1097/AOG.0000000000002372.

7. Zambrano MD, Miller EC. Maternal stroke: An update. *Curr Atheroscler Rep.* 2019 June 22;21(9):33. doi: 10.1007/s11883-019-0798-2. PMID: 31230137; PMCID: PMC6815220.

8. Aroor S, Singh R, Goldstein LB. BE-FAST (Balance, eyes, face, arm, speech, time): Reducing the proportion of strokes missed using the FAST mnemonic. *Stroke.* 2017;48(2):479–481. doi: 10.1161/STROKEAHA.116.015169.

9. Teleb MS, Ver Hage A, Carter J, Jayaraman MV, McTaggart RA. Stroke vision, aphasia, neglect (VAN) assessment—A novel emergent large vessel occlusion screening tool: Pilot study and comparison with current clinical severity indices. *J Neurointerv Surg.* 2017 February;9(2):122–126. doi: 10.1136/neurintsurg-2015-012131. Epub 2016 February 17. PMID: 26891627; PMCID: PMC5284468.

10. Beume LA, Hieber M, Kaller CP, Nitschke K, Bardutzky J, Urbach H, Weiller C, Rijntjes M. Large vessel occlusion in acute stroke. *Stroke.* 2018 October;49(10):2323–2329. doi: 10.1161/STROKEAHA.118.022253. PMID: 30355088.

11. Kothari RU, Pancioli A, Liu T, Brott T, Broderick J. Cincinnati Prehospital Stroke Scale: Reproducibility and validity. *Ann Emerg Med.* 1999;33(4):373–378. doi: 10.1016/s0196-0644(99)70299-4.

12. Warner JJ, Harrington RA, Sacco RL, Elkind MSV Guidelines for the Early Management of Patients with Acute Ischemic Stroke: 2019 update to the 2018 Guidelines for the Early Management of Acute Ischemic Stroke. *Stroke.* 2019;50(12):3331–3332. doi: 10.1161/STROKEAHA.119.027708.

13. Ladhani NNN, Swartz RH, Foley N, et al. Canadian Stroke Best Practice Consensus Statement: Acute Stroke Management during pregnancy. *Int J Stroke.* 2018;13(7):743–758. doi: 10.1177/1747493018786617.

14. Gartman EJ. The use of thrombolytic therapy in pregnancy. *Obstet Med.* 2013;6(3):105–111. doi: 10.1177/1753495X13488771.

15. Connolly ES Jr, Rabinstein AA, Carhuapoma JR, Derdeyn CP, Dion J, Higashida RT, Hoh BL, Kirkness CJ, Naidech AM, Ogilvy CS, Patel AB, Thompson BG, Vespa P; American Heart Association Stroke Council; Council on Cardiovascular Radiology and Intervention; Council on Cardiovascular Nursing; Council on Cardiovascular Surgery and Anesthesia; Council on Clinical Cardiology. Guidelines for the management of aneurysmal subarachnoid hemorrhage: A guideline for healthcare professionals from the American Heart Association/American Stroke Association. *Stroke.* 2012 June;43(6):1711–1737. doi: 10.1161/STR.0b013e3182587839. Epub 2012 May 3. PMID: 22556195.

16. Hemphill JC 3rd, Greenberg SM, Anderson CS, Becker K, Bendok BR, Cushman M, Fung GL, Goldstein JN, Macdonald RL, Mitchell PH, Scott PA, Selim MH, Woo D; American Heart Association Stroke Council; Council on Cardiovascular and Stroke Nursing; Council on Clinical Cardiology. Guidelines for the management of spontaneous intracerebral hemorrhage: A guideline for healthcare professionals from the American Heart Association/American Stroke Association. *Stroke.* 2015 July;46(7):2032–2060. doi: 10.1161/STR.0000000000000069. Epub 2015 May 28. PMID: 26022637.

17. Carney N, Totten A, O'Reilly C, et al. Brain Trauma Foundation. Website. https://braintrauma.org/guidelines/guidelines-for-the-management-of-severe-tbi-4th-ed. Published September 2016. Accessed October 19, 2020.

18. Frontera JA. *Decision making in neurocritical care.* Thieme; 2009.

19. Brown MA, Magee LA, Kenny LC, Karumanchi SA, McCarthy FP, Saito S, Hall DR, Warren CE, Adoyi G, Ishaku S; International Society for the Study of Hypertension in Pregnancy (ISSHP). The hypertensive disorders of pregnancy: ISSHP classification, diagnosis and management recommendations for international practice. *Pregnancy Hypertens.* 2018 July;13:291–310. doi: 10.1016/j.preghy.2018.05.004. Epub 2018 May 24. PMID: 29803330.

20. Saposnik G, Barinagarrementeria F, Brown RD Jr, Bushnell CD, Cucchiara B, Cushman M, deVeber G, Ferro JM, Tsai FY; American Heart Association Stroke Council and the Council on Epidemiology and Prevention. Diagnosis and management of cerebral venous thrombosis: A statement for healthcare professionals from the American Heart Association/American Stroke Association. *Stroke.* 2011 April;42(4):1158–1192. doi: 10.1161/STR.0b013e31820a8364. Epub 2011 February 3. PMID: 21293023.

# Post-Arrest Care

11

## 11.1 INTRODUCTION

This chapter discusses the 2020 AHA guidelines for immediate post-arrest care in addition to recommendations specific to pregnant or postpartum patients.[1] Continuation of effective post-arrest care can lead to an improved likelihood of survival to discharge; therefore, it is critical for practitioners to know the immediate next steps after ROSC or death. This chapter also reviews factors to consider when deciding to stop resuscitation efforts during a maternal code and the recommended steps to take after a maternal death.

## 11.2 LEARNING OBJECTIVES

Learner will appropriately

- Review the 2020 AHA guidelines for immediate post-arrest care in the adult patient.
- Describe appropriate timing, criteria, and steps to ensure maternal hemodynamic stability immediately following ROSC.
- Review the Post-ROSC Checklist.
- Describe appropriate timing and criteria for targeted temperature management (TTM).
- Describe appropriate indication for extracorporeal cardiopulmonary resuscitation (ECPR) and organ transplantation with determination of circulatory death.

## 11.3 IMPORTANCE OF POST-ARREST CARE

Two-thirds of nonpregnant patients in the hospital who have cardiac arrest do not survive to discharge,[2,3] and for OH cardiac arrest, survival to discharge is only 6.8%. Pregnant people have better outcomes, with 58.9% surviving to discharge[4-6] often with limited, or no, sequelae after cardiac arrest. Many pregnant patients receive prolonged CPR (some upward of 55 minutes or more) and ECPR during their care.[7-15] Providers must be aware of the critical pregnancy-specific considerations that occur immediately following ROSC and the steps to take after a death from MCA.

DOI: 10.1201/9781003299288-12

## 11.4 STANDARD POST-RETURN OF SPONTANEOUS CIRCULATION CHECKLIST AFTER MATERNAL CARDIAC ARREST

Follow the principles of ABCDEFGH after ROSC:

**A**irway
**B**reathing
**C**irculation
**D**isability[16]
**E**CPR
**E**tiology
**F**etus
**G**ather
**H**ead

See Table 11.2 and Appendices E and F for the Post-ROSC Care Checklists.

## 11.5 <u>A</u>IRWAY

After an MCA, most patients will have an advanced airway in place. If they were not intubated prior to ROSC, intubation should now be performed, with continuous waveform capnography monitoring. It is also reasonable to consider stomach decompression with placement of an orogastric or nasogastric tube to reduce the risk of aspiration. A chest radiograph is recommended to ensure proper ET tube placement, regardless of when the tube was placed.

## 11.6 <u>B</u>REATHING

Post-ROSC, continue to avoid hyperventilation and maintain oxygenation status >94%. Initial ventilation settings should be set to standard settings. Oxygenation can be controlled via positive end-expiratory pressure (PEEP) and fraction of inspired oxygen ($FiO_2$) adjustments. It is crucial to minimize over-oxygenation and maintain normocarbia (end-tidal $CO_2$ 30–40 mm Hg or $PaCO_2$ 35–45 mm Hg) unless otherwise indicated.

## 11.7 <u>C</u>IRCULATION

One of the essential pregnancy-specific modifications in the post-arrest patient is to **continue LUD if the patient remains pregnant**. If ROSC is achieved in the field, put the patient in full left lateral tilt or continue left uterine displacement until they can be positioned into a left lateral tilt. If the patient is in the hospital, perform LUD until they are transported to the ICU. Here, place the patient on a rotator bed or place a wedge under their left hip. However best accomplished, continued LUD is critical to avoid rearrest.

In the post-arrest phase, providers should establish central and arterial lines and maintain normotension using IV fluids and vasopressors as needed. At least one large-bore IV (preferably two) should be above the diaphragm if the patient remains pregnant. The goals of vasopressor therapy are to maintain a mean arterial pressure (MAP) of ≥65 mm Hg, preferably >80 mm Hg, and systolic blood pressure (SBP) of ≥90 mm Hg. Prompt correction of hypotension can reduce mortality rates. Several studies have shown improved neurologic outcomes with higher MAPs, especially in the initial post-ROSC period.[17]

Another critical component of post-ROSC care is the use of a 12-lead electrocardiogram (ECG). If the ECG indicates a coronary etiology of arrest (such as STEMI or non-ST-segment elevation myocardial infarction [NSTEMI]), emergent coronary angiography is recommended even if comatose.[18] If acute myocardial infarction is suspected or confirmed in the pregnant or recently and newly postpartum patient, coronary angiography is recommended, similar to the nonpregnant patient.[19]

If ECG does not show evidence of a cardiac event, it is reasonable to consider POC-US to evaluate for other possible etiologies of an arrest. In addition to the physical exam and clinical findings, use POC-US to evaluate for possible massive pulmonary embolism, tension pneumothorax, or pericardial tamponade. If the patient is stable, consider further imaging, such as CT, to rule out pulmonary embolism.

Stroke should always be considered as a possible cause of cardiac arrest. SAH is associated with neurogenic myocardial stunning,[20] myocardial infarction, and arrhythmias.[21] Occlusion of the basilar artery can also cause sudden loss of consciousness, convulsive activity, and respiratory arrest.[22] For this reason, Obstetric Life Support recommends brain imaging with noncontrast head CT and, if possible, CT angiography in the emergency department as soon as the patient is stabilized. This helps to rule out intracranial hemorrhage or large cerebral artery occlusion prior to initiation of targeted temperature management.

Other clinical markers of adequate perfusion, such as urine output and cardiac output, remain undefined even in the nonpregnant population, and no targeted metrics are recommended at this time. However, accurate inputs and outputs should be monitored and recorded using an indwelling urinary catheter.

Additional post-arrest labs should include arterial blood gas, lactic acid, and others as indicated based on the most likely etiology of the MCA. In post-MCA patients, avoid hypoglycemia and manage glucose for critical care patients, with no alterations for pregnant or postpartum mothers.

# 11.8  DISABILITY

## 11.8.1  Targeted Temperature Management

TTM is recommended for the neuroprotection of post-ROSC patients who are comatose. TTM is not required if the patient is following commands. Limited case reports describe the use of TTM in post-ROSC pregnant patients with good outcomes; thus, TTM is recommended in this population.[23] The 2020 AHA guidelines for cardiac arrest in pregnancy recommend a constant temperature between 32°C and 36°C for TTM.

If patients are at increased risk for bleeding or have intracranial hemorrhage, set a temperature closer to 36°C,[24] with lower temperatures more beneficial in patients who exhibit seizures or cerebral edema.[25]

TTM is recommended for at least 24 hours post-ROSC. Studies demonstrate that patients who undergo at least 24 hours of TTM have better neurologic outcomes, due in part to avoidance of fever.[26]

The 2020 AHA guidelines do not recommend TTM via cold IV fluid replacement for patients who are being transported post-ROSC following an OH arrest. TTM started in the OH setting does not improve survival to discharge and has been shown to increase the risk of pulmonary edema and rearrest.[27]

## 11.8.2  Prevention of Major Disability in Mechanically Ventilated Patients in the Intensive Care Unit

Ventilator-associated pneumonia (VAP) results from microaspiration of pathogenic bacteria from the oropharynx and upper airways. VAP affects approximately 15% of mechanically ventilated patients in the ICU. VAP typically occurs between 48 hours and 10 days of mechanical ventilation.[28] Table 11.1 lists the risk factors and most important pathogens associated with VAP, including antibiotic-resistant organisms.[28]

**TABLE 11.1**  Risk Factors and Common Pathogens Isolated in VAP in Pregnant and Postpartum Patients[28]

| Risk factors | • History of abdominal surgery<br>• Functional debilitation (e.g., prolonged immobilization or hospitalization) |
|---|---|
| Pathogens | • *Pseudomonas aeruginosa*<br>• Methicillin-sensitive *Staphylococcus aureus*<br>• Methicillin-resistant *S. aureus* (MRSA)<br>• Listeria |

Infection with a drug-resistant organism markedly increases morbidity and mortality in VAP. The risk factors for post-ROSC VAP infection with a drug-resistant organism in pregnancy and postpartum patients include

- prior IV antibiotic treatment within the previous 90 days,
- septic shock at time of VAP,
- ARDS preceding VAP,
- hospitalization for ≥5 days prior to the occurrence of VAP, and
- acute renal replacement therapy prior to VAP onset.

Use of high-dose corticosteroids, such as betamethasone used for fetal lung maturity, increase the risk of *Legionella* and *Pseudomonas* infections.[28]

VAP bundles have been advocated to reduce the risk of developing VAP and decreased mortality. While pregnancy was not an included criterion in the studies of VAP bundles, these simple measures should also be followed in pregnant or postpartum patients post-ROSC. The recommendations from VAP bundles include elevating the head of the bed at least 30°, interrupting daily sedation, assessing readiness to extubate, using subglottic secretion drainage, and avoiding scheduled ventilator circuit changes.[27] Because proton pump inhibitors raise the pH of the stomach contents and promote colonization with potentially pathogenic organisms, stress ulcer prevention remains a balance of risk between GI bleeding and development of VAP.[29] Recent randomized trials have also shown that oral chlorhexidine washes are associated with increased mortality in nonpregnant, non–cardiac surgery patients. Based on this evidence, the Intensive Care Society does not recommend using oral chlorhexidine in non–cardiac surgery patients, and the National Institute for Health and Care Excellence (NICE) has recently withdrawn oral chlorhexidine washes from its VAP prevention recommendations.[30]

## 11.8.3 The Post-ROSC Patient Who Is Delivered

Guidelines and recommendations for post-arrest care in patients who are delivered, typically by RCD, are largely based on case studies. It is reasonable to apply nonpregnant post-arrest checklist therapies to a patient who has undergone an RCD and achieves ROSC.

Because a patient's risk of bleeding is significantly higher after MCA and RCD due to postoperative changes and the recent pregnancy, TTM may be considered at higher temperatures to decrease the chances of significant bleeding.

## 11.8.4 The Post-ROSC Patient Who Remains Undelivered

Routine post-arrest care measures, such as TTM and VAP bundles, should be implemented in the undelivered patient as indicated. While data are limited on maternal-fetal dyad who undergo TTM after ROSC, TTM is currently recommended in these patients if they would otherwise qualify.

If the patient achieved ROSC prior to RCD or is <20 weeks, place her in the full left lateral decubitus position by placing a wedge under her left hip or perform continuous LUD. This will help to minimize the risk of rearrest.

## 11.8.5 Seizure Prevention

The prevalence of post-arrest seizures is as high as 22%. If seizures occur post-ROSC, electroencephalogram (EEG) monitoring is recommended.[31] Importantly, as many as 12% of patients develop nonconvulsive status epilepticus after cardiac arrest, and outcomes are extremely poor in this population.[32] Consequently, OBLS recommends early consultation with a neurologist in all patients after cardiac arrest, prompt brain imaging, and consideration of continuous EEG monitoring in comatose patients undergoing TTM.[33] Use anticonvulsants as recommended for status epilepticus protocols. In post-arrest patients who remain pregnant, use similar seizure protocols, with benzodiazepines recommended as first-line therapy. Patients with neurologic complications like stroke or status epilepticus need to be managed at a facility that can provide appropriate care given these needs.

## 11.9 EXTRACORPOREAL CARDIOPULMONARY RESUSCITATION

The 2020 AHA pregnancy guidelines do not specifically address using ECPR in cases of refractory MCA. Based on multiple case reports of MCA and successful outcomes with ECPR, OBLS recommends considering the application of ECPR for refractory CPR during MCA, regardless of delivery status. Teams caring for patients in MCA should consider early notification of the ECPR team(s) closest to their facility.

## 11.10 ETIOLOGY

Use the BAACC TO LIFE mnemonic to identify the possible cause of arrest. Teams must consider the risk of rearrest and can optimize treatment when having identified the proper etiology quickly.

## 11.11 FETUS

If the patient is considered ≥23 weeks pregnant (viable) and undelivered, perform continuous LUD after ROSC is achieved and during TTM. Continuous fetal monitoring can be completed in the ICU while the patient is intubated. Intermittent fetal monitoring occurring at several discrete times during the day may be an alternative monitoring plan, depending on maternal or fetal status. If a nonreassuring fetal heart rate tracing develops during either continuous or intermittent monitoring, providers should consider the possibility of impending maternal decompensation, and the patient should be emergently evaluated. There should be a low threshold for delivery in the post-arrest patient with maternal or fetal decompensation, and this may need to occur in the ICU setting. An RCD kit should be maintained at the patient's bedside.

### 11.11.1 Post-Arrest Medications and Fetal Toxicity

While concerns about fetal toxicity and teratogenicity (disruption of development resulting in birth defects) are highest in the first trimester, indicated medications and treatments should continue to be used to optimize post-arrest care of the patient. No necessary treatments or imaging studies should be withheld due to pregnancy concerns. If reasonable alternatives exist that are safer in pregnancy, it is acceptable to use these drugs preferentially in pregnant post-ROSC patients.

### 11.11.2 Antepartum Corticosteroids and Magnesium Sulfate for Neuroprotection

If the pregnant post-arrest patient is between 23 and 0/7 and 36 and 6/7 weeks gestation (i.e., viable to late preterm in their pregnancy), a 48-hour course of antepartum steroids (e.g., betamethasone 12 mg IM q 24 hours × 2 doses) is recommended unless contraindications exist. Antepartum steroids accelerate fetal lung maturity and thus increase the chances of neonatal survival in cases of spontaneous or indicated preterm births (which could occur in cases of rearrest resulting in RCD, or maternal decompensation resulting in the need for delivery). If the post-arrest patient is between 23 and 0/7 and 31 and 6/7 weeks gestation, it is also recommended to start IV magnesium sulfate to improve fetal neurologic outcomes (decrease rates of cerebral palsy) if delivery becomes necessary (or imminent).[34] The dose of magnesium sulfate is 6 g IV bolus over 15–20 minutes, followed by 2 g/hr.[35]

Magnesium sulfate for fetal neuroprotection is typically given for 4 hours prior to anticipated or imminent delivery and can be stopped after 12–24 hours if delivery is no longer imminent. It should not be administered longer than 72 hours. If there is a concern for imminent delivery after stopping the magnesium sulfate in a patient who is <32 weeks, readminister IV magnesium sulfate at that time. At 32 weeks and beyond, magnesium sulfate is not given for neuroprotection in preterm deliveries.

# 11.12 GATHER

Communicating with the team involved with maternal resuscitation and with the patient's family members is a critical component of post-arrest care. Strategies on communication and debriefs with the healthcare team and family members are covered in more detail in Chapter 12.

# 11.13 HEAD

Perhaps one of the most critical—and overlooked—steps in post-arrest care is to evaluate the brain. Patients with unknown etiology for arrest should have a CT head completed before admission to the floor/ICU. The presence and type of stroke would significantly affect the patient's post-arrest care treatment plan. It is also challenging to obtain the scan quickly once admitted. OBLS recommends head imaging whether the patient remains pregnant or not. Please refer to Chapter 10 on stroke for further workup recommendations.

**TABLE 11.2**   Standard Post-ROSC Checklist Using ABCDEFGH

| ABCDEFGH | RESPONSE | DOSE AND RECOMMENDATIONS | PREGNANCY-SPECIFIC CONSIDERATIONS |
|---|---|---|---|
| **A**irway | • Intubate, if not already<br>• Place orogastric (OG) or nasogastric (NG) tubes | • Vent settings: 6–8 mL/kg<br>• Avoid hyperventilation | • Same as nonpregnant<br>• Same as nonpregnant |
| **B**reathing | • Maintain $O_2$ saturation >94%<br>• Maintain normocarbia-continuous wave capnography<br>• Maintain normocarbia-continuous wave capnography | • Manage via PEEP and $FiO_2$<br>• Avoid hypoxia or hyperoxia | • Same as nonpregnant<br><br>• *Capnography has limited data in post-arrest pregnant patients, and more data are required for firm recommendations<br>• Recommend $PaCO_2$ 28–32 mm Hg for patients who remain pregnant<br>• In post-arrest patient s/p RCD, management of acid-base status will be dictated by serial ABG evaluation |
| **C**irculation | • 12-lead ECG<br><br>• Maintain normovolemia (SBP >90, MAP >65, ideally >80)<br>• Monitor appropriately | • Emergent coronary angiography for concern for myocardial infarction<br>• N/A<br><br>• Central line<br>• Arterial line<br>• POC-US<br>• Serial labs (including lactic acid)<br>• Indwelling urinary catheter<br>• Consider further imaging if warranted | • Same as nonpregnant<br><br>• Same as nonpregnant<br><br>• There should be at least two lines above the diaphragm if the patient remains pregnant |
| **D**isability | • TTM<br><br>• Prevention of stress ulcer<br>• Prevention of deep venous thrombosis | • 32°C–36°C<br>• Maintain TTM for at least 24 hours post-arrest<br>• Histamine-2 blocker<br>• Sequential compression devices, anticoagulation | • Do not start during transport for out-of-hospital with ROSC<br>• Same as nonpregnant<br>• Same as nonpregnant |

(Continued)

**TABLE 11.2**   Standard Post-ROSC Checklist Using ABCDEFGH (Continued)

| ABCDEFGH | RESPONSE | DOSE AND RECOMMENDATIONS | PREGNANCY-SPECIFIC CONSIDERATIONS |
|---|---|---|---|
| | • Prevention of ventilator-associated pneumonia | • Elevate head of the bed at least 30° <br> • Interrupt daily sedation and assess for readiness to extubate <br> • Use subglottic secretion drainage <br> • Avoid scheduled ventilator circuit changes[27] | • Same as nonpregnant |
| **EC**PR | • ECPR for refractory MCA | • N/A | • If circulatory determination of death, approach family about organ donation desires |
| **E**tiology | • BAACC TO LIFE post-arrest care aid | • N/A | • Depends on suspected cause of arrest |
| **F**etus | • Continuous fetal monitoring | • ≥23–24 weeks | • Begin as soon as possible after ROSC achieved and pregnancy at 23–24 weeks <br> • Emergency cesarean delivery may need to be considered in the setting of nonreassuring fetal status or rearrest |
| | • Prepare for delivery | • Betamethasone 12 mg IM every 24 hr x 2 <br> • Magnesium sulfate 6g IV bolus over 15–20 min, then 2 g/hr | • Always maintain RCD kit at patient's bedside <br> • Alert team of the possibility of a bedside cesarean delivery or RCD <br> • Administer corticosteroids if gestational age 23+0–36+6 weeks gestation <br> • Consider IV magnesium sulfate for fetal neuroprotection if gestational age 23+0 to 31+6 weeks and delivery is imminent (ideally administered at least 4 hours prior to delivery) |
| **G**ather | • Debrief with code response team and family members | • N/A | • Use techniques such as SPIKES or the ALIVE AT FIVE MCA debrief tool |
| **H**ead | • Obtain brain imaging early in post-arrest care treatment to evaluate for possible stroke <br> • CT head or MRI head <br> • Do not delay scan waiting for MR | | • Do not avoid radiation due to concerns for pregnancy <br> • Avoid gadolinium for MR imaging |

**KEY POINTS**

- Following MCA, intubate the patient and start continuous waveform capnography.
- **ABCDEFGH** is a useful mnemonic to remember post-arrest care steps following ROSC during a maternal cardiac arrest event.
- It is important to debrief the care team and family after MCA.

## 11.14  WHEN TO CEASE RESUSCITATION EFFORTS

Deciding when to stop CPR in a pregnant patient is a difficult decision for the care team to make. While indications to start CPR are straightforward and covered in all basic CPR courses, indications to discontinue CPR efforts are less clear. There is no agreed-upon clinical decision aid or algorithm to assist teams about when to stop resuscitative efforts.

**TABLE 11.3**   Potential Barriers to Ceasing Resuscitation Efforts

| |
|---|
| Family members present |
| Institutional pressure to reduce mortality rates |
| Pregnancy, increased emotions, and loss of potentially more than one life |
| Poor communication |
| Technological imperative |
| Young age of patient |

There are many real and perceived barriers to stopping resuscitative efforts that may be even more pronounced when caring for pregnant people, with two lives in the balance. Table 11.3 lists some of the barriers that practitioners may encounter.

## 11.14.1  CEASE–Clinical Features and Effectiveness

The mnemonic **CEASE** serves as a framework to gather information. **CEASE** assists team leaders in decisions about stopping resuscitation efforts and in communicating with surviving family members[17]:

Clinical features
Effectiveness
Ask
Stop
Explain

Table 11.4 lists key clinical prearrest and resuscitation factors when considering when to stop resuscitative efforts during MCA. Resuscitation factors include clinical features that may impact CPR effectiveness in the pregnant or postpartum patient. These factors must be considered or corrected by the team leader before stopping a code.

## 11.14.2  CEASE–Ask–Share Information among Team Members

Communication and information sharing among team members are essential when making the difficult decision to discontinue resuscitative efforts. Members from the interdisciplinary team may have relevant knowledge about the patient. For example, a nurse knows that the pregnant patient had metastatic colon cancer, about which the code lead was aware. This may result in less aggressive efforts and earlier cessation of maternal resuscitation efforts. The team leader needs to be proactive in their attempts to obtain information from all team members before stopping a code on a pregnant patient. It is helpful to call a brief huddle to ask the team for additional information or ideas.

## 11.14.3  CEASE–Stop the Code

After gathering all relevant information, the team leader may decide to stop a code because further attempts at resuscitation are futile. Mounting evidence suggests that family presence during resuscitation may be beneficial for the family. Chapter 12 outlines how to support families during, and debrief after, a code.

## 11.14.4  CEASE–Explain What Has Happened to the Family

It is important to talk with the family members with compassion about what has occurred, including the events of the code and the potential cause of MCA and death. Team members involved in the MCA will also benefit from debriefing, recognition, and support for the natural emotional distress that can accompany caring for critically ill patients. Family and team members may react in different ways to the potential loss of the mother and/or fetus(es), including sadness, anger, disbelief, despair, guilt, or loneliness. Such emotions are normal and support and compassion should be provided.

Debriefing techniques for family and team members and awareness of the second victim are covered in more detail in Chapter 12.

**TABLE 11.4**    Clinical Factors to Consider When Stopping Resuscitation Efforts

| | CLINICAL FEATURE | CONSIDERATIONS IN PREGNANCY |
|---|---|---|
| Prearrest factors | Age | Pregnant people are frequently younger and healthier than the nonpregnant arrest population and thus may be able to survive long periods of resuscitation |
| | Cancer, metastatic or hematologic cancer | Metastatic and hematologic cancers may present in later stages during pregnancy, and may be more difficult to manage and thus act more aggressively |
| | Neurologic status Altered mental status | No evidence for differences |
| | Medical non-cardiac diagnosis<br>• Pneumonia<br>• Hypotension<br>• Renal insufficiency/failure<br>• Acute stroke<br>• Septicemia<br>• Respiratory insufficiency | Pregnant people may have *reversible* causes of cardiac arrest that are easier to treat and recover from:<br>• Respiratory insufficiency<br>• Lidocaine toxicity<br>• Opioid overdose<br>• High spinal<br>• Magnesium toxicity |
| | Major trauma | No evidence for differences |
| | Witnessed arrest | No evidence for differences |
| | Initial rhythm<br>• Ventricular fibrillation<br>• Pulseless ventricular tachycardia | No evidence for differences |
| | Return of pulse within 10 minutes of chest compressions | No evidence for differences |
| Resuscitation factors | Duration of arrest (conflicting data about direction of effect) | Pregnant people may be able to survive longer periods of resuscitation than the general arrest population |
| | Full chest recoil after each compression<br>Minimize compression interruptions<br>Avoid excessive ventilation | Chest compression effectiveness may be hindered by large, dense breasts and the irrational fear of hurting the patient and fetus |
| | Application of LUD | Reduces aortocaval compression and increases CPR effectiveness; uncertain if late application of this technique may improve survival |
| | Performance of RCD | Maternal mortality is increased with longer intervals between the time of arrest and RCD |
| | Application of ECPR | Cases of fetal survival reported as long as 25 minutes from the time of arrest and maternal survival reported as long as 40 minutes from the time of arrest[36]<br>Evidence suggests that survival is improved if ECPR is applied in the setting of refractory cardiac arrest<br>ECPR has been applied as long as 100 minutes from the time of maternal cardiac arrest with good neurologic outcomes |

Adapted from Torke et al.[17]

In line with ALS and ACLS, OBLS recommends documenting the timeline of events. Once a decision is made to stop resuscitative efforts, the team leader must call out the date and time of death. Another team member should document this in the patient's chart.

**KEY POINTS**
- **CEASE** assists team leaders in gathering information for the decision to stop CPR.
- Assess the following when considering stopping a code: age, cancer status (metastatic or hematologic cancer), neurologic status, medical non-cardiac diagnoses, and major trauma.
- Barriers to stopping a code during MCA include young age, emotional loss of fetus(es), institutional pressure to reduce mortality rates, poor communication, and technological imperative.

# 11.15  DETERMINATION OF DEATH AND ORGAN PROCUREMENT

There are few studies on the determination of death and organ procurement for pregnant patients in cardiac arrest. As reported in multiple case reports, pregnant patients can make a remarkable recovery with limited or no sequelae, even with prolonged resuscitation attempts. Situations remain when the providers must make a difficult decision on when to end a code in a pregnant or postpartum person.

The AHA 2020 maternal cardiac arrest guidelines offer several prognostic factors that should be considered for pregnant patients who experience MCA. Providers should wait a minimum of 72 hours post-ROSC **and** post–targeted temperature management (TTM) before offering predictions on the outcomes. If concern for oversedation during TTM is present (which is not uncommon due to slower metabolism of sedatives while undergoing TTM), it is reasonable to wait up to 5 days post-TTM. If other conditions are present, such as brain herniation, terminal disease, or other obviously nonsurvivable conditions, it is not necessary to wait for 72 hours following ROSC and TTM. Table 11.5 lists predictors of poor outcomes in patients who do not undergo TTM. All these predictors of poor outcomes have false-positive rates ranging from 0 to 17%. Only absent pupillary light reflex (i.e., pupils are fixed and dilated) at 72–108 hours was associated with a 0% false-positive rate.[18]

Table 11.6 lists predictors of poor outcomes in patients who underwent TTM. These predictors of poor outcomes had false-positive rates ranging from 0 to 10%. Similar to patients who did not undergo TTM, only absent pupillary light reflex revealed the most consistent and lowest false-positive rate (0–1%).

Other predictors such as status myoclonus (continuous, prolonged, and generalized myoclonus) during the first 72 hours have also resulted in poor outcomes. The presence of **any** type of myoclonus, however, is not a reliable predictor of outcomes. Blood levels of neuron-specific enolase and S-100B **should not** be used alone as predictors of outcome.

## 11.15.1  Organ Procurement

Evidence is limited on outcomes of organ procurement in the setting of MCA. However, there are promising studies demonstrating improved rates of viable organ procurement with the addition of ECPR.[37–47] Thus, it is reasonable to consider ECPR for organ donation in the setting of brain death following MCA in qualified patients.

The 2020 AHA cardiac arrest guidelines recommend that all patients with brain death following ROSC be evaluated for possible organ donation.[28] Patients who do not experience ROSC may be considered for liver or kidney procurement. Any discussion of organ donation must agree with the patients' and their families' wishes, as well as with hospital ethics guidelines.

**TABLE 11.5**  Predictors of Poor Outcomes in Patients Who Do Not Undergo Targeted Temperature Management

| |
|---|
| Absent pupillary light reflex 72 hours after cardiac arrest |
| Absent corneal reflex at 24 and 48 hours after cardiac arrest |
| Extensor posturing **or** no pain stimulus withdrawal at 72 hours (this is the least reliable predictor and should not be the only predictor used) |
| Persistent burst suppression on electroencephalogram after 72 hours (in combination with other predictors) |
| Bilateral absence of nitrous oxide (NO$_2$) waveform at 24–72 hours after arrest CT head with diffuse cerebral edema at 72 hours |

**TABLE 11.6**  Predictors of Poor Outcomes in Patients Who Did Undergo Targeted Temperature Management

| |
|---|
| Bilateral absent pupillary light reflex at 72–108 hours |
| Bilateral absent corneal reflex at 72–108 hours |
| Extensor posturing or no pain stimulus withdrawal at 36–108 hours (this is the least reliable and should not be the only predictor used) |
| Persistent absence of EEG reactivity to external stimuli at 72 hours after arrest Persistent burst suppression on EEG after **rewarming** |
| Bilateral absent NO$_2$ waveform during TTM or absence after rewarming |

**KEY POINTS**

- Providers should wait for a minimum of 72 hours post-ROSC **and** post-TTM before offering predictions on outcomes following MCA.
- Absent pupillary light reflex revealed the most consistent and lowest false-positive rate for predicting poor outcomes following MCA.
- It is reasonable to consider continuing ECPR application to facilitate organ donation in the setting of brain death following MCA in otherwise qualified and consented patients.

**Case Vignette**

A 28-year-old patient at 35 weeks gestation with a history of Wolff-Parkinson-White disease collapses while at her OB clinic appointment. Clinic staff effectively initiate OBLS and call EMS providers who transport the patient to the ED. ED staff is notified to assemble the maternal cardiac arrest team. Her OB provider, who rode in the ambulance with her, performs a STAT resuscitative cesarean delivery upon entry to the ED. CPR continues, and return of spontaneous circulation is achieved. She is intubated by anesthesia, surgery is completed in the OR, and she is transferred to the ICU for immediate post-arrest care.

**REVIEW QUESTIONS**

**Q.** What are the immediate next steps that need to be considered after return of spontaneous circulation?

**A.** Immediately following ROSC, treat the patient following **ABCDEFGH**: **A**irway, **B**reathing, **C**irculation, **D**isability, **E**CPR, **E**tiology, **F**etus, **G**athering, and **H**ead. Steps include:
- Intubate if not already in situ
- Check ventilator settings
- Consider cardiac catheterization (as indicated), TTM, seizure/DVT/stress ulcer prophylaxis, ECPR, fetal monitoring (if still pregnant)
- Debrief the team and family

**Q.** What are the immediate next steps if a patient does not survive an MCA?

**A.** If a patient does not survive MCA, follow the principles of **CEASE**: **C**linical features, **E**ffectiveness, **A**sk, **S**top, **E**xplain. Consider talking with the family about the option of organ donation.

# CHAPTER 11. PRACTICE QUESTIONS

1. Which mnemonic is useful to providers immediately after sustained ROSC?
   - A. ABCDEFGH
   - B. 12345
   - C. STAY ALIVE
   - D. JUMP START

2. EMS providers observe ROSC after performing four cycles of CPR on a pregnant person with BMV. However, the patient remains unresponsive without respiratory effort. What is the BEST next step in airway management?
   - A. Continue BMV as long as there is sustained ROSC
   - B. Place laryngeal mask airway and nasogastric tube
   - C. Perform endotracheal intubation
   - D. Discontinue BMV as long as there is sustained ROSC

3. Providers should wait for a minimum of how many hours post-ROSC and post-TTM before offering predictions on the outcome following maternal cardiac arrest in a patient not on sedation and whose conditions are considered survivable?
   - A. 24
   - B. 38

C. 72
D. 96

4. As the code lead, you decide to stop a code after 60 minutes of resuscitation attempts because one of your team members tells you the pregnant patient has metastatic colon cancer. To which category in the mnemonic **CEASE** does this correspond?
   A. Clinical features
   B. Effectiveness
   C. Ask
   D. Explain

5. As the code lead, you consider stopping a code after 30 minutes of no ROSC following multiple gunshot wounds in a pregnant patient with twins at 16 weeks gestation. The team does not want to stop, and one member begins to cry. You understand the team's reluctance and identify this response as normal because of which of the following?
   A. Technological imperative to improve outcomes
   B. Emotional response to loss of the pregnant patient and fetuses
   C. Institutional pressure to reduce the maternal mortality rate
   D. Poor communication among the team members

# CHAPTER 11. ANSWERS

1. **ANSWER: A.** The mnemonic useful to providers immediately after sustained ROSC is
   **ABCDEFGH**: Airway, Breathing, Circulation, Disability, ECPR, Fetus, Gather, and Head.
2. **ANSWER: C.** Following MCA, most patients will already have an advanced airway in place. If they have not been intubated prior to ROSC, intubation should be performed, and continuous waveform capnography started. It is also reasonable to consider stomach decompression via orogastric or nasogastric tube to reduce the risk of aspiration. An X-ray is recommended to ensure proper ET tube placement.
3. **ANSWER: C.** Providers should wait for a minimum of 72 hours post-ROSC and post-TTM before offering predictions on the outcome. If concern for oversedation during TTM is present (which is not uncommon due to slower metabolism of sedatives while undergoing TTM), it is reasonable to wait 5 days post-ROSC and post-TTM. If other conditions are present such as brain herniation, terminal disease, or other obviously nonsurvivable conditions, it is not necessary to wait for 72 hours.
4. **ANSWER: C.** The mnemonic **CEASE** assists team leaders in gathering information on making a decision to stop CPR. The "Ask" step involves communication and information sharing among team members when considering stopping a code. There are factors that some of the team members may know that will impact this decision.
5. **ANSWER: B.** Barriers to stopping a code during MCA include young age of the patient, emotional loss of fetus(es), institutional pressure to reduce mortality rates, poor communication, and technological imperative. Team members may react in different emotional ways to the potential loss of the mother and/or fetus(es), including sadness, anger, disbelief, despair, guilt, or loneliness.

# CHAPTER 11. REFERENCES

1. Panchal AR, Bartos JA, Cabañas JG, et al. Part 3: Adult basic and advanced life support: 2020 American Heart Association guidelines for cardiopulmonary resuscitation and emergency cardiovascular care. *Circulation*. 2020;142(16_suppl_2). doi: 10.1161/cir.0000000000000916.
2. McNally B, Robb R, Mehta M, et al. Out-of-hospital cardiac arrest surveillance—Cardiac arrest registry to enhance survival (CARES), United States, October 1, 2005–December 31, 2010. *MMWR Surveill Summ*. 2011;60(8):1–19.
3. Girotra S, Nallamothu B, Spertus J, et al. Trends in survival after in-hospital cardiac arrest. *N Engl J Med*. 2012;367(20):1912–1920. doi: 10.1056/NEJMoa1109148.

4. Mhyre JM, Tsen LC, Einav S, et al. Cardiac arrest during hospitalization for delivery in the United States, 1998–2011. *Anesthesiology*. 2014. doi: 10.1097/ALN.000000000000015.

5. Anast N, Kwok J, Carvalho B, Lipman S, Flood P. Intact survival after obstetric hemorrhage and 55 minutes of cardiopulmonary resuscitation. *A & A Case Rep*. 2015 July 1;5:9–12. doi: 10.1213/XAA.0000000000000163.

6. Mogos MF, Salemi JL, Spooner KK, McFarlin BL, Salihu HM. Differences in mortality between pregnant and nonpregnant women after cardiopulmonary resuscitation. *Obstet Gynecol*. 2016;12(4):880–888. doi: 10.1097/AOG.0000000000001629.

7. Fernandes P, Allen P, Valdis M, Guo L. Successful use of extracorporeal membrane oxygenation for pulmonary embolism, prolonged cardiac arrest, post-partum: A cannulation dilemma. *Perfusion*. 2015;30(2). doi: 10.1177/0267659114555818.

8. Imaeda T, Nakada T, Abe R, Tateishi Y, Oda S. Veno-arterial extracorporeal membrane oxygenation for *Streptococcus pyogenes* toxic shock syndrome in pregnancy. *J Artif Organs*. 2016;19:200. doi: 10.1007/s10047-015-0884-3.

9. Krumnikl JJ, Toller WG, Prenner G, Metzler H. Beneficial outcome after prostaglandin-induced post-partum cardiac arrest using levosimendan and extracorporeal membrane oxygenation. *Acta Anaesthesiol Scand*. 2006;50(6):768–770.

10. Hosono K, Matsumura N, Matsuda N, Fujiwara H, Sato Y, Konishi I. Successful recovery from delayed amniotic fluid embolism with prolonged cardiac resuscitation. *Indian J Obstet Gynecol Res*. 2011;37(8). doi: 10.1111/j.1447-0756.2010.01470.x.

11. Marty T, Hilton L, Spear K, Greyson K. Postcesarean pulmonary embolism, sustained cardiopulmonary resuscitation, embolectomy, and near-death experience. *Obstet Gynecol*. 2005. doi: 10.1097/01.AOG.0000164054.53501.96.

12. Arlt M, Philipp A, Lesalnieks I, Kobuch R, Graf B. Successful use of a new hand-held ECMO system in cardiopulmonary failure and bleeding shock after thrombolysis in massive post-partal pulmonary embolism. *Perfusion*. 2009;24(1):49–50. doi: 10.1177/0267659109106295.

13. Biderman P, Carmi U, Setton E, Fainblut M, Bachar O, Einav S. Maternal salvage with extracorporeal life support, lessons learned at a single center. *Anesthesia & Analgesia*. 125(4):1275–1280. doi: 10.1213/ANE.0000000000002262.

14. Kivlehan SM. *The post-ROSC checklist*. Academic Life in Emergency Medicine. Website. www.aliem.com/2017/04/post-rosc-checklist/. Updated 2017.

15. Müller M, Jürgens J, Redaèlli M, Klingberg K, Hautz WE, Stock S. Impact of the communication and patient hand-off tool SBAR on patient safety: A systematic review. *BMJ*. doi: 10.1136/bmjopen-2018-022202.

16. Callaway CW, Donnino MW, Fink EL, Geocadin RG, et al. Part 8: Post-cardiac arrest care: 2015 American Heart Association guidelines update for cardiopulmonary resuscitation and emergency cardiovascular care. *Circulation*. 2015;132(18 Suppl 2):465–482. doi: 10.1161/CIR.0000000000000262.

17. Torke AM, Bledsoe P, Wocial LD, Bosslet GT, Helf PR. CEASE: A guide for clinicians on how to stop resuscitation efforts. *Ann Am Thorac Soc*. 2015;12(3):440–445. doi: 10.1513/AnnalsATS.201412-552PS.

18. Pecher S, Williams E. Out-of-hospital cardiac arrest in pregnancy with good neurological outcome for mother and infant. *Int J Obstet Anesth*. 2017;29:81–84. doi: 10.1016/j.ijoa.2016.11.002.

19. Lavinio A, Scudellari A, Gupta AK. Hemorrhagic shock resulting in cardiac arrest: Is therapeutic hypothermia contraindicated? *Minerva Anestesiol*. 2012;78:969–970.

20. Kerro A, Woods T, Chang JJ. Neurogenic stunned myocardium in subarachnoid hemorrhage. *J Crit Care*. 2017;38:27–34. doi: 10.1016/j.jcrc.2016.10.010.

21. Ahmadian A, Mizzi A, Banasiak M. Cardiac manifestations of subarachnoid hemorrhage. *Heart Lung Vessel*. 2013;5(3):168–178.

22. Otsuji R, Uno J, Motoie R. Basilar artery occlusion with "seizures" as a presenting symptom: Three cases treated using mechanical thrombectomy. *World Neurosurg*. 2018;117:32–39 doi: 10.1016/j.wneu.2018.05.227.

23. Corry JJ, Dhar R, Murphy T, Diringer MN. Hypothermia for refractory status epilepticus. *Neurocrit Care*. 2008;9:189–197. doi: 10.1007/s12028-008-9092-9.

24. Link MS, Berkow LC, Kudenchuk PJ, et al. Part 7: Adult advanced cardiovascular life support: 2015 American Heart Association guidelines update for cardiopulmonary resuscitation and emergency cardiovascular care. *Circulation*. 2015;132(2):444–464. doi: 10.1161/CIR.0000000000000261.

25. Kim F, Nichol G, Maynard C, Hallstrom A, et al. Effect of prehospital induction of mild hypothermia on survival and neurological status among adults with cardiac arrest: A randomized clinical trial. *JAMA*. 2014;311:45–52. doi: 10.1001/jama.2013.282173.

26. Kalil AC, Metersky ML, Klompas M, et al. Management of adults with hospital-acquired and ventilator-associated pneumonia: 2016 clinical practice guidelines by the Infectious Diseases Society of America and the American Thoracic Society. *Clin Infect Dis*. 2016;Sep 1;63(5):e61–e111. doi: 10.1093/cid/ciw353.

27. Hellyer TP, Ewan V, Wilson P, Simpson AJ. The Intensive Care Society recommended bundle of interventions for the prevention of ventilator-associated pneumonia. *J Intensive Care Soc*. 2016;17(3):238–243. doi: 10.1177/1751143716644461.

28. Jeejeebhoy FM, Zelop CM, Lipman S, et al. Cardiac arrest in pregnancy: A scientific statement from the American Heart Association. *Circulation*. 2015;132:1747–1773. doi: 10.1161/CIR.0000000000000300.

29. Magnesium sulfate before anticipated preterm birth for neuroprotection. Committee Opinion No. 455. American College of Obstetricians and Gynecologists. *Obstet Gynecol*. 2010;115:669–671.

30. NICE. Technical patient safety solutions for ventilator-associated pneumonia in adults. *NICE*. 2008. Website. http://guidance.nice.org.uk/PSG00

31. Pecher S, Williams E. Out-of-hospital cardiac arrest in pregnancy with good neurological outcome for mother and infant. *Int J Obstet Anesth*. 2017;29:81–84. doi: 10.1016/j.ijoa.2016.11.002.

32. Rittenberger JC, Popescu A, Brenner RP, Guyette FX, Callaway C. Frequency and timing of nonconvulsive status epilepticus in comatose post-cardiac arrest subjects treated with hypothermia. *Neurocrit Care*. 2012;16:114–122. doi: 10.1007/s12028-011-9565-0.

33. Limotai C, Ingsathit A, Thadanipon K, McEvoy M, Attia J, Thakkinstian A. How and whom to monitor for seizures in an ICU: A systematic review and meta-analysis. *Crit Care Med*. 2019 Apr;47(4):e366–e373. doi: 10.1097/CCM.0000000000003641.

34. Bataillard A, Hebrard A, Gaide-Chevronnay L, Casez M, Dessertaine G, Durand M, Chavanon O, Albaladejo P. Extracorporeal life support for massive pulmonary embolism during pregnancy. *Perfusion*. 2016;31(2):169–171. doi: 10.1177/0267659115586578.

35. Rouse DJ, Hirtz DG, Thom E, Vaner MW, et al. A randomized, controlled trial of magnesium sulfate for the prevention of cerebral palsy. *NEJM*. 2008;359:895–905. doi: 10.1056/NEJMoa0801187.

36. LoMauro A, Aliverti A, Frykholm P, et al. Adaptation of lung, chest wall, and respiratory muscles during pregnancy: Preparing for birth. *J Appl Physiol*. 2019;127(6):1640–1650. doi: 10.1152/japplphysiol.00035.2019.

37. Fang Z, Van Diepen S, Royal Alexandra Hospital and University of Alberta Hospital Cardiac Arrest Teams. Successful inter-hospital transfer for extracorporeal membrane oxygenation after an amniotic fluid embolism induced cardiac arrest. *Can J Anaesth*. 2016 Apr;63(4):507–8. doi: 10.1007/s12630-015-0548-z.

38. Fernandes P, Allen P, Valdis M, Guo L. Successful use of extracorporeal membrane oxygenation for pulmonary embolism, prolonged cardiac arrest, post-partum: A cannulation dilemma. *Perfusion*. 2015;30(2). doi: 10.1177/0267659114555818.

39. Huang KY, Li YP, Lin SY, Shih JC, Chen YS, Lee CN. Extracorporeal membrane oxygenation application in post-partum hemorrhage patients: Is post-partum hemorrhage contraindicated? *J Obstet Gynecol Res*. 2017. doi: 10.1111/jog.13426.

40. Kim HY, Jeon HJ, Yun JH, Lee JH, Lee GG, Woo SC. Anesthetic experience using extracorporeal membrane oxygenation for cesarean section in the patient with peripartum cardiomyopathy: A case report. *Korean Journal of Anesthesiology*. 2014;66(5):392–397. doi: 10.4097/kjae.2014.66.5.392.

41. Seong GM, Kim SW, Kang HS, Kang HW. Successful extracorporeal cardiopulmonary resuscitation in a postpartum patient with amniotic fluid embolism. *Thorac Dis*. 2018. doi: 10.21037/jtd.2018.03.06.

42. van Zwet CJ, Rist A, Haeussler A, Graves K, Zollinger A, Blumenthal S. Extracorporeal membrane oxygenation for treatment of acute inverted takotsubo-like cardiomyopathy from hemorrhagic pheochromocytoma in late pregnancy. *A & A Case Reports*. 2016;7(9):196–199. doi: 10.1213/XAA.0000000000000383.

43. Imaeda T, Nakada T, Abe R, Tateishi Y, Oda S. Veno-arterial extracorporeal membrane oxygenation for *Streptococcus pyogenes* toxic shock syndrome in pregnancy. *J Artif Organs*. 2016;19:200. doi: 10.1007/s10047-015-0884-3.

44. Moore SA, Dietl CA, Coleman DM. Extracorporeal life support during pregnancy. *J Thorac Cardiovasc Surg*. 2016;15(4):1154. doi: 10.1016/j.jtcvs.2015.12.027.

45. McDonald C, Laurie J, Janssens S, Zazulak C, Kotze P, Shekar K. Successful provision of inter-hospital extracorporeal cardiopulmonary resuscitation for acute post-partum pulmonary embolism. *Int J Obstet Anesth*. 2017;30:65–68. doi: 10.1016/j. ijoa.2017.01.003.

46. Takacs ME, Damisch KE. Extracorporeal life support as salvage therapy for massive pulmonary embolus and cardiac arrest in pregnancy. *J Emerg Med*. 2018;55(1):121–124. doi: 10.1016/j.jemermed.2018.04.009.

47. Bataillard A, Hebrard A, Gaide-Chevronnay L, Casez M, Dessertaine G, Durand M, Chavanon O, Albaladejo P. Extracorporeal life support for massive pulmonary embolism during pregnancy. *Perfusion*. 2016;31(2):169–171. doi: 10.1177/0267659115586578.

# Communication during Maternal Cardiac Arrest

**12**

## 12.1 INTRODUCTION

Coordinating resuscitation efforts during MCA is a challenge for medical teams. Application of teamwork principles is essential to optimize response and outcomes. This chapter outlines the fundamental principles of communication to maximize team response to MCA.

## 12.2 LEARNING OBJECTIVES

Learner will appropriately

- Describe the guiding principles of team-based care.
- Describe the framework, competencies, and principles of TeamSTEPPS® as they apply to MCA.
- Describe the components of a multiteam system for patient care in MCA, including core, contingency, coordinating, and ancillary teams.
- Describe the importance of assigning roles during MCA, including
  - Code leader who utilizes available cognitive aids/algorithms
  - Code recorder/timekeeper, who keeps time and records a timeline of events
- Describe and demonstrate standard tools used for optimizing communication during a multidisciplinary team care for patients with MCA.
- Describe and demonstrate how to communicate with family members during and after the event.
- Describe and demonstrate how to debrief the team.

## 12.3 GUIDING PRINCIPLES OF TEAM-BASED CARE

MCA is one of the most complex and clinically challenging resuscitations. The additional tasks of LUD and RCD make effective teamwork and communication that much more critical.

Team-based care is defined as "the provision of health services to individuals, families and their communities by at least two healthcare providers who work collaboratively with patients and their families to accomplish shared goals to achieve coordinated, high-quality care."[1] Specifically, the guiding principles of team-based care include the following:[1]

- The patient and families are central to and **actively engaged** as members of the healthcare team. It is essential to keep the family informed of the status of the patient during the resuscitation.
- The team has a **shared mental model**.
- **Role clarity** is essential to team effectiveness and team functioning.
- All **team members are accountable** for their practice and to the team.
- **Effective communication** is the key to quality team performance.
- **Team leadership** is situational and dynamic. Clearly define team leaders during MCA. This role is fluid, with multiple teams and clinicians participating in the maternal and neonatal resuscitation.

DOI: 10.1201/9781003299288-13

## 12.3.1 TeamSTEPPS® Framework, Competencies, and Principles

TeamSTEPPS® is a communication framework designed to optimize team performance across healthcare systems and improve patient safety. Its strategies and communication tools can be effectively integrated into managing MCA or other high-risk scenarios. TeamSTEPPS is founded on a framework that includes knowledge, attitude, and performance of the team, which subsequently guides optimal clinical outcomes.

Competencies include

- **Knowledge** (shared mental model)
- **Attitudes** (mutual trust and team orientation)
- **Performance** (adaptability, accuracy, productivity, efficiency, and safety)[2]

All team members must have a shared understanding, or mental model, of the situation and goals of the team's efforts. One technique used to establish and ensure a shared mental model is to hold a team huddle or brief before starting procedures. Huddles can help to facilitate open communication and teamwork among team members. Though a prearrest huddle for a sudden MCA is not always feasible, communication during the event becomes even more critical to optimizing clinical outcomes. TeamSTEPPS has five key principles, based on team structure and the following four skills[2]:

- **Communication**—This is a structured process by which information is clearly and accurately exchanged among team members.
- **Leadership**—This is the ability to maximize the activities of team members by ensuring that team actions are understood, changes in information are shared, and team members have the necessary resources.
- **Situation monitoring**—This is a process of actively scanning and assessing situational elements to gain information or understanding, or to maintain awareness to support team functioning.
- **Mutual support**—This is an ability to anticipate and support team members' needs through accurate knowledge about their responsibilities and workload.

The TeamSTEPPS framework is shown in Figure 12.1, with the four skills at the core of the framework. The arrows demonstrate the interdependence between the four skills and the team-related outcomes of knowledge, attitudes, and performance. These skills and outcomes are critical for optimizing maternal outcomes during MCA. Encircling the four skills is the team structure, which is described next.

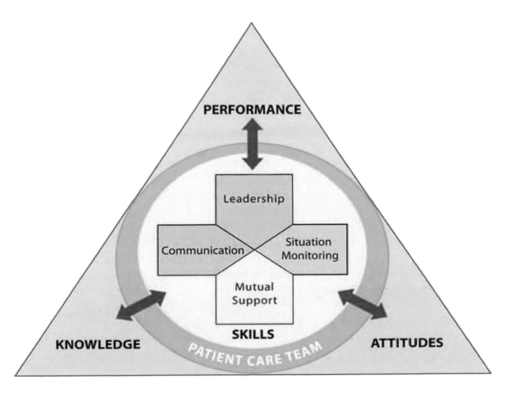

**FIGURE 12.1**   TeamSTEPPS® framework.[3]

**TABLE 12.1**  TeamSTEPPS® Team Competency Outcomes[3]

| KNOWLEDGE | ATTITUDES | PERFORMANCE |
|---|---|---|
| • Shared mental model | • Mutual trust<br>• Team orientation | • Adaptability<br>• Accuracy<br>• Productivity<br>• Efficiency<br>• Safety |

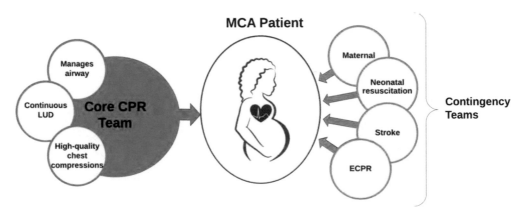

**FIGURE 12.2**  Maternal cardiac arrest teams and responsibilities.

# 12.4 MATERNAL CARDIAC ARREST TEAM STRUCTURE

MCAT structure requires the identification of the appropriate teams and team members, which is especially critical for MCA. Team coordination is vital to ensure optimal outcomes in MCA. Working interdependently, the **core CPR team** is responsible for maintaining chest compressions, LUD, and airway management. At the same time, **multiple contingency teams** are responsible for performing RCD, subsequent neonatal resuscitation, and ECPR, if indicated (Figure 12.2).

Each team has a leader who must ensure effective communication within their own team and between the contingency teams and ancillary services such as the blood bank, laboratory, and interpreters. The MCAT is also responsible for ensuring all other teams are trained, ready, and available.

OBLS also recommends designating a code leader and a recorder. The code leader should be a team member with a solid understanding of OBLS. This includes leading with the OBLS cognitive aid and algorithms and modifying CPR as recommended for pregnant patients. Cognitive aids and algorithms should be available to all EMS personnel and on code carts where MCA is most likely to occur in the hospital, including the ED, labor and delivery, ORs, and ICUs. The code leader is responsible for assigning roles during a code: situation monitoring, calling out orders, and mobilizing additional resources and team members as needed. This role may need to shift during a maternal code, depending on who is on the team and which team members have the best understanding of the modifications of CPR for a pregnant patient. For example, an OB may be the code leader initially. The OB may then hand over the lead to the anesthesiologist so they as the OB can perform the RCD. Communication using call-outs and check-backs ensures all team members understand that leader roles have changed (further described in the next section).

The other designated and critical team member is the code recorder or timekeeper. The code recorder should be exclusively tasked with keeping time and calling out time intervals every 30 seconds for the entire team to hear. This team member is also responsible for documenting a timeline of critical events, including time of arrest, shocks administered, medications given (including doses and route of administration), time of RCD or other critical procedures (such as ECPR), and time of ROSC or death. This timeline should become a permanent part of the patient's medical records and may be referenced when debriefing the team or family.

**KEY POINTS**

- TeamSTEPPS is a communication framework designed to optimize team performance across healthcare systems and improve patient safety, which can be used to improve team communication and functioning in emergencies.
- TeamSTEPPS competencies include
  - Knowledge (shared mental model)
  - Attitudes (mutual trust and team orientation)
  - Performance (adaptability, accuracy, productivity, efficiency, and safety)
- Successful management of MCA includes two sets of teams. First, is the core team responsible for BLS and ACLS. Second are the contingency teams, principally responsible for performing RCD, neonatal resuscitation, and ECPR, if indicated. Teams work interdependently and toward successful resuscitation of the patient.
- Teams responding to MCA should designate a team leader and a recorder who can keep time and record events.

**TABLE 12.2**   Example: Facility Notification—SBAR

| |
|---|
| *Situation*: "Medic 101 transporting a priority one OB Arrest Alert. ETA of 5." |
| *Background*: "24-year-old pregnant person in MCA following a motor vehicle crash. CPR in progress with LUD. Her fundus appears to be 2 cm above the umbilicus." |
| *Assessment*: "Resuscitative cesarean delivery may be required." |
| *Recommendation/Request*: "Request OB and neonatal resuscitation teams be present at the ED upon arrival." |

TeamSTEPPS can be applied in a variety of clinical scenarios. Useful tools to coordinate optimal team communication during OBLS include situation, background, assessment, recommendation (SBAR), call-outs, and check-backs, which are described in the next section.

# 12.5 SITUATION, BACKGROUND, ASSESSMENT, AND RECOMMENDATION/REQUEST

SBAR is a technique for communicating critical information that requires immediate attention and action concerning a patient's condition. This communication is brief and directed toward the essential clinical components of the patient's status. Code teams can use this technique within their team or with contingency team members. SBAR is useful when EMS providers are communicating with the hospital before the patient arrives. OBLS recommends that EMS crews and hospitals develop an **OB Arrest Alert** program that helps team members to keep communications brief. Calling the hospital and indicating an **OB Arrest Alert** immediately prompts the OB and neonatal teams to be present at the ED upon the crew's arrival.

SBAR can also be an effective way to reduce communication errors in medicine and improve patient safety. OBLS recommends using SBAR during MCA to promote effective multiteam coordination and communication to optimize outcomes. Consistent use of proven communication tools and strategies provides the best possible outcomes.[4]

# 12.6 CALL-OUTS

Call-outs are used to communicate important or critical information during patient care. They are called out loud for the entire team to hear without an identified receiver. Call-outs ensure that team members are made aware of information that may influence the next steps of the resuscitation. They direct responsibility for a specific task to the person responsible for executing it.

**TABLE 12.3**   Example: Call-Outs during MCA

| |
|---|
| *Leader*: "Abdominal ultrasound findings?" |
| *Team member*: "Intrauterine pregnancy consistent with 26 weeks gestation." |
| *Leader*: "Cardiac rhythm?" |
| *Team member*: "Nonshockable rhythm." |
| *or* |
| *Leader*: "Khayah, I need you to pick up the blood from the blood bank." |
| *Team member (Khayah)*: "Leaving now to pick up blood from the blood bank." |

**TABLE 12.4**   Example: Check-Back during MCA

| |
|---|
| *Leader*: "Give 0.1 mg epinephrine IV push." |
| *Team member*: "Drawing up and giving 0.1 mg epinephrine IV push now." |
| *Leader*: "Correct. Give epinephrine now." |

# 12.7 CHECK-BACKS

Check-backs provide closed-loop communication to ensure that information communicated by the sender is understood by the receiver as intended. Check-backs include three steps:

1. Sender initiates the message.
2. Receiver accepts the message and provides feedback.
3. Sender double-checks to ensure the message was received as intended.

# 12.8 SITUATION-BACKGROUND-ASSESSMENT-RECOMMENDATION AND CALL-OUTS FOR THE MATERNAL TEAM ENTERING A MATERNAL CARDIAC ARREST EVENT—THE 5A's

When responding to an MCA, the maternal team should announce themselves so that the core team is aware of their arrival. The core must then provide SBAR to situate the arriving team. Use OBLS's **5A's** to remember the critical information exchange that should occur between teams (Figure 12.3).

**5 A's**

**A**nnounce – yourself or team
    "Dr. Mishra from OB" or "Maternal team is here"
**A**sk – how many minutes since MCA and if ROSC
**A**ssess – uterine fundus
**A**sk – RCD kit/scalpel and neonatal team
**A**ct – perform RCD as indicated

**FIGURE 12.3**   The 5A's used to situate the maternal team arriving to a maternal cardiac arrest.

**KEY POINTS**

- SBAR stands for situation, background, assessment, and recommendation/request and is used when providing a summary of the patient's condition to a new team/member.
- Keep SBAR brief and directed toward the essential clinical components of the patient's status.
- Call-outs increase awareness for the entire team.
- Check-backs improve closed-loop communication and accuracy of orders given/received.
- Use the 5A's to orient the core and contingency teams during a maternal cardiac arrest.

## 12.9 COMMUNICATION OF MATERNAL CARDIAC ARREST AND OUTCOMES TO THE FAMILY

Communication with the family during an MCA is important. Ideally, one person is assigned to communicate with the family, explain interventions, and answer questions. Regardless of the outcome of the MCA, the team should review the event and management with the family and discuss next steps or interventions.

While many providers have been trained to remove family members from the room during emergency situations, newer data suggest that family members should be allowed to stay with their family member during emergencies. This allows them to witness the tremendous efforts and resources that are used on behalf of the patient and may provide some closure in the event of death.[5]

Several tools are available for debriefing adverse outcomes to patients and their families.[6] One of these is SPIKES, an evidence-based, validated communication tool used for delivering bad news, or adverse outcomes, to patients and their family members. This tool is composed of a structured format consisting of six steps, through which the provider progresses when delivering difficult or serious news (Figure 12.4).[6]

The following case vignette illustrates the steps to share serious news. Table 12.5 shows each element, including a description for each category and example statements based on the case vignette.

Setting – make a connection
Perception – ask before you tell
Invitation – check first
Knowledge – small, bite sized, non-technical information
Emotion – allow emotional expression
Summary

**FIGURE 12.4**  SPIKES.

### Case Vignette

EMS providers transport to the ED a 24-year-old person, pregnant at an unknown gestational age, following a collapse. They provide BMV, LUD, high-quality chest compressions, and have peripheral IV access. En route, the crew lead notified the ED core team lead that the patient's brother said he did not know how many weeks the pregnancy was.

Using SBAR, the crew lead calls an OB Arrest Alert.

**S**: OB Arrest Alert.
**B**: 24 y/o person with suspected pregnancy of unknown gestational age in cardiac arrest. They suffered an acute collapse and arrest while shopping.

**A**: CPR in progress with LUD.
**R**: Have the OBLS code team ready for a potential RCD.

The MCAT and contingency teams were all contacted, informed, and are standing by in the ED upon EMS arrival. Transport time to the ED was 10 minutes. A code recorder is designated, and high-quality CPR is continued by the ED team. A primary survey is performed by the ED provider (code leader) without interrupting chest compressions, LUD, or ventilation.

The maternal (contingency) team leader performs an ultrasound (while LUD is maintained) and identifies and immediately communicates to the code leader that a pregnancy with a biparietal diameter consistent with 26 weeks gestation is noted. The code leader determines and communicates that the patient's cardiac rhythm is nonshockable, and the maternal team informs the core team that RCD is indicated.

While LUD is momentarily interrupted, an RCD is performed by the maternal contingency team leader. Delivery of the neonate and placenta is accomplished less than 1 minute after skin incision while chest compressions continue. The neonate is handed to the pediatric team (contingency) in attendance in the ED, and the maternal (contingency) team leader rapidly closes the hysterotomy incision. Due to the sudden onset of the collapse, concern for pulmonary embolism is heightened, and point-of-care ultrasound is performed revealing a large saddle pulmonary embolus. The ECPR team is then activated.

After several days of ECPR, the patient regains consciousness and has little sequelae. Team leadership remains situational and dynamic during this scenario with all team members demonstrating a shared vision with clearly defined roles and timely communication to other teams which helps to ensure optimal patient outcomes.

## REVIEW QUESTIONS

**Q.** Which teams are considered contingency in an MCAT?
**A.** The maternal, neonatal, stroke, and ECPR teams are contingency teams in an MCAT.
**Q.** What is the core CPR team responsible for during MCA resuscitation?
**A.** The core CPR team is responsible for maintaining chest compressions, LUD, and airway management.
**Q.** What is an example of a call-out in the vignette?
**A.** An example of a call-out is when the maternal team leader communicated to the core leader that the pregnancy was >20 weeks.
**Q.** Based on the presentation of this 24-year-old patient, what potential causes of cardiac arrest are of most concern?
**A.** Using BAACC TO LIFE as a guide and based on the patient's collapse, she is at most risk for pulmonary embolism or cardiac causes such as acute myocardial infarction, cardiomyopathy, or an abnormal rhythm such as Wolff-Parkinson-White. A point-of-care ultrasound can be used to evaluate for embolism, cardiac function, or other causes of MCA as resources and training allow.

**TABLE 12.5**   SPIKES Protocol for Sharing Difficult News with Family Members

| MAJOR CATEGORY | REQUIREMENTS | EXAMPLE FROM CASE VIGNETTE |
|---|---|---|
| **Setting** | | |
| | Find a private location, where confidentiality can be maintained. | |
| | Make a connection and establish rapport immediately. If this is the first visit, introduce yourself and ensure the family member acknowledges you prior to you discussing any medical information. | "Hello Mr. Ember, my name is Dr. Mishra. It's been a rough morning. How are you holding up?" |
| **Perception** | | |
| | Assess family's perception or understanding of medical situation. | "What do you understand about what's happened to Lani?" or "Has anyone told you about what is going on with Lani?" |
| **Invitation** | | |
| | Ask permission before giving the news. | "I would like to discuss what I know is happening with Lani so far. Is that okay?" |

**TABLE 12.5**  (Continued)

| MAJOR CATEGORY | REQUIREMENTS | EXAMPLE FROM CASE VIGNETTE |
|---|---|---|
| **Knowledge** | | |
| Warning Shot | Give a clear and concise warning that you are about to share serious news. | "I have some serious news to share." |
| Headline | Direct communication of adverse outcome; describe what happened in clear terms. | "Lani suddenly collapsed at the mall. Their heart stopped beating and EMS providers did CPR. EMS brought Lani here, where we delivered the baby via a cesarean. We did this procedure to help Lani. We're giving them both more care in the ICU." |
| **PAUSE AND WAIT** | | |
| **Wait 3+ seconds to allow the receiver a chance to digest what has been said** | | |
| **Emotion** | | |
| First statement after sharing the difficult news | Provide empathetic statement for adverse outcome. | "I know this is not what you expected to hear today." |
| **Summary/Next Steps** | | |
| Ask for permission | Discus plan only after family member asks or gives permission to discuss next steps. | "Do you want me to discuss next steps for Lani and your baby's care?" |
| Next steps | Suggest a plan for the next step(s). | "Let's talk about how Lani and baby are doing now, and what we will be doing for them going forward." |

**KEY POINTS**

- Communicate difficult news to family members both **during** the event (if adequate staff are available) and **as soon as** the patient is stable or after death.
- Family members may benefit from staying with the patient and witnessing efforts to revive their loved one. This must not interfere with the healthcare team's efforts.
- Use an evidence-based, validated communication tool for sharing serious or difficult news with patients and their family members.
- SPIKES is a structured format to communicate with a patient's family members. SPIKES consists of six steps: Setting, Perception, Invitation, Knowledge, Emotion, and Summary.
- When sharing difficult or serious news with family members, pause when speaking and assess the patient/family's understanding of the situation.
- Team members may have an emotional response to an adverse patient outcome and should be debriefed and offered support.

## 12.10 DEBRIEFING THE TEAM AFTER MATERNAL CARDIAC ARREST

Communication with the team that assisted in the resuscitation efforts is critical to

- Review the events that occurred
- Identify any system issues that need to be addressed
- Reduce the possibility of "second victim" effects on the team

OBLS recommends holding a team debrief as soon as possible after the event and including as many team members as possible. Teams should refer to their institution's policy regarding debrief and may consider including a member from risk management or the hospital attorney. Holding the debrief soon after the event will provide the clearest recollection of details from the team and allow for the healing process to begin. Designate a team leader who can lead the debrief using one of the available debriefing tools.[7]

The ALIVE @ 5® Maternal Cardiac Arrest Debrief Tool (Figure 12.5) highlights the many unique steps required for MCA resuscitation and provides a framework to debrief the system and communication events contributing to the teams' success or

**ALIVE** @ 5 - Maternal Cardiac Arrest Debrief Tool

| **A**CTIVATE OBLS | ☐ **CALLS MCAT**<br>☐ Lowers head of bed and inserts backboard<br>☐ Performs continuous high-quality compressions<br>☐ Changes compressors every 2 min<br>☐ Immediately resumes compressions after shock<br>☐ Establishes airway: breaths or BMV<br>☐ Applies AED or defibrillator correctly<br>    ○ Avoids breast tissue with lateral pad<br>    ○ Accurately assesses rhythm<br>☐ Defibrillates every 2 min, if indicated<br>☐ Obtains crash cart and RCD kit quickly<br>☐ Removes fetal monitoring, if applicable<br>☐ Calls for contingency teams (i.e., NICU, ECPR, CT surgeon, MAST)<br>☐ Team leader guides resuscitation with OBLS cognitive aid<br>    ○ Assigns timekeeper<br>    ○ Uses BAACC TO LIFE to guide management based on cause<br>    ○ Orders medications as indicated |
|---|---|
| **L**EFT UTERINE<br>DISPLACEMENT (LUD) | ☐ Applies continuous LUD if fundus @ umbilicus until RCD<br>☐ Performs POC-US on reproductive age female |
| **I**V PLACEMENT/<br>**I**NTUBATE EARLY | ☐ Places IV/IO above diaphragm<br>☐ Anticipates difficult airway/obtains advanced airway equipment<br>☐ Applies advanced airway techniques, if necessary<br>☐ 2 attempts at intubation<br>☐ Uses size 6-7 ETT<br>☐ Attempts supraglottic airway x2 if unsuccessful<br>☐ Attempts surgical airway if unsuccessful |
| **V**ENTILATE/ **V**ERIFY | ☐ Maintains effective ventilation<br>    ○ Chin lift/jaw thrust, 100% $O_2$ at 15L/min<br>☐ Ventilates at correct rate<br>    ○ If not intubated: 30 compressions : 2 breaths<br>    ○ If intubated: breath every 5-6 sec<br>☐ Verifies arrival of RCD equipment and contingency teams<br>(i.e., NICU, ECPR, CT surgeon, MAST) |
| **E**VACUATE UTERUS | ☐ Performs RCD if no ROSC and fundus @ umbilicus<br>☐ RCD by 5 min at site of arrest |
| Debrief *teamwork* with 3 S's: **S**BAR (orientation), **S**ituational awareness, **S**ystem issues<br>Debrief *communication* with 3 C's: **C**all-outs, **C**heck-backs, and overall team **C**ommunication | |

Abbreviations: AED: automated external defibrillator, BMV: bag-mask ventilation, CPR: cardiopulmonary resuscitation, CT: cardiothoracic, ECPR: extracorporeal CPR, ETT: endotracheal tube, IV: intravenous, IO: intraosseous, L: liter, LUD: left uterine displacement, min: minute, $O_2$: oxygen, OBLS: Obstetric Life Support, MAST: maternal stroke team, MCAT: maternal cardiac arrest team, NICU: neonatal intensive care unit, RCD: resuscitative cesarean delivery, ROSC: return of spontaneous circulation, sec: second

V. 12/23/2020

**FIGURE 12.5** ALIVE @ 5 Maternal Cardiac Arrest Debrief Tool IH.

challenges. The team leader can use the 3Ss (SBAR, Situational awareness, System challenges/highlights) and 3C's (Call-outs, Check-backs, and overall Communication) to debrief the system and communication events that occurred during the code response.

At the beginning of the debrief, set the stage for a blame-free environment so team members are engaged, feel respected, and are comfortable sharing their feelings and thoughts. The outline provided in Figure 12.6 helps team leaders to establish this safe space.

It is important to use a confidentiality or quality improvement/peer-review statement at the beginning of the debrief as the debrief conversation is considered confidential information. During the debrief, it is important to ensure all staff participating understand which conversations will be kept confidential and those which are discoverable (such as conversations outside of the debriefing or quality improvement process). Having risk management present to help navigate the legal aspect of the debrief can help to ensure all parties are informed and aware of these differences.

Don't blame
Everyone's opinions matter
Be open to discussion including constructive criticism, disagreements
Respect one another
Identify what went well
Engage all team members
Feelings matter

**FIGURE 12.6**   DEBRIEF mnemonic—set the stage for a debrief.

**KEY POINTS**
- Hold a team debrief as soon as possible after the event to identify what went well and what could be improved.
- Effective debriefing requires setting the stage for a **blame-free environment** so team members do not feel threatened, and can freely share observations, suggestions for improvement, and their feelings about what happened.
- Use the ALIVE AT FIVE Maternal Cardiac Arrest Debriefing Tool to guide team debriefs. This checklist outlines the many unique aspects required for MCA resuscitation.

# CHAPTER 12. PRACTICE QUESTIONS

1. The EMS team leader calls in, "Medic 101 transporting a priority one OB Arrest Alert. ETA of 5." They receive the following response, "Copy. OB Arrest Alert. Teams will be in the ED upon your arrival." Which of the following BEST describes this form of TeamSTEPPS communication?
   A. SBAR
   B. Cross-monitoring
   C. Shared mental model
   D. Closed-loop communication/Check-back

2. In the SPIKES model, after telling the family the headline that the patient has died, the provider's next step should be to:
   A. Pause for at least 3 seconds
   B. Make empathetic statement
   C. Discuss next steps
   D. Provide a glass of water

3. EMS providers transport to the ED a reproductive-age person who has sustained multiple gunshot wounds. The trauma leader performs an extended Focused Assessment of Sonography for Trauma exam including ultrasound of the abdominal/pelvic region where pregnancy is confirmed. The fundus is palpated near the level of the umbilicus. The charge nurse calls for the OB and neonatal team, and they arrive 5 minutes later. The trauma code leader tells the contingency team that the patient is pregnant, and fundus is above the umbilicus, and they have sustained multiple gunshot wounds. They recommend a resuscitative cesarean delivery as CPR has been ongoing for 15 minutes. Which of the following BEST describes this form of communication?
   A. SBAR
   B. DEBRIEF
   C. Cross-monitoring
   D. Closed-loop communication

4. Attempts to resuscitate a pregnant person at term are unsuccessful following a motor vehicle collision. The senior crew leader approaches the patient's partner and asks them if they have been told what is happening. This BEST exemplifies which step when sharing serious news?
   A. Setting
   B. Perception

C. Knowledge
D. Invitation

5. Which of the following is the most critical step in a team debrief following an adverse event?
   A. Waiting for at least a day before debriefing to give the team time to process and think about the event
   B. Setting a blame-free environment prior to the debriefing
   C. Making sure the debrief is efficient by asking closed-ended questions
   D. Immediately creating a list of which team members made mistakes during the resuscitation

# CHAPTER 12. ANSWERS

1. **ANSWER: D.** Check-backs provide closed-loop communication to ensure that information communicated by the sender is understood by the receiver as intended. Check-backs include three steps: (1) sender initiates the message, (2) receiver accepts the message and provides feedback, and (3) sender double-checks to ensure the message was received as intended.
2. **ANSWER: A.** Using SPIKES, a provider **pauses** after sharing that the patient has died. This allows the receiver time to hear and digest the news. Pause for at least 3+ seconds.
3. **ANSWER: A.** SBAR is a technique for communicating critical information that requires immediate attention and action concerning a patient's condition. This technique is used within a team (such as a core team) or with contingency team members. Conversely, this tool is essential when EMS provides communication before the patient arrives at the hospital. Keep this communication extremely brief and directed toward the essential clinical components of the patient's status.
4. **ANSWER: B.** The "perception" step of SPIKES is used to assess the patient/family's perception or understanding of the medical situation.
5. **ANSWER: B.** It is important to set the stage for a blame-free environment during the debrief so team members are engaged, feel respected, and are comfortable sharing their feelings. Follow the principles of DEBRIEF to recall the important aspects of setting the stage:
   • **D**on't blame
   • **E**veryone's opinion matters
   • **B**e open to discussion including constructive criticism, disagreements
   • **R**espect one another
   • **I**dentify what went well
   • **E**ngage all team member
   • **F**eelings matter

# CHAPTER 12. REFERENCES

1. Executive summary: Collaboration in practice: Implementing team-based care: Report of the American College of Obstetricians and Gynecologists' Task Force on Collaborative Practice. *Obstet Gynecol.* 2016;127(3):612–617. doi: 10.1097/AOG.0000000000001304. https://www.acog.org/clinical/clinical-guidance/task-force-report/articles/2016/collaboration-in-practice-implementing-team-based-care. Accessed March 12, 2023.
2. Agency for Healthcare Research and Quality. *TeamSTEPPS® 2.0.* Website. www.ahrq.gov/teamstepps/instructor/index.html. Updated 2019. Accessed September 3, 2019.
3. Keebler JR, Dietz AS, Lazzara EH, Benishek LE, Almeida SA, Toor PA, King HB, Salas E. Validation of a teamwork perceptions measure to increase patient safety. *BMJ Qual Saf.* 2014;23(9):718–726. doi: 10.1136/bmjqs-2013-001942.
4. Müller M, Jürgens J, Redaèlli M, Klingberg K, Hautz WE, Stock S. Impact of the communication and patient hand-off tool SBAR on patient safety: A systematic review. *BMJ.* doi: 10.1136/bmjopen-2018-022202.
5. Goldberger ZD, Nallamothu BK, Nichol G, Chan PS, Curtis JR, Cooke CR. American Heart Association's get with the guidelines. Policies allowing family presence during resuscitation and patterns of care during in-hospital cardiac arrest. *Circ Cardiovasc Qual Outcomes.* 2015. doi: 10.1161/CIRCOUTCOMES.114.001272.
6. Bailea WF, Buckmanb R, Lenzia R, Globera G, Bealea EA, Kudelkab AP. SPIKES: A six-step protocol for delivering bad news: Application to the patient with cancer. *Oncologist.* 2000;5(4):302–311. doi: 10.1634/theoncologist.5-4-302.
7. Kessler DO, Cheng A, Mullan PC. Debriefing in the emergency department after clinical events: A practical guide. *Ann Emerg Med.* 2015. doi: 10.1016/j.annemergmed.2014.10.019.

# Putting It All Together

# 13

## 13.1 INTRODUCTION

This scenario-based chapter provides opportunities to apply knowledge of maternal physiology, as well as skills gained from studying the *Obstetric Life Support Manual*.

## 13.2 SCENARIO ONE

The patient is a 22-year-old person involved in a head-on collision with a tree as an unrestrained driver. They are wearing a medical alert bracelet for type II diabetes. EMS providers extricate the unresponsive person, and an ECG shows sinus tachycardia without a pulse. They begin high-quality CPR. A crew member is unable to definitely palpate a uterine fundus due to the person's body habitus. The crew lead uses SBAR to communicate with the nearest tertiary care facility.

---

**PUTTING IT ALL TOGETHER**

**What is the patient's cardiac rhythm?**
~ PEA

**What is considered high-quality CPR?**
~ Chest compressions at the rate of 100–120/min and with the ratio of 30:2 (compressions: breaths), or continuous chest compressions with ventilations delivered every 5–6 seconds.

**What should EMS providers consider when evaluating an unconscious reproductive-age person?**
~ Are they or could they be pregnant? Is there a palpable uterine fundus? If so, where is its location in relation to the umbilicus?

**What is the best facility for EMS providers to transport this patient?**
~ The head injury means EMS should transport the patient to a tertiary care center/major trauma center.

---

The patient's injuries appear extensive. EMS providers transport the patient to the nearest tertiary care center. Upon arrival to the ED, the patient's cardiac rhythm remains in PEA. Providers give several rounds of IV epinephrine and continue high-quality CPR. Given their concerns of a difficult airway because of the patient's obesity, EMS providers ventilated with a supraglottic airway. One crew member is concerned that ventilation is not adequate because of the lack of chest rise and decreased breath sounds on the right.

---

**PUTTING IT ALL TOGETHER**

**How is PEA treated? What if the patient is pregnant?**
~ PEA is treated with CPR and epinephrine. Epinephrine is used in pregnant patients at the same dose and timing as nonpregnant patients.

**ACLS guidelines recommend what dose of epinephrine?**
~ 1 mg every 3–5 minutes

---

DOI: 10.1201/9781003299288-14

**At this point, what are the possible causes of the cardiac arrest/PEA?**
~ Consider the BAACC TO LIFE mnemonic. The MCA has multiple potential causes, including complications of diabetes (although less likely in this scenario), trauma (severe closed head injury, spinal cord/neck injury, tension pneumothorax, cardiac tamponade), and hypovolemia due to trauma.
**What is the most likely cause for unilateral decreased breath sounds?**
~ This suggests tension pneumothorax due to trauma and should be evaluated further.

While continuing high-quality CPR, the senior emergency attending performs a rapid Optimal Sequence Intubation. Decreased breath sounds persist. The team suspects tension pneumothorax and places a chest tube. Immediately, a lot of blood releases, and breath sounds improve. Another provider performs an eFAST exam.

## PUTTING IT ALL TOGETHER

**What is the treatment for tension pneumothorax?**
~ Definitive treatment in the hospital is chest tube placement. Needle decompression may be considered in the field if pneumothorax is strongly suspected at that time. Chest tube/needle decompression should be performed in the fourth intercostal space in the midaxillary line.
**How should a practitioner perform an eFAST exam on people of reproductive age with unknown pregnancy status?**
~ Perform an abdominopelvic POC-US, if available, to evaluate for the possibility of pregnancy. Do so in the T fashion: sweep across the upper abdomen and then down the midline. If intrauterine pregnancy is found, apply fundal palpation. If the uterus is not palpable due to body habitus, use a POC-US to assess for BPD or FL. A BPD of ≥45 mm and FL of ≥30 mm correspond to a pregnancy at 20 weeks. This can cause significant aortocaval compression and reduce the effectiveness of CPR.
~ Responders should immediately apply continuous LUD.

Because of the patient's age, a team member performs an abdominopelvic POC-US that shows an intrauterine pregnancy. Given the patient's obesity, it is hard to palpate for the fundal height, so the provider quickly obtains a fetal BPD of 50 mm.

## PUTTING IT ALL TOGETHER

**What is your best next step?**
~ Call the MCAT.
**Who are members of the MCAT?**
~ The MCAT is composed of CORE and CONTINGENCY teams. The core team is responsible for OBLS resuscitation. Contingency teams are responsible for obstetric evaluation/RCD, stroke care, neonatal resuscitation following RCD, and ECPR, if indicated. An example of various contingency team members includes:
  ~ OB/GYNs, Anesthesiologist, L&D RN, critical care MD, NICU or pediatric team, respiratory therapist, neurologist
  ~ Adult ECPR team, if available
The CORE and CONTINGENCY teams operate interdependently. The code team leader may alternate depending on where in the OBLS algorithm care is currently being given. For instance, the ED physician may start as code lead until the OB/GYN arrives. The ED physician continues leading chest compressions while the OB/GYN assess pregnancy and determines if RCD is indicated. Once RCD is started, the OB/GYN may turn code lead to the Anesthesiologist to perform the RCD.
**Once pregnancy ≥20 weeks is confirmed, what are the next steps after calling the MCAT?**
~ Apply continuous LUD (BPD is >45 mm, suggesting pregnancy >20 weeks, which could cause significant aortocaval compression)
~ Prepare for immediate RCD
~ Obtain IV access above the diaphragm if not already done
~ Consider the BAACC TO LIFE mnemonic for possible causes of MCA

The designated code leader assigns one team member to call for the OBLS code team, another to initiate LUD, a third team member to obtain the RCD kit and crash cart, and a fourth team member to start recording events and keeping time. Each person provides a verbal check-back of their role with the code leader. EMS providers have already placed two 16-gauge antecubital IV lines. Crystalloid fluids are being administered. The team has a high index of concern for significant neurologic injury. Due to the patient's history of diabetes, point-of-care glucose is checked and found to be 35 mg/dL. At this time, the RCD kit has arrived at the ED. The on-call OB/GYN has not yet arrived.

## PUTTING IT ALL TOGETHER

**What is the appropriate treatment for the patient's hypoglycemia?**
~ 20–50 mL of 50% glucose solution (D50) as an IV bolus, or subcutaneous or intramuscular injection of glucagon 0.5–1.0 mg.
~ If D50 is unavailable or not immediately available, 10% dextrose solutions (D10) via 50 mL boluses for a total of 250 mL can be considered.

**What are the possible arrest causes?**
~ Hypoglycemia most likely led to altered mental status, leading to the collision. The patient was unrestrained and suffered significant trauma, leading to closed head injury and hypovolemia due to hemorrhage into the chest cavity from broken ribs.

**Who should perform the RCD?**
~ Any physician trained in RCD, to include OB/GYN, ED physicians, Family Medicine or general/trauma surgeons.

**What type of incision should be used for RCD?**
~ Use a vertical midline skin incision for RCD. Vertical incisions are fast, associated with less blood loss with ROSC, and allow for extension for maximum exposure of the abdomen and pelvis. A vertical uterine incision allows for improved access to smaller gestations and decreases fetal manipulation in the event the fetus is still viable and premature. If the delivering provider is an OB provider, uterine incision may be left to their discretion. However, a vertical skin incision is always recommended in a traumatic MCA.

The emergency physician quickly starts the RCD via vertical skin incision and then removes the fetus and placenta from the uterus. The total time from arrest to incision is approximately 20 minutes. The waiting neonatal team immediately assumes care of the newborn. At that time, the attending OB/GYN arrives in the ED and assumes surgical care of the patient. The patient remains unconscious after several additional rounds of high-quality CPR and epinephrine doses. ROSC is achieved.

## PUTTING IT ALL TOGETHER

**What is the post-arrest care/evaluation for this patient?**
~ The patient's injuries require further assessment and treatment by the multidisciplinary team. As she suffered a significant head injury, neurosurgery and trauma teams should be involved.
~ Once stabilized from an injury standpoint, she is a candidate for TTM.

**What is the recommended length of time for TTM?**
~ 24–72 hours

**What are some of the signs used to determine brain death?**
~ The most consistent findings with brain death are absent pupillary light and absent corneal reflexes after 72–108 hours.

**What are considerations or conversations that the medical team should have with the family in the event of concern for brain death?**
~ Organ donation/procurement
~ Follow SPIKES to optimize communication.

**In the event of organ procurement, what are some considerations for improved organ procurement success?**
~ Initiate ECPR for organ procurement.

Once the surgery is complete, both the trauma and neurosurgery teams fully evaluate the patient due to the concern for a significant head injury. After closing the head injury, neurosurgery admits the patient to the ICU for 72 hours of TTM. With no bilateral pupillary light and corneal reflexes, they keep the patient on life support. The team finds the same reflexes upon repeat neurologic exam at 110 hours. After extensive counseling with the care team, the family chooses to remove life support and donate the organs. The team starts the patient on ECMO for organ procurement before they withdraw life support.

# 13.3  SCENARIO TWO

The patient is a 38-year-old gravida 2, para 1 at 39 weeks gestation, admitted in active labor with cervical dilation at 6 cm. Their pregnancy has been uncomplicated, and they have no medical problems or surgical history. Upon admission, vital signs and labs are as expected, and the team places a single right antecubital 18-gauge IV and an epidural after an IV fluid bolus. Approximately 20 minutes after the epidural is placed, the patient's water spontaneously breaks with clear amniotic fluid. A vaginal exam determines 8-cm dilation. The patient reports feeling acutely short of breath during the cervical check and is increasingly uncomfortable laying reclined. Oxygen saturation is rapidly declining to 90%. The team gives 2 L oxygen by face mask. The patient is afebrile; blood pressure is 75/45 mm Hg (previously 100/70), and pulse 120 beats per minute.

## PUTTING IT ALL TOGETHER

**What are the red flags? What is the proper response/next best step based on maternal warning score systems?**
~ Acute change in status involving the respiratory system and in vital signs to include $O_2$ desaturation, hypotension, and tachycardia.
  ~ This should trigger immediate provider evaluation at the bedside.
**What is a developing differential for the patient's acute change in status?**
~ BAACC TO LIFE: anesthesia, AFE, PE underlying/unknown cardiac disease, pulmonary edema from fluid overload.
**What are the best next steps?**
~ Maternal resuscitation to include bedside evaluation, $O_2$ supplementation, maternal repositioning.
~ Call a rapid response team.

Late decelerations are noted on the fetal heart rate monitor, and an OB rapid response is called. The on-call anesthesiologist and the OB/GYN come quickly to the bedside and administer ephedrine. BP improves briefly, and the patient reports it is increasingly hard to catch their breath. Oxygen saturation drops to 85%. The team places the patient on a non-rebreather mask and gives 15 L $O_2$. Fetal monitoring continues to show late decelerations. Shortly after the OB/GYN enters the L&D department, the patient says they "feel really funny" and begins hemorrhaging from the vagina.

## PUTTING IT ALL TOGETHER

**What is now higher on your differential?**
~ AFE/DIC
**What is the best next step in management?**
~ Initiate massive transfusion protocol
~ Call the MCAT
**Who is part of the MCAT?**
~ OB/GYN, anesthesiology, L&D RNs, NICU/pediatric team, critical care RN/MD, respiratory therapy, blood bank

The patient loses consciousness soon after starting to bleed. The team detects fetal bradycardia. They initiate the massive transfusion protocol. The patient becomes apneic and pulseless. An OBLS code is called, and continuous chest compressions are performed with breaths delivered by BMV every 6 seconds. The bed is flattened, and a backboard is placed under the patient to facilitate chest compressions.

**PUTTING IT ALL TOGETHER**

**What are the best next steps after calling an OBLS code?**
~ Initiate high-quality CPR, continuous LUD, obtain the crash cart and RCD kit, IV placement above the diaphragm, obtain a secure airway, and prepare for resuscitative cesarean delivery.
**These steps are occurring simultaneously and as equipment and people allow, in sequence.**
**Where should the patient be moved for RCD?**
~ The patient should not be moved. Perform RCD at the place of arrest for an IH MCA.

Anesthesia personnel remain at the bedside and continue using BMV while waiting for the crash cart and intubation equipment. The respiratory technician arrives and hands a 6-mm endotracheal tube to the anesthesiologist. The anesthesiologist secures a definitive airway on the first attempt and maintains adequate ventilation at 10–12 breaths per minute. Compressions are continued at a rate of 100–120 per minute. The OB/GYN calls for an RCD kit and instructs two team members to continue LUD and high-quality chest compressions.

A second large-bore IV is placed in the left antecubital region, and crystalloid fluid is administered.

The OB/GYN performs RCD via midline vertical skin incision in the labor room immediately upon receiving a scalpel. The newborn is handed off to the waiting pediatricians. The total time from arrest to delivery of the newborn is approximately 7 minutes. Shortly after evacuation of the uterus, ROSC is achieved, and the patient continues hemorrhaging from the vagina. As the OB/GYN quickly closes the uterus and administers uterotonics as well as tranexamic acid, the team notes bleeding from multiple sites, including the IV sites. The blood appears watery. B-lynch procedure and uterine artery ligation are attempted with no improvement in vaginal bleeding.

**PUTTING IT ALL TOGETHER**

**What condition has developed? How is it managed?**
~ DIC, which is managed with massive transfusion protocol.
**What is the ratio of blood products (packed red blood cells [PRBC]:fresh frozen plasma [FFP]:platelets) used during massive transfusion?**
~ Ratios vary between institutions. Common ratios include 6:6:1, 4:4:1, and 1:1:1. Whole blood is also being used in select places across the United States.
**What is the next best step If bleeding is not improved with uterotonics/tranexamic acid, and other surgical corrections such as B-lynch procedure and uterine artery ligation?**
~ A lifesaving hysterectomy must be considered for refractory hemorrhage after correction of DIC.

Bleeding continues. The OB/GYN proceeds with a supracervical cesarean hysterectomy. Bleeding improves following the hysterectomy and cardiovascular rearrest occurs. Chest compressions are resumed. At the next rhythm check, the patient is in pulseless ventricular tachycardia, and a 150 Joule shock is administered. The patient begins to show signs of right heart straining with ARDS. The ECPR team is called.

**PUTTING IT ALL TOGETHER**

**What rhythms are considered shockable rhythms?**
~ Pulseless ventricular tachycardia or ventricular fibrillation
**What are the criteria for starting ECPR?**
~ Respiratory failure
~ Refractory CPR
Relative contraindications for ECPR include coagulopathy, hemorrhagic shock/instability, and trauma due to inability to anticoagulate. While data are limited, several case studies have shown that recovery from AFE and resulting ARDS is rapidly improved with ECPR, even despite DIC.

The ECPR team cannulates the patient according to protocol. Due to hemorrhagic shock from DIC, they do not start anticoagulation but give a higher rate of flow during ECMO. After 3 days on ECMO, the patient becomes alert and responsive. ECMO is discontinued.

After 10 more days of hospitalization, the patient recovers and is discharged without sequelae. Their newborn is discharged from the NICU on day 5 of life with no significant sequelae.

# 13.4  SCENARIO THREE

EMS providers are called to an apartment building. A concerned neighbor called 911 after listening to a baby cry constantly for 2 hours and hearing no response to their to knocking on the door.

The crew surveys the scene after forceful entry to the apartment. They see a person about 20 years of age lying on the floor and hear an infant wailing in the crib. The adult has recent vomit around the mouth, a faint heartbeat with agonal breathing, and an incision on the lower abdomen that appears to be healing.

## PUTTING IT ALL TOGETHER

**What are the most likely diagnoses?**
~ Think BAACC TO LIFE for the postpartum patient: Clot/cerebrovascular (pulmonary embolism), Overdose (drug), Cardiovascular disease (cardiomyopathy, other), and Ions (diabetic ketoacidosis or hypoglycemia in patient with diabetes)

EMS providers are concerned about a possible opioid overdose due to the patient's postpartum status, recent surgery (presumed cesarean delivery), and weak pulse with agonal breathing.

## PUTTING IT ALL TOGETHER

**What is the best next step once opioid overdose is suspected?**
~ Naloxone administration and airway management.
**What CPR considerations should be taken for postpartum patients?**
~ Basic Life Support/Advanced Cardiac Life Support are unchanged as in other nonpregnant patients, but physiology may not have returned to baseline until 8–12 weeks following delivery. The patient remains at risk for cardiovascular complications (such as cardiomyopathy and hypertensive disorders), homicide, mood disorders leading to suicide attempts, and opioid addiction or overdose up to 1 year after delivery.

EMS crew members establish an IV and immediately give the patient a dose of naloxone. BMV is attempted but unsuccessful. The team suctions the patient's mouth for vomit, then intubates, and successfully secures the patient's airway with continuous wave capnography reading 35–40 mm Hg. A point-of-care glucose is 110 mg/dL. Heart rate is bradycardic, pulse is weak, and the patient remains unresponsive. A second dose of naloxone is administered. The patient's vital signs improve, respiratory effort is minimal, and airway is maintained. The team transports the patient to the nearest hospital with ICU capabilities, where they are admitted for respiratory failure secondary to presumed opioid overdose. The patient is extubated the following day and begins to recover.

Once awake and alert, the patient shares that they were experiencing severe postpartum depression and feelings of hopelessness and helplessness. They felt their baby would be better if they were dead and so they took the remaining postoperative pain narcotic medication at once. Voluntarily, the patient accepts inpatient therapy for severe postpartum depression. Antidepressant medications assist with recovery. The family reunites following completion of inpatient therapy.

# 13.5  SCENARIO FOUR

A 28-year-old person presents to the ED of a community hospital complaining of a severe headache and saying they gave birth 6 days ago to their first full-term baby after an uncomplicated pregnancy. The patient has a history of migraines but reports that "this one is different." Ibuprofen and acetaminophen provided no relief. Initial check shows blood pressure is 155/98 but on recheck is 140/85. Patient reports of a "blind spot" on the right side similar with prior migraines. The team treats the migraine with IV fluids and ketorolac. Feeling a little better, the patient requests to go home to be with their baby.

**PUTTING IT ALL TOGETHER**

**What red flag features are present in this postpartum patient?**
~ Remember SCAN ME: Sudden/Severe/Seizure, Change in position/quality, Altered mental status, Neurologic deficits/Nausea and vomiting, Medications without relief, Elevated blood pressure (hypertension) or temperature (fever). This patient has five red flags: severe, change in quality, neurologic deficit (vision changes), medications without relief, and elevated blood pressure.

**Should the patient be discharged home?**
~ No. This patient has multiple red flag features and should have brain imaging and a neurologic and OB// GYN consultation. Even if neurologic evaluation is reassuring, this patient should likely be admitted for treatment of postpartum preeclampsia with severe features.

The patient agrees to stay for a head CT and a telehealth consultation with the neurologist on call. However, while waiting for the scanner, the patient begins crying and becomes confused and agitated. After vomiting and losing consciousness, they have generalized shaking which stops spontaneously after 1 minute. The patient remains unresponsive. Blood pressure is now 180/110. The ED physician intubates for airway protection, starts a propofol drip, and then calls OB/GYN consult. The OB consultant recommends starting a magnesium drip for treatment of postpartum eclampsia. Blood pressure remains in the 160/90 range after initiation of magnesium.

**PUTTING IT ALL TOGETHER**

**What should be the next step in management?**
~ While the diagnosis of postpartum eclampsia is likely correct, the patient should still have immediate brain imaging to exclude brain hemorrhage.

The patient undergoes brain imaging with a noncontrast head CT which reveals a 30-cc left occipital intracerebral hemorrhage, diffuse convexity subarachnoid hemorrhage, and multiple areas of brain edema. While the ED physician is on the phone with the radiologist, the nurse reports that the patient has some jerking movements. On examination, the patient is lying flat on the CT scanner table and has intermittent bucking, with stiffening and extension of both arms. Blood pressure is now 200/110, and heart rate is in the 40s.

**PUTTING IT ALL TOGETHER**

**What immediate action should the team take?**
~ The patient is extensor posturing and has hypertension and bradycardia, all signs of increased intracranial pressure with impending brain herniation. The staff should immediately move the patient from the scanner table and elevate the head of the bed with the neck midline.

**What are the next steps in management?**
~ Start nicardipine drip for goal systolic BP <140. Patient remains unresponsive.
~ Call stat neurology and neurosurgical consults.
~ Place central or intraosseous line.
~ Administer either mannitol 1 g/kg (can be given peripherally with filter) or 30 mL of 23.4% hypertonic saline through the central line.
~ Consider reversal agents (platelets, DDAVP) given intracranial hemorrhage and recent nonsteroidal anti-inflammatory drug administration, and likely need for neurosurgical procedures.
~ Obtain CT angiogram of head and neck to evaluate for underlying vascular lesions.

The extensor posturing movements stop as soon as the head of the bed is elevated. A nicardipine drip is started, and the blood pressure rapidly lowers to <140 systolic. A central line, arterial line, and Foley catheter are placed, and 70 g of mannitol is given. The neurologist and neurosurgeon evaluate the patient and recommend transfer to a tertiary care facility with a neurocritical care unit. After transfer to the regional medical center with a neuro-ICU, maternal-fetal medicine specialists consult on eclampsia management. Cerebrovascular imaging reveals diffuse multifocal arterial vasospasm consistent with postpartum angiopathy. The patient undergoes clot evacuation of an occipital hemorrhage, and the brain edema resolves after treatment of eclampsia. Once home, physical and occupational therapy assist with neurologic deficits, including visual field cut, mild right-sided weakness, and cognitive deficits.

# CHAPTER 13. REFERENCE

1. Aissi James S, Klein T, Lebreton G, Nizard J, Chommeloux J, Bréchot N, Pineton de Chambrun M, Hékimian G, Luyt CE, Levy B, Kimmoun A, Combes A, Schmidt M. Amniotic fluid embolism rescued by venoarterial extracorporeal membrane oxygenation. *Crit Care*. 2022;26(1):96. doi: 10.1186/s13054-022-03969-3. PMID: 35392980; PMCID: PMC8988404.

# Appendix A: Abbreviations

| | | | | |
|---|---|---|---|---|
| ABG | Arterial blood gas | ECMO | Extracorporeal membrane oxygenation |
| ACCD | Automated chest compression device | ECPR | Extracorporeal cardiopulmonary resuscitation |
| ACLS | Advanced Cardiac Life Support | ED | Emergency department |
| ACOG | American College of Obstetricians and Gynecologists | EEG | Electroencephalogram |
| | | eFAST | Extended Focused Assessment of Sonography for Trauma |
| ACS | Acute coronary syndrome | EMS | Emergency medical services |
| AED | Automated external defibrillators | Eq/L | Equivalent per liter |
| AFE | Amniotic fluid embolism | ERAS | Enhanced recovery after surgery |
| AHA | American Heart Association | ERV | Expiratory reserve volume |
| AI/AN | American Indian/Alaska Native | ET tube | Endotracheal tube |
| AIM | Alliance for Innovation on Maternal Health | ETCO$_2$ | End-tidal CO$_2$ |
| AIS | Acute ischemic stroke | EWS | Early warning systems |
| ALI | Acute lung injury | FFP | Fresh frozen plasma |
| ALS | American Red Cross Advanced Life Support | FiO$_2$ | Fraction of inspired oxygen |
| aPTT | Activated partial thromboplastin time | FL | Femur length |
| ARDS | Acute respiratory distress syndrome | FRC | Functional reserve capacity |
| ASA | American Stroke Association | GABA | Gamma-aminobutyric acid |
| ATLS | Advanced Traumatic Life Support | GAS | Group A streptococcal |
| AVPU | Alert, verbal, pain, unresponsive | GFR | Glomerular filtration rate |
| BP | Blood pressure | GI | Gastrointestinal |
| BPD | Biparietal diameter | HELLP | Hemolysis, Elevated Liver Enzymes, and Low Platelets |
| BLS | Basic Life Support | | |
| BMI | Body mass index | HR | Heart rate |
| BMP | Basic metabolic panel | ICH | Intracerebral/intracranial hemorrhage |
| BMV | Bag mask ventilation | ICNARC | Intensive Care National Audit and Research Centre |
| BNP | B-type natriuretic peptide | | |
| CABG | Coronary artery bypass graft | ICP | Intracranial pressure |
| CBC | Complete blood count | ICU | Intensive care unit |
| CEMACH | Confidential Enquiry into Maternal and Child Health | IHCA | In-hospital cardiac arrest |
| | | IH | In-hospital |
| CMP | Comprehensive metabolic panel | IM | Intramuscular |
| CMQCC | California Maternal Quality Care Collaborative | INR | International normalized ratio |
| | | IO | Intraosseous |
| CNS | Central nervous system | IPV | Intimate partner violence |
| CO | Cardiac output | ISSHP | International Society for the Study of Hypertension in Pregnancy |
| CPB | cardiopulmonary bypass | | |
| CPR | Cardiopulmonary resuscitation | IV | Intravenous |
| CRNA | Certified Registered Nurse Anesthetist | JVD | Jugular venous distention |
| Cryo | Cryoprecipitate | K | Potassium |
| CT | Computed tomography | L&D | Labor and Delivery |
| CTA | Computed tomography angiography | LMWH | Low-molecular-weight heparin |
| CTV | Computed tomography cerebral venography | LoMC | Levels of Maternal Care |
| CVD | Cardiovascular disease | LUD | Left uterine displacement |
| CVST | Cerebral venous sinus thrombosis | LVO | Large vessel occlusion |
| DBP | Diastolic blood pressure | MAOI | Monoamine oxidase inhibitors |
| DIC | Disseminated intravascular coagulation | MAP | Mean arterial pressure |
| DKA | Diabetic ketoacidosis | MAST | Maternal Stroke Team |
| DVT | Deep vein thrombosis | MCA | Maternal cardiac arrest |
| ECG | Electrocardiogram | | |

| | | | |
|---|---|---|---|
| **MCAT** | MCA teams | **PPCM** | Peripartum cardiomyopathy |
| **MEOWS** | Modified Early Obstetric Warning System | **PPH** | Postpartum hemorrhage |
| **MEWS** | Modified Early Warning System | **PPV** | Positive predictive value |
| **mEq/L** | Milliequivalents per Liter | **PRBC** | Packed red blood cells |
| **MI** | Myocardial infarction | **PRES** | Posterior reversible encephalopathy syndrome |
| **MEWT** | Maternal Early Warning Trigger | **PRMR** | Pregnancy-related mortality ratio |
| **mg/dL** | Milligrams per deciliter | **PRN** | When necessary |
| **mm Hg** | Millimeters of mercury | **P-SCAD** | Pregnancy-associated SCAD |
| **mmol/L** | Millimoles per liter | **PT/INR** | Prothrombin time/International normalized ratio |
| **mOsmol/kg** | Milliosmoles (one-thousandth of an osmole) per kilogram of water | **PT/PTT** | Prothrombin time/Partial thromboplastin time |
| **MRA** | Magnetic resonance angiogram | **qSOFA** | Quick Sequential Organ Failure Assessment Score |
| **MRI** | Magnetic resonance imaging | | |
| **MRV** | Magnetic resonance venography | **RCD** | Resuscitative cesarean delivery |
| **NEWS** | National Early Warning System | **RCVS** | Reversible cerebral vasoconstriction syndrome |
| **NG** | Nasogastric | **RPF** | Renal plasma flow |
| **NICE** | National Institute for Health and Care Excellence | **ROSC** | Return of spontaneous circulation |
| | | **rtPA** | Recombinant tissue plasminogen activator |
| **NICU** | Newborn intensive care unit | **RV** | Residual volume |
| **NIHSS** | National Institutes of Health Stroke Scale | **SAH** | Subarachnoid hemorrhage |
| **NO$_2$** | Nitrous oxide | **SBAR** | Situation, Background, Assessment, Recommendation |
| **NSTEMI** | Non-ST-elevation myocardial infarction | | |
| **OBLS** | Obstetric Life Support | **SBP** | Systolic blood pressure |
| **OB/GYN** | Obstetricians and gynecologist | **SCAD** | Spontaneous coronary artery dissection |
| **OG** | Orogastric | **S.O.S.** | Sepsis in Obstetric Score |
| **OH** | Out-of-hospital | **SMM** | Severe maternal morbidity |
| **OHCA** | Out-of-hospital cardiac arrest | **SSC** | Surviving Sepsis Campaign |
| **OR** | Operating room | **STEMI** | ST-elevation myocardial infarction |
| **PaCO$_2$** | Partial pressure of carbon dioxide | **SV** | Stroke volume |
| **PANS** | Peripheral/autonomic nervous system | **SVR** | Systemic vascular resistance |
| **PCC** | Prothrombin complex concentrates | **TID** | Three times a day |
| **PCI** | Percutaneous coronary intervention | **T-MCA** | Traumatic Maternal Cardiac Arrest |
| **PE** | Pulmonary embolism | **TTM** | Targeted temperature management |
| **PEA** | Pulseless electrical activity | **tPA** | Tissue plasminogen activator |
| **PEEP** | Positive end-expiratory pressure | **TV** | Tidal volume |
| **PETCO$_2$** | End-tidal carbon dioxide (also called ETCO$_2$) | **TXA** | Tranexamic acid |
| **PFO** | Patent foramen ovale | **UFH** | Unfractionated heparin |
| **pg/mL** | Picograms/mL | **U.S.** | United States |
| **PIERS** | Preeclampsia Integrated Estimate of Risk | **VAP** | Ventilator-associated pneumonia |
| **PO** | Orally | **VF/VT** | Ventricular fibrillation/Ventricular tachycardia |
| **POC-US** | Point-of-care ultrasound | **VTE** | Venous thromboembolism |

# Appendix B: OBLS Mnemonics

## ABCDEFGH

**Purpose**: remember post-arrest care steps following ROSC during maternal cardiac arrest
**Location**: Chapter 11, Sections 11.4–11.13

Airway
Breathing
Circulation
Disability
ECPR
Etiology
Fetus
Gather
Head

## ALIVE @ 5

**Purpose**: recall the steps to care for maternal patients in cardiac arrest
**Location**: Chapter 6, Figure 6.7

Activate OBLS
Left uterine displacement
IV placement above diaphragm/Intubate early
Ventilate/Verify equipment and personnel
Evacuate uterus by 5 minutes

## BAACC TO LIFE®

**Purpose**: recall the major categories of MCA
**Location**: Chapter Introduction, 4,
　　　　　Sections 4.1–4.14

Bleeding
Anesthesia
AFE
Cardiovascular/cardiomyopathy
Clot/cerebrovascular
Trauma
Overdose (magnesium sulfate/opioids/other)
Lung injury/ARDS
Ions (glucose/K⁺)
Fever (sepsis)
Emergency hypertension/eclampsia

## CEASE

**Purpose**: to recall the clinical factors to consider when stopping resuscitation efforts
**Location**: Chapter 11, Section 11.14

Clinical features
Effectiveness
Ask
Stop
Explain

## DEBRIEF

**Purpose**: to set the stage for a debrief. Create blame-free environment so team members are engaged, feel respected, and are comfortable sharing their feelings and thoughts
**Location**: Chapter 12, Section 12.10

Don't blame
Everyone's opinion matters
Be open to discussion including constructive criticism, disagreements
Respect one another
Identify what went well
Engage all team members
Feelings matter

## SCAN ME

**Purpose**: recall "red flag" headache features, any one of which should prompt a rapid neurologic evaluation and consideration of brain imaging
**Location**: Chapter 9, Section 9.4.7 and Chapter 10, Section 10.4

Sudden/Severe/Seizure
• "Thunderclap" or "worst headache of my life"
Change in position or quality
• Worse in supine position
• Change in quality from usual headache/migraine
Altered mental status
Neurologic deficits/Nausea and vomiting
• Dizziness, vision changes, weakness/numbness, speech difficulties
Medications without relief
Elevated blood pressure (hypertension) or temperature (fever)

# Appendix C: Resources

---

## CHAPTER 1

---

- Black Mamas Matter Alliance: https://blackmamasmatter.org/
- Moms Rising: www.momsrising.org/
- Institute for Healthcare Improvement: www.ihi.org/communities/blogs/how-to-reduce-implicit-bias

---

## CHAPTER 9

---

- The California Maternal Quality Care Collaborative has generously given us permission to include their materials and informative tools (permission August 29, 2019), including the following:
    - A preeclampsia toolkit: www.cmqcc.org/resources-tool-kits/toolkits/preeclampsia-toolkit
    - A toolkit to help institutions with timely identification of and quick response to postpartum hemorrhage: www.cmqcc.org/resources-tool-kits/toolkits/ob-hemorrhage-toolkit
    - Resources for management of postpartum hemorrhage: www.cmqcc.org/resource/ob-hem-emergency-management-plan-checklist
    - Table demonstrating how to differentiate normal versus abnormal signs/symptoms of pregnancy in people with and without underlying cardiac disease: https://www.cmqcc.org/resources-toolkits/toolkits/improving-health-care-response-cardiovascular-disease-pregnancy-and
- The NYHA functional classification is available at: www.heart.org/HEARTORG/Conditions/Heartfailure/about heartfailure/classes-of-Heart-Failure_UCM_306328 Article.jsp (permission requested)
- The Hour-1 Bundle is available at:
    - https://www.sccm.org/SurvivingSepsisCampaign/Guidelines/Adult-Patients (permission requested)

# Appendix D: American Heart Association Opioid-Associated Emergency Algorithm for Healthcare Providers

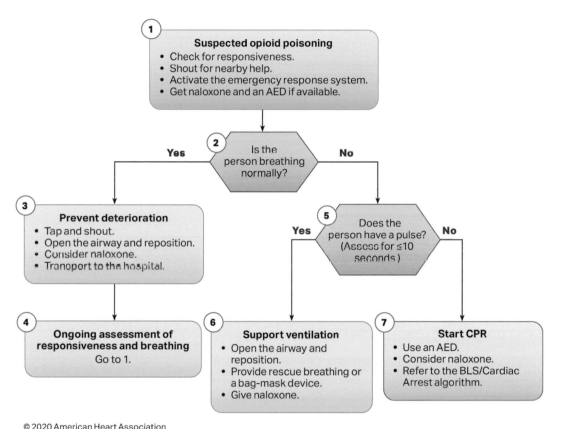

**1**
**Suspected opioid poisoning**
- Check for responsiveness.
- Shout for nearby help.
- Activate the emergency response system.
- Get naloxone and an AED if available.

**2** Is the person breathing normally?

Yes — No

**3**
**Prevent deterioration**
- Tap and shout.
- Open the airway and reposition.
- Consider naloxone.
- Transport to the hospital.

**5** Does the person have a pulse? (Assess for ≤10 seconds.)

Yes — No

**4**
**Ongoing assessment of responsiveness and breathing**
Go to 1.

**6**
**Support ventilation**
- Open the airway and reposition.
- Provide rescue breathing or a bag-mask device.
- Give naloxone.

**7**
**Start CPR**
- Use an AED.
- Consider naloxone.
- Refer to the BLS/Cardiac Arrest algorithm.

© 2020 American Heart Association

# Appendix E: Post-ROSC Care Checklist IH

## AIRWAY

- ❏ Intubate (if not already)
- ❏ Vent setting: 6–8mL/kg
- ❏ Avoid hyperventilation
- ❏ Place OG/NG

## BREATHING

- ❏ Oxygen saturation > 94%
- ❏ Maintain via PEEP and $FiO_2$
- ❏ Avoid hypoxia or hyperoxia
- ❏ Continuous wave capnography
- ❏ $ETCO_2$: 30–40 mm Hg
- ❏ $PACO_2$ Pregnant: 28–32 mm Hg
- ❏ $PACO_2$ Not pregnant: 35–45 mm Hg

## CIRCULATION

- ❏ 12-lead EKG
- ❏ Maintain SBP > 90, MAP > 65, but ideally > 80
- ❏ IV Fluids: 1–2 L NS/LR
- ❏ Serial labs (include lactic acid)
- ❏ Indwelling urinary catheter
- ❏ POC-US for etiology
- ❏ Central/arterial line
- ❏ First-line pressor: Norepinephrine 0.1–0.5 mcg/kg/min
- ❏ Alternate: Epinephrine 0.1–0.5 mcg/kg/min or Dopamine 5–10 mcg/kg/min
- ❏ Indwelling urinary catheter

## DISABILITY

- ❏ Targeted Temperature Management
  - ❏ 32–36°C for at least 24 hr
- ❏ Mechanical compression or anticoagulation for DVT prevention

- ❏ $H_2$ blocker for ulcer prevention
- ❏ Seizure treatment if indicated

## ECPR

- ❏ Refractory CPR
- ❏ Organ donation if circulatory determination of death

## FETUS

- ❏ If 23+0–36+6 weeks: continuous external fetal monitoring ASAP after ROSC + betamethasone 12 mg IM q24 hours X 2
- ❏ If 23+0–31+6 weeks: IV magnesium sulfate (unless otherwise contraindicated) for fetal neuroprotection

After RCD
- ❏ Perioperative antibiotics
- ❏ Cefazolin: 1–2 grams IV
- ❏ Penicillin allergy: Clindamycin 900 mg IV + Gentamicin 5 mg/kg IV

## FIND CAUSE

- ❏ BAACC TO LIFE (see reverse side)
- ❏ Multidisciplinary coordination

## GATHER

- ❏ Debrief with code response team and family members

## HEAD

- ❏ Obtain CT or MRI head early to evaluate for possible stroke

# BAACC TO LIFE

**B**leeding
- [ ] Diagnosis: inspect vagina, uterus
  - [ ] Treat: uterotonics, balloon tamponade, TXA, surgery, IR

**A**nesthesia
- [ ] High spinal: supportive
- [ ] Lidocaine overdose: IV lipids

**A**FE
- [ ] Supportive
- [ ] A-OK: atropine 1 mg, ondansetron 8 mg, ketorolac 30 mg

**C**ardiovascular
- [ ] MI: emergent angiography
- [ ] PPCM: POC-US

**C**lot
- [ ] VTE: CT angiogram, POC-US
  - [ ] Treat: Anticoagulation, catheter-directed TPA, surgery
- [ ] ECMO
- [ ] Stroke: CT head, EEG, MRI
- [ ] TPA, aspirin, anticoagulation

**T**rauma
- [ ] r/o abruption: OB ultrasound, coagulation factors, fibrinogen, KB

**O**verdose (opioids, IV drugs)
- [ ] Mag OD: stop infusion, calcium gluconate
- [ ] Opioid OD: naloxone

**L**ung injury
- [ ] PE: CXR
  - [ ] Treat: Lasix
- [ ] ARDS: CT chest
  - [ ] Treat: PEEP

**I**atrogenic/ions
- [ ] POC glucose

**F**ever
- [ ] Lactate
- [ ] IV antibiotics

**E**mergency HTN/Eclampsia
- [ ] Antihypertensives
  - [ ] IV Labetalol: 20 mg1/n40 mg1/n80 mg1/n80 mg (q10 min)
  - [ ] IV Hydralazine: 5 mg1/n10 mg1/n10 mg (q20 min)
  - [ ] Immediate-release oral nifedipine: 10 mg1/n 20 mg1/n20 mg (q20 min)
- [ ] Anticonvulsants: magnesium sulfate

# Appendix F: Post-ROSC Care Checklist OH

**Checklist Purpose:** OH team lead uses checklist to direct post-ROSC care elements.

| | Post-ROSC Actions |
|---|---|
| ❑ | Verifies ROSC |
| ❑ | Evaluates AVPU |
| ❑ | Manages airway and gives breaths every 6-8 seconds, as needed |
| ❑ | Maintains LUD |
| ❑ | Obtains and transmits 12-lead ECG |
| ❑ | Maintains vascular access and administers fluids |
| ❑ | Evaluates for causes |

# Appendix G: Venous Thromboembolism Prophylaxis Following Stroke

## VENOUS THROMBOEMBOLISM PROPHYLAXIS FOLLOWING STROKE

| STROKE TYPE | RECOMMENDED PROPHYLAXIS |
|---|---|
| Ischemic stroke | • Intermittent pneumatic compression devices beginning the day of hospital admission<br>• Consider LMWH or unfractionated heparin (UFH)<br>• In patients who received tPA, LMWH or UFH may be considered after imaging obtained 24 hours following tPA administration confirms no intracranial hemorrhage |
| Intracranial hemorrhage | • Intermittent pneumatic compression devices beginning the day of hospital admission<br>• Low-dose subcutaneous LMWH or UFH after documentation of cessation of bleeding for 1–4 days |
| Subarachnoid hemorrhage | • Intermittent pneumatic compression devices beginning the day of hospital admission and continuing until ruptured aneurysm (if present) is secured |

Abbreviations: LMWH, low-molecular-weight heparin; UFH, unfractionated heparin.

# Appendix H: Megacode Checklist OH Basic

**OBLS MEGACODE CHECKLIST - Out-of-Hospital BASIC**

**Name of Team Leader** _____     **Scenario** _____

**Directions**: For each participant, use the scale provided and circle the number indicating the extent to which they completed the action. Items with * are critical components. *Participants may score 0 on only two critical components.*

| Step | Assessment/Action | Done Correctly = 5<br>Done Poorly or Delayed = 3<br>Not Done = 0<br>N/A | | | | |
|------|-------------------|:---:|:---:|:---:|:---:|:---:|
| | **RESUSCITATION** | | | | | |
| 1 | Performs primary survey | 5 | 3 | 0 | N/A | |
| 2 | Recognizes cardiac arrest* | **5** | **3** | **0** | **N/A** | |
| 3 | Calls for additional resources as needed | 5 | 3 | 0 | N/A | |
| 4 | Places patient on hard surface/safe location | 5 | 3 | 0 | N/A | 1 min |
| 5 | Initiates high-quality chest compressions* | **5** | **3** | **0** | **N/A** | |
| 6 | Establishes and maintains effective ventilation (as staffing allows)* | **5** | **3** | **0** | **N/A** | |
| 7 | Ventilates at an appropriate rate and depth | 5 | 3 | 0 | N/A | |
| 8 | Assesses possibility of pregnancy/assesses uterine fundus relationship to umbilicus | 5 | 3 | 0 | N/A | |
| 9 | Performs LUD* | **5** | **3** | **0** | **N/A** | |
| 10 | Anticipates potential need for RCD | 5 | 3 | 0 | N/A | |
| 11 | Places defibrillation pads avoiding breast tissue | 5 | 3 | 0 | N/A | |
| 12 | Assesses cardiac rhythm with AED after 1 cycle of CPR | 5 | 3 | 0 | N/A | 2-5 mins |
| 13 | Defibrillates if indicated by AED, clears patient prior to shock* | **5** | **3** | **0** | **N/A** | |
| 14 | Directs preparation for and transport of patient to most appropriate facility (OB Arrest Alert)* | 5 | 3 | 0 | N/A | |
| 15 | Applies ACCD correctly, if used | 5 | 3 | 0 | N/A | |
| | **A. Resuscitation SUBTOTAL (Items 1-15)** | | | | | |
| | **POST-ROSC CARE** | | | | | |
| 16 | Verifies ROSC | 5 | 3 | 0 | N/A | |
| 17 | Evaluates AVPU scale (alert, verbal, pain, unresponsive) | 5 | 3 | 0 | N/A | |
| 18 | Maintains airway and gives breaths every 6 seconds, as needed | 5 | 3 | 0 | N/A | POST-ROSC CARE |
| 19 | Maintains LUD | 5 | 3 | 0 | N/A | |
| 20 | Obtains and transmits 12-lead ECG | 5 | 3 | 0 | N/A | |
| 21 | Maintains vascular access and administers fluids | 5 | 3 | 0 | N/A | |
| 22 | Evaluates for causes | 5 | 3 | 0 | N/A | |
| | **B. Post-ROSC SUBTOTAL (Items 16-22)** | | | | | |

| Step | Assessment/Action | Done Correctly = 5 Done Poorly or Delayed = 3 Not Done = 0 N/A | | | |
|---|---|---|---|---|---|
| | **TEAM PERFORMANCE** | | | | |
| 23 | Performs continuous LUD throughout resuscitation | 5 | 3 | 0 | N/A |
| 24 | Rotates personnel performing chest compressions and LUD every 2 min | 5 | 3 | 0 | N/A |
| 25 | Minimizes chest compression interruptions (< 10 sec delay) | 5 | 3 | 0 | N/A |
| 26 | Designated team member guides resuscitation with OBLS cognitive aid (ALIVE at 5) | 5 | 3 | 0 | N/A |
| | **C. Team Performance SUBTOTAL (Items 23-26)** | | | | |

TEAM PERF

| Step | How well did the TEAM | Perfect = 5    Good = 4 Average = 3    Poor = 2 Unacceptable = 1 | | | | |
|---|---|---|---|---|---|---|
| | **COMMUNICATION/TEAMWORK** | | | | | |
| 27 | Use SBAR to orient team members as they arrived? | 5 | 4 | 3 | 2 | 1 |
| 28 | Call for ADDITIONAL ASSISTANCE in a timely manner? | 5 | 4 | 3 | 2 | 1 |
| 29 | Utilize CLOSED-LOOP communication? | 5 | 4 | 3 | 2 | 1 |
| 30 | Maintain SITUATIONAL AWARENESS? | 5 | 4 | 3 | 2 | 1 |
| 31 | Utilize PATIENT FRIENDLY language and tone | 5 | 4 | 3 | 2 | 1 |
| Step | **Rate** | | | | | |
| 32 | OVERALL team communication | 5 | 4 | 3 | 2 | 1 |
| 33 | OVERALL team performance | 5 | 4 | 3 | 2 | 1 |
| | **D. Communication/Teamwork SUBTOTAL (Items 27-33)** | | | | | |

| | **SCORING** | Subtotals |
|---|---|---|
| A | Resuscitation | |
| B | Post ROSC | |
| C | Team Performance | |
| D | Total Communication/Teamwork | |
| E | Subtotal (add A + B + C + D) | |
| F | **Total points possible** | 165 |
| G | N/A adjustment (multiply # of N/A by 5) | |
| H | Adjusted total points (F minus G) | |
| I | Overall weighted score (divide E by H) | |
| J | Number of critical components* scored 0 (#1-22) | |

**SUMMARY**

PASS = Overall score > 74%  and no critical components scored 0.
Circle YES or NO.

| YES | NO |
|---|---|

Instructor Signature:

_____

Instructor Name and Date:

_____

Instructor potential?      **YES**      **NO**

2021.06.15

# Appendix I: Megacode Checklist OH Advanced

**OBLS MEGACODE CHECKLIST - Out-of-Hospital Advanced**

Name of Team Leader _____     Scenario _____

**Directions**: For each participant, use the scale provided and circle the number indicating the extent to which they completed the action. Items with * are critical components. *Participants may score 0 on only two critical components.*

| Step | Assessment/Action | Done Correctly = 5 Done Poorly or Delayed = 3 Not Done = 0 N/A | | | | |
|---|---|---|---|---|---|---|
| | | **RESUSCITATION** | | | | |
| 1 | Performs primary survey | 5 | 3 | 0 | N/A | |
| 2 | Recognizes cardiac arrest* | 5 | 3 | 0 | N/A | |
| 3 | Calls for additional resources as needed | 5 | 3 | 0 | N/A | |
| 4 | Places patient on hard surface/safe location | 5 | 3 | 0 | N/A | 1 min |
| 5 | Initiates high-quality chest compressions* | 5 | 3 | 0 | N/A | |
| 6 | Establishes and maintains effective ventilation (as staffing allows) * | 5 | 3 | 0 | N/A | |
| 7 | Ventilates at an appropriate rate | 5 | 3 | 0 | N/A | |
| 8 | Assesses possibility of pregnancy/assesses uterine fundus relationship to umbilicus | 5 | 3 | 0 | N/A | |
| 9 | Performs left uterine displacement* | 5 | 3 | 0 | N/A | |
| 10 | Anticipates potential need for resuscitative cesarean delivery | 5 | 3 | 0 | N/A | |
| 11 | Places defibrillation pads avoiding breast tissue | 5 | 3 | 0 | N/A | |
| 12 | Assesses cardiac rhythm after 1 cycle of CPR | 5 | 3 | 0 | N/A | |
| 13 | Defibrillates if indicated, clears patient prior to shock* | 5 | 3 | 0 | N/A | 2-5 mins |
| 14 | Inserts IV or IO above diaphragm | 5 | 3 | 0 | N/A | |
| 15 | Administers epinephrine | | | | | |
| | a. non-shockable: immediately | 5 | 3 | 0 | N/A | |
| | b. shockable: after two shocks | 5 | 3 | 0 | N/A | |
| 16 | Recognizes and treats reversible etiologies for maternal cardiac arrest, if applicable (e.g., Narcan for opioid overdose, etc.) | 5 | 3 | 0 | N/A | |
| 17 | Directs preparation for and transport of patient to most appropriate facility (OB Arrest Alert)* | 5 | 3 | 0 | N/A | |
| 18 | Applies ACCD correctly, if used | 5 | 3 | 0 | N/A | |
| | **A. Resuscitation SUBTOTAL (Items 1-18)** | | | | | |
| | | **POST-ROSC CARE** | | | | |
| 19 | Verifies return of spontaneous circulation (ROSC) | 5 | 3 | 0 | N/A | |
| 20 | Evaluates AVPU | 5 | 3 | 0 | N/A | |
| 21 | Maintains airway and gives breaths every 6 seconds, as needed | 5 | 3 | 0 | N/A | POST-ROSC CARE |
| 22 | Maintains left uterine displacement | 5 | 3 | 0 | N/A | |
| 23 | Obtains and transmits 12-lead ECG | 5 | 3 | 0 | N/A | |
| 24 | Maintains vascular access and administers fluids | 5 | 3 | 0 | N/A | |
| 25 | Evaluates for causes | 5 | 3 | 0 | N/A | |
| | **B. Post-ROSC SUBTOTAL (Items 19-25)** | | | | | |

| Step | Assessment/Action | Done Correctly = 5 Done Poorly or Delayed = 3 Not Done = 0 N/A | | | | |
|---|---|---|---|---|---|---|
| | **TEAM PERFORMANCE** | | | | | |
| 26 | Performs continuous LUD throughout resuscitation | 5 | 3 | 0 | N/A | |
| 27 | Rotates personnel performing chest compressions and LUD every 2 min | 5 | 3 | 0 | N/A | |
| 28 | Minimizes chest compression interruptions (< 10 sec delay) | 5 | 3 | 0 | N/A | TEAM PERF |
| 29 | Designated team member guides resuscitation with OBLS cognitive aid (ALIVE at 5) | 5 | 3 | 0 | N/A | |
| 30 | Keeps time of cardiac arrest and log of times/interventions | 5 | 3 | 0 | N/A | |
| 31 | Performs continuous high-quality CPR/OBLS until ROSC or higher level of care transfer achieved | 5 | 3 | 0 | N/A | |
| 32 | Uses BAACC TO LIFE for differential diagnosis | 5 | 3 | 0 | N/A | |
| | **C. Team Performance SUBTOTAL (Items 26-32)** | | | | | |

| Step | How well **did the TEAM** | Perfect = 5   Good = 4 Average = 3   Poor = 2 Unacceptable = 1 | | | | |
|---|---|---|---|---|---|---|
| | **COMMUNICATION/TEAMWORK** | | | | | |
| 33 | Use SBAR to orientt eam members as they arrived? | 5 | 4 | 3 | 2 | 1 |
| 34 | Call for ADDITIONAL ASSISTANCE in a timely manner? | 5 | 4 | 3 | 2 | 1 |
| 35 | Utilize CLOSED-LOOP communication? | 5 | 4 | 3 | 2 | 1 |
| 36 | Maintain SITUATIONAL AWARENESS? | 5 | 4 | 3 | 2 | 1 |
| 37 | Utilize PATIENT FRIENDLY language and tone | 5 | 4 | 3 | 2 | 1 |
| **Step** | **Rate** | | | | | |
| 38 | OVERALL team communication | 5 | 4 | 3 | 2 | 1 |
| 39 | OVERALL team performance | 5 | 4 | 3 | 2 | 1 |
| | **D. Communication/Teamwork SUBTOTAL (Items 33-39)** | | | | | |

| | **SCORING** | Subtotals |
|---|---|---|
| A | Resuscitation | |
| B | Post-ROSC | |
| C | Team Performance | |
| D | Total Communication/Teamwork | |
| E | Subtotal (add A + B + C + D) | |
| F | **Total points possible** | 195 |
| G | N/A adjustment (multiply # of N/A by 5) | |
| H | Adjusted total points (F minus G) | |
| I | Overall weighted score (divide E by H) | |
| J | Number of critical components* scored 0 (#1-21) | |

**SUMMARY**

PASS = Overall score > 74% and no critical components scored 0.
Circle YES or NO.

| YES | NO |
|---|---|

Instructor Signature:

_____

Instructor Name and Date:

_____

Instructor potential?     YES     NO

# Appendix J: Megacode Checklist IH

**OBLS MEGACODE CHECKLIST - In-Hospital**

Name of Team Leader _____     Scenario _____

**Directions**: For each participant, use the scale provided and circle the number indicating the extent to which they completed the action. Items with * are critical components. *Participants may score 0 on only two critical components.*

| Step | Assessment/Action | Done Correctly = 5 Done Poorly or Delayed = 3 Not Done = 0 N/A | | | | |
|------|-------------------|---|---|---|---|---|
| **RESUSCITATION** | | | | | | |
| 1 | Recognizes unstable vital signs in pregnant patient | 5 | 3 | 0 | N/A | |
| 2 | Recognizes cardiac arrest* | 5 | 3 | 0 | N/A | |
| 3 | Activates MCAT | 5 | 3 | 0 | N/A | |
| 4 | Positions patient flat and places backboard | 5 | 3 | 0 | N/A | |
| 5 | Initiates high-quality chest compressions* | 5 | 3 | 0 | N/A | **1 min** |
| 6 | Establishes and maintains effective ventilation* | 5 | 3 | 0 | N/A | |
| 7 | Ventilates at appropriate rate | 5 | 3 | 0 | N/A | |
| 8 | Assesses possibility of pregnancy/assesses uterine fundus relationship to umbilicus | 5 | 3 | 0 | N/A | |
| 9 | Performs and maintains LUD throughout resuscitation* | 5 | 3 | 0 | N/A | |
| 10 | Gathers equipment for RCD | 5 | 3 | 0 | N/A | |
| 11 | Places defibrillation pads avoiding breast tissue | 5 | 3 | 0 | N/A | |
| 12 | Assesses cardiac rhythm after 1 cycle of CPR | 5 | 3 | 0 | N/A | |
| 13 | Removes fetal monitors | 5 | 3 | 0 | N/A | |
| 14 | Defibrillates if indicated, clears patient before shock* | 5 | 3 | 0 | N/A | |
| 15 | Inserts IV or IO above diaphragm | 5 | 3 | 0 | N/A | **2-5 mins** |
| 16 | Administers epinephrine: a. non-shockable: immediately | 5 | 3 | 0 | N/A | |
| | b. shockable: after two shocks | 5 | 3 | 0 | N/A | |
| 17 | Recognizes and treats reversible etiologies for MCA, if applicable (e.g., calcium gluconate for magnesium toxicity, Narcan for opioid overdose) | 5 | 3 | 0 | N/A | |
| 18 | Completes RCD by 5 min at site of arrest* | 5 | 3 | 0 | N/A | |
| 19 | Minimizes chest compression interruptions (< 10 sec delay) | 5 | 3 | 0 | N/A | **5+ mins** |
| 20 | Timely notification of contingency teams (i.e., ECPR, MAST, vascular surgeon) | 5 | 3 | 0 | N/A | |
| 21 | Verifies ROSC | 5 | 3 | 0 | N/A | |
| **A. Resuscitation SUBTOTAL (Items 1-21)** | | | | | | |
| **POST-ROSC CARE** | | | | | | |
| 22 | Discusses post-arrest care elements following ROSC to establish next steps in management | 5 | 3 | 0 | N/A | |
| 23 | Secures airway and gives breaths every 6 seconds, as needed | 5 | 3 | 0 | N/A | |
| 24 | Maintains LUD, if pregnant | 5 | 3 | 0 | N/A | **POST-ROSC CARE** |
| 25 | Maintains vascular access and administers fluids | 5 | 3 | 0 | N/A | |
| 26 | Uses BAACC TO LIFE to consider potential etiology(ies) | 5 | 3 | 0 | N/A | |
| 27 | Manages wounds (closure, antibiotics) | 5 | 3 | 0 | N/A | |
| 28 | Orders head CT prior to transfer to ICU, ifi indicated | 5 | 3 | 0 | N/A | |
| **B. Post-ROSC Care SUBTOTAL (Items 22-28)** | | | | | | |

| TEAM LEADER PERFORMANCE | | | | | |
|---|---|---|---|---|---|
| Step | Assessment/Action | Done Correctly = 5<br>Done Poorly or Delayed = 3<br>Not Done = 0<br>N/A | | | |
| 29 | Effectively guides resuscitation, focusing on high-quality chest compressions and continuous LUD | 5 | 3 | 0 | N/A |
| 30 | Effectively delineates responsibilities to team members | 5 | 3 | 0 | N/A |
| 31 | Ensures team member keeps time of cardiac arrest and logs times/interventions | 5 | 3 | 0 | N/A |
| 32 | Ensures contingency teams are present and working together effectively | 5 | 3 | 0 | N/A |
| 33 | Recommends debrief w/ OBLS debrief tool | 5 | 3 | 0 | N/A |
| C. Team Leader Performance SUBTOTAL (Items 29-33) | | | | | |

LEAD PERF

| COMMUNICATION/TEAMWORK | | | | | | |
|---|---|---|---|---|---|---|
| Step | How well did the TEAM | Perfect = 5    Good = 4<br>Average = 3    Poor = 2<br>Unacceptable = 1 | | | | |
| 34 | Use SBAR to orientt eam members as they arrived? | 5 | 4 | 3 | 2 | 1 |
| 35 | Call for ADDITIONAL ASSISTANCE in a timely manner? | 5 | 4 | 3 | 2 | 1 |
| 36 | Utilize CLOSED-LOOP communication? | 5 | 4 | 3 | 2 | 1 |
| 37 | Maintain SITUATIONAL AWARENESS? | 5 | 4 | 3 | 2 | 1 |
| 38 | Utilize PATIENT FRIENDLY language and tone | 5 | 4 | 3 | 2 | 1 |
| | Rate | | | | | |
| 39 | OVERALL team communication | 5 | 4 | 3 | 2 | 1 |
| 40 | OVERALL team performance | 5 | 4 | 3 | 2 | 1 |
| D. Communication/Teamwork SUBTOTAL (Items 34-40) | | | | | | |

| SCORING | | |
|---|---|---|
| | | Subtotals |
| A | Resuscitation | |
| B | Post-ROSC | |
| C | Team Performance | |
| D | Total Communication/Teamwork | |
| E | Subtotal (add A + B + C + D) | |
| F | Total points possible | 200 |
| G | N/A adjustment (multiply # of N/A by 5) | |
| H | Adjusted total points (F minus G) | |
| I | Overall weighted score (divide E by H) | |
| J | Number of critical components* scored 0 (#1-21) | |

**SUMMARY**

PASS = Overall score > 74%  and no critical components scored 0.
Circle YES or NO.

| YES | NO |
|---|---|

Instructor Signature:

_____

Instructor Name and Date:

_____

Instructor potential?   YES          NO

2021.03.18

# Appendix K: Institutional Preparedness

## INSTITUTIONAL PREPAREDNESS

I. Resuscitative cesarean delivery hospital preparation toolkit
   A. Quick highlight checklists
   B. Algorithms
   C. Cognitive aids
   D. Figures showing different incisions and how to perform
   E. Multiple choice of incision type with different scenarios
   F. Naming instruments needed for delivery
   G. Location of delivery (at place of arrest in-hospital)
   H. Video simulation of resuscitative cesarean delivery
      1. Voiceover of ≥20 weeks, professionals who perform this procedure, 4 minutes to incision (2 cycles of CPR)/5 incision minutes to delivery
      2. Voiceover for resuscitative cesarean delivery/video simulation

# Appendix L: OBLS Drug List

| MEDICATION | DOSE | ROUTE | INDICATION | CONTRAINDICATIONS | | CONSIDERATIONS |
|---|---|---|---|---|---|---|
| | | | | ABSOLUTE | RELATIVE | |
| **Atropine** | 0.5–1 mg or 0.04 mg/kg IV q5 min | IV IM | Sinus bradycardia | Acute myocardial infarction, angina, bleeding, cardiac arrhythmias, cardiac disease, coronary artery disease, heart failure, hypertension, hyperthyroidism, hypersensitivity, mitral stenosis, myocardial infarction, tachycardia, thyrotoxicosis | Narrow-angle glaucoma, tachycardia, asthma, GI obstruction, severe ulcerative colitis, toxic megacolon, bladder outlet obstruction | Maximum dose: 3 mg<br><br>Likely ineffective treatment for bradycardia in the setting of heart transplant patients |
| **Carboprost tromethamine** | 250 mcg q 1–3 hours | IM | Postpartum hemorrhage | Pulmonary (e.g., asthma), cardiovascular, renal, or hepatic disease, hypersensitivity. | Hypertension, acute pelvic inflammatory disease | The total dose administered of carboprost tromethamine should not exceed 2 mg and continuous administration of the drug for more than two days is not recommended |
| **Dilute epinephrine (1:10,000)** | 0.5 mg (5 mL) IV q3–5 min | IV/IO | Cardiac arrest | None in life-threatening situations | Nonanaphylactic shock, narrow-angle glaucoma, thyrotoxicosis, diabetes, hypertension, cardiovascular disease, sulfite hypersensitivity | |
| **Ephedrine** | 5–10 mg | IV bolus | Severe hypotension/ shock | Hypersensitivity | Caution with renal disease | Maximum total cumulative dose: 50 mg |

*(Continued)*

(Continued)

| MEDICATION | DOSE | ROUTE | INDICATION | CONTRAINDICATIONS ABSOLUTE | CONTRAINDICATIONS RELATIVE | CONSIDERATIONS |
|---|---|---|---|---|---|---|
| Lipid emulsion | Patients >70 kg: 100 mL bolus of 20% lipid emulsion over 1–3 min, followed 0.25 mL/kg/min infusion (max 200–250 mL) minutes<br><br>Patients <70 kg: 1.5 mL/kg (of lean body weight) bolus of 20% lipid emulsion followed by a 0.25 mL/kg/minute infusion | IV | Local anesthetic systemic toxicity | Abnormal lipid metabolism, lipid nephrosis, acute pancreatitis, hypersensitivity | Documented severe egg allergy, impaired lipid metabolism and lipid storage disorders, severe hyperlipidemia<br><br>A blood coagulation disorder, moderate to severe liver disease, compromised pulmonary function | |
| Methylergo-novine | 0.2 mg q2–4 hr PRN; not to exceed 5 doses | IM | Postpartum hemorrhage/uterine atony | Hypertension, heart disease, hypersensitivity, mitral valve stenosis, stroke, liver disease | Sepsis, vascular disease | Avoid IV administration |
| Misoprostol | 800–1000 mcg | PO or PR | Postpartum hemorrhage/uterine atony | Hypersensitivity, known bleeding disorder, concurrent anticoagulant therapy | Renal impairment | Use of misoprostol in the setting of postpartum hemorrhage is accepted by ACOG, however is technically off-label use of this medication<br><br>Abortifacient: do not use for uterine bleeding in the setting of pregnant uterus |
| Oxytocin | 30 units/500 mL; set the infusion pump rate to 334 mL/hour for 30 minutes (10 units in 167 mL), then reduce the rate to 95 mL/hour (remaining 20 units) over 3.5 hours<br><br>10 U IM if no IV access | IV, IM | Postpartum hemorrhage/uterine atony | Hypersensitivity | Cardiovascular disease/ myocardial ischemia | In the setting of maternal cardiac arrest, oxytocin may precipitate rearrest. Titrate slowly as needed |
| Packed red blood cells (PRBC) | Massive transfusion protocol, e.g., 1:1:1 (units PRBC:FFP:Platelet) | IV | Postpartum hemorrhage | Cross-type mismatch | | |
| Phenylephrine | Hypotension from anesthesia: 40–100 mcg q1–2 min PRN, not to exceed total dose of 200 mcg<br><br>For shock: 0.5–2 mcg/kg/min, titrate to desired MAP | IV | Severe hypotension/ shock | Sulfite hypersensitivity, stroke/ intracranial bleed, hypertension, cardiac disease, Concomitant use of monoamine oxidase inhibitors (MAOI) | Septic shock (unless norepinephrine is associated with arrhythmia; or needed as salvage therapy) | Continuous IV infusion: If blood pressure is below the target goal, start a continuous IV infusion with an infusion rate of 10–35 mcg/min; not to exceed 200 mcg/min |

| Drug | Dose | Route | Indication | Contraindications | | |
|---|---|---|---|---|---|---|
| **Tranexamic acid** | 1 g in 10 mL (100 mg/mL) IV at 1 mL per min | IV | Postpartum hemorrhage | Hypersensitivity, active intravascular clotting, subarachnoid hemorrhage, active thromboembolic disease, DIC | Visual defects, seizures | May consider an additional 1 g if bleeding continues after 30 minutes of 1st dose |

**Indication: Acute Ischemic Stroke**

| Drug | Dose | Route | Indication | Contraindications | | |
|---|---|---|---|---|---|---|
| **Alteplase (rtPA)** | ≤67 kg: 15 mg IVP bolus over 1–2 minutes, **then** 0.75 mg/kg IV infusion over 30 minutes (not to exceed 50 mg), and **then** 0.5 mg/kg IV over next 60 minutes (not to exceed 35 mg over 1 hr); >67 kg (100 mg total dose infused over 1.5 hr): 15 mg IVP bolus over 1–2 minutes, **then** 50 mg IV infusion over next 30 minutes, and **then** remaining 35 mg over next 60 minutes | IV | Acute ischemic stroke | Current or prior intracranial hemorrhage · Subarachnoid hemorrhage suspected · Active internal bleeding · Stroke within 3 months except when within 4.5 hours · Recent (within 3 months) intracranial or intraspinal surgery or serious head trauma · Presence of intracranial conditions that may increase the risk of bleeding (e.g., some neoplasms, arteriovenous malformations, aneurysms) · Bleeding diathesis · Current severe uncontrolled hypertension · Acute myocardial infarction or pulmonary embolism · Significant closed head or facial trauma with radiographic evidence of brain injury or facial trauma within 3 months | Cardiogenic shock, traumatic or prolonged CPR, major surgery within past 3 weeks, internal bleeding within past 4 weeks, active peptic ulcer disease, noncompressible vascular puncture, current use of anticoagulants | May also be used in the setting of pulmonary embolism (hemodynamically stable): 100 mg IV infusion over 2 hr |
| **Protamine sulfate** | 1 mg per 100 U of heparin | IV | Coagulopathy due to heparin infusion or with subcutaneous heparin | Hypersensitivity | History of past protamine exposure, vasectomy, fish allergies, and insulin-controlled diabetes | Maximum single dose 50 mg |
| **Protamine sulfate (off-label)** | ≤8 hr from last dose: protamine sulfate 1 mg per 1 mg of enoxaparin (maximum single dose 50 mg) | IV | Coagulopathy due to heparin infusion or with subcutaneous heparin | Hypersensitivity | History of past protamine exposure, vasectomy, fish allergies, and insulin-controlled diabetes. | |
| **Prothrombin complex concentrates (PCC)** | Based on pretreatment INR obtained close to time of dosing | IV | Coagulopathy due to current therapy with vitamin K antagonist | History of disseminated intravascular coagulation, history of MI/angina/PVD/stroke/VTE in last 3 months | | |

*(Continued)*

(Continued)

| MEDICATION | DOSE | ROUTE | INDICATION | CONTRAINDICATIONS ABSOLUTE | CONTRAINDICATIONS RELATIVE | CONSIDERATIONS |
|---|---|---|---|---|---|---|
| **Vitamin K** | 5–10 mg | IV | Coagulopathy due to current therapy with vitamin K antagonist | Hypersensitivity | | Maximum rate of infusion is 1 mg/min. For severe coagulopathy, administer with clotting factors or plasma |
| **Indication: Amniotic Fluid Embolism/Right-Heart Failure** | | | | | | |
| Sildenafil | PO: 5 mg or 20 mg TID; administer 4–6 hr apart. IV: 2.5-mg or 10-mg bolus TID if patient is temporarily unable to take PO | IV/PO | Pulmonary arterial hypertension | Hypersensitivity. Soluble guanylate cyclase (sGC) stimulators (e.g., riociguat); concomitant use can cause hypotension. Coadministration with nitrates. Use of protease inhibitors | Hypotension; history of vision loss; hepatic impairment | |
| Dobutamine | 0.5–5 mcg/kg/min IV continuous infusion initially, then 2–20 mcg/kg/min; not to exceed 40 mcg/kg/min | | Cardiac decompensation/cardiogenic shock | Hypersensitivity (or hypersensitivity to sulfites) including corn, hypertrophic cardiomyopathy with outflow tract obstruction, uncorrected hypovolemia | Cardiac arrythmias, coronary artery disease/hypertension, renal failure | Not effective in the setting of aortic stenosis. Correct electrolyte imbalances prior to use to limit risk of arrhythmia |
| Milrinone | 50 mcg/kg loading dose by IV push over 10 minutes, then 0.125–0.75 mcg/kg/min IV | IV | Congestive heart failure | Hypersensitivity | Severe heart failure, severe pulmonary hypertension, acute renal failure, end-stage renal disease | Correct electrolyte imbalances prior to use to limit risk of arrhythmia |
| Inhaled nitric oxide | 5–10 ppm | Inhaled | Pulmonary arterial hypertension | Severe left ventricular dysfunction, congenital heart disease with ductal dependent systemic circulation (e.g., interrupted aortic arch, critical aortic stenosis, hypoplastic left heart syndrome) | | |
| Iloprost (Inhaled prostacyclin) | Initial: 2.5 mcg inhaled, if well-tolerated, **then** 5 mcg subsequent doses. 6–9 times/day PRN; >q2 hr while awake. Maintenance: 2.5–5 mcg/dose; not to exceed 45 mcg/day | Inhaled | Pulmonary arterial hypertension | None | Relative: worsening cardiogenic pulmonary edema, active hemorrhage, renal dysfunction | |

## Indication: Amniotic Fluid Embolism/Right-Heart Failure

| | | | | | |
|---|---|---|---|---|---|
| IV prostacyclin | | 1 ng/kg/min infusion pump over 24–48 hours; titrate 1–2 ng/kg/min q 15 min or longer, until desired effect | Hypersensitivity; chronic use in patients with CHF due to left ventricular systolic dysfunction; development of pulmonary edema during initial infusion | Risk factors for bleeding | Abrupt withdrawal (including interruptions in drug delivery) or sudden large reductions in dosage may result in symptoms associated with rebound pulmonary hypertension, including dyspnea, dizziness, and asthenia; in clinical trials, death attributable to interruption of therapy reported; avoid abrupt withdrawal |
| Norepinephrine | IV | Initial: 0.05 mcg/kg/min; usual dosage: 0.05–0.4 mcg/kg/min<br><br>Non-weight based: 5–30 mcg/min IV infusion; titrate to effect (typically MAP >65) | Post-cardiac arrest shock; acute severe hypotension | Hypersensitivity, peripheral or mesenteric thrombosis; sulfite hypersensitivity (certain formulations) | During halothane or cyclopropane anesthesia; preexisting hyperthyroidism or hypertension; patients on MAO inhibitors → Antidote for extravasation ischemia: to prevent sloughing and necrosis in areas where extravasation has taken place, infiltrate areas promptly with 10–15 mL of saline solution containing 5–10 mg of phentolamine mesylate for injection |

## Indication: Cardiac Arrest

| | | | | | |
|---|---|---|---|---|---|
| Amiodarone | IV | 300 mg IV or intraosseous push after epinephrine if no initial response to defibrillation<br><br>May follow initial dose with 150 mg IV q3–5 min | Cardiac arrest; pulseless ventricular fibrillation/ventricular tachycardia | Hypersensitivity (to amiodarone or iodine but **not** shellfish or contrast dye)<br>Severe sinus node dysfunction, 2°/3° AV block or bradycardia causing syncope (except with functioning artificial pacemaker), cardiogenic shock | Hepatitis; pulmonary interstitial abnormalities; thyroid abnormalities → Pulmonary and hepatotoxicities can occur with amiodarone use |
| **Dilute epinephrine (1:10,000)** | IV/IO | 1 mg IV q3–5 min | Cardiac arrest | Narrow-angle glaucoma | None |

*(Continued)*

(Continued)

| MEDICATION | DOSE | ROUTE | INDICATION | CONTRAINDICATIONS ABSOLUTE | CONTRAINDICATIONS RELATIVE | CONSIDERATIONS |
|---|---|---|---|---|---|---|
| **Dopamine** | 1–5 mcg/kg/min IV (**low dose**): May increase urine output and renal blood flow<br><br>5–15 mcg/kg/min IV (**medium dose**): May increase renal blood flow, cardiac output, heart rate, and cardiac contractility<br><br>20–50 mcg/kg/min IV (**high dose**): May increase blood pressure and stimulate vasoconstriction; may not have a beneficial effect in blood pressure; may increase risk of tachyarrhythmias<br><br>May increase infusion by 1–4 mcg/kg/min at 10–30 min intervals until optimum response obtained | IV | Treatment of hypotension, low cardiac output, poor perfusion of vital organs; used to increase mean arterial pressure in septic shock patients who remain hypotensive after adequate volume expansion | Hypersensitivity to dopamine, pheochromocytoma, ventricular fibrillation, uncorrected tachyarrhythmias, acidosis | Concomitant use of phenytoin (hypotension, bradycardia) or oxytocin (hypertension stroke) | |
| **Lidocaine** | 1–1.5 mg/kg slow IV bolus over 2–3 minutes<br><br>May repeat doses of 0.5–0.75 mg/kg in 5–10 minutes up to 3 mg/kg total if refractory VF or pulseless VT<br><br>Continuous infusion: 1–4 mg/min IV after return of perfusion<br><br>Administer 0.5 mg/kg bolus and reassess infusion if arrhythmia reappears during constant infusion<br><br>If IV not feasible may use IO/ET | IV/IO | Cardiac arrest; pulseless ventricular tachycardia | Hypersensitivity to lidocaine or amide-type local anesthetic Adams-Stokes syndrome, SA/AV/ intraventricular heart block in the absence of artificial pacemaker CHF, cardiogenic shock, 2nd and 3rd degree heart block (if no pacemaker is present), Wolff-Parkinson–White syndrome | | |

**Indication: Heart Attack**

| Drug | Dose | Route | Indication | Contraindications | Precautions | Notes |
|---|---|---|---|---|---|---|
| **Alteplase (rtPA)** | ≤67 kg: 15 mg IVP bolus over 1–2 minutes, **then** 0.75 mg/kg IV infusion over 30 minutes (not to exceed 50 mg), and **then** 0.5 mg/kg IV over next 60 minutes (not to exceed 35 mg over 1 hr)<br><br>>67 kg (100 mg total dose infused over 1.5 hr): 15 mg IVP bolus over 1–2 minutes, **then** 50 mg IV infusion over next 30 minutes, and **then** remaining 35 mg over next 60 minutes | IV | Acute MI | See Contraindications in Acute Ischemic Stroke section | | See Contraindications in Acute Ischemic Stroke section |
| **Aspirin** | 160–325 mg PO; chew non-enteric-coated tablet; If unable to take PO, may give 300–600 mg suppository PR | PO or PR | Acute coronary syndrome | Hypersensitivity to aspirin or NSAIDs; aspirin-associated hypersensitivity reactions include aspirin-induced urticaria, asthma/rhinitis/nasal polyps, gastrointestinal bleed/peptic ulcer disease, head trauma, bleeding disorder | G6PD deficiency, renal impairment, preexisting liver disease, systemic lupus erythematosus, heart failure, acid/base imbalance | |
| **Beta-blocker (Metoprolol)** | 5 mg rapid IV q5 min, up to 3 doses; then, begin PO therapy 15–30 minutes after last IV, 50 mg q6 hr for 48 hours, then 50–100 mg PO q12 hr | IV | Acute MI | Asthma or obstructive airway disease, severe bradycardia, 2°/3° heart block (without pacemaker), cardiogenic shock, bronchial asthma, uncompensated cardiac failure, hypersensitivity, sinus bradycardia, sick sinus syndrome without permanent pacemaker; conditions associated with prolonged and severe; severe peripheral arterial circulatory disorder | 1st degree heart block, chronic heart failure, ischemic heart disease, myasthenia gravis (use with caution) | Use can lead to AV block (first, second, or complete) |
| **Clopidogrel** | STEMI: 300 mg loading dose; 75 mg/day PO for up to 12 months; STEMI: 75 mg/day PO | PO | NSTEMI/STEMI | Hypersensitivity; active bleeding (ex: GI bleed, SAH/intracranial bleed) | Renal disease, liver impairment, poor metabolizers (patients who are homozygous for nonfunctional alleles of the CYP2C19 gene) | Coordinate with cardiology re: fibrinolytic therapy and reperfusion |
| **Fentanyl** | 1–2 mcg/kg IV bolus or 25–100 mcg/dose loading dose, followed by 25–50 mcg Q 30–60 min or 1–2 mcg/kg/hr by continuous IV infusion or 25–200 mcg/hr | IV | Analgesia | Hypersensitivity, acute/severe asthma, respiratory depression, gastrointestinal obstruction | Obstructive sleep apnea, drug addiction, seizure disorder, renal or liver disease | |

*(Continued)*

(Continued)

| MEDICATION | DOSE | ROUTE | INDICATION | CONTRAINDICATIONS ABSOLUTE | CONTRAINDICATIONS RELATIVE | CONSIDERATIONS |
|---|---|---|---|---|---|---|
| **Heparin** | Adjunct to fibrinolytic for STEMI or NSTEMI: bolus 60–70 units/kg (max: 5000 units), **then** initial IV infusion of 12–15 units/kg/hr (max: 1000 units/hr) | IV | Unstable angina/ NSTEMI | Hypersensitivity; thrombocytopenia; history of heparin-induced thrombocytopenia, uncontrollable active bleeding, renal dysfunction, uncontrolled or severe hypertension | Hyperkalemia, products containing benzyl alcohol (preservative) is contraindicated in pregnant/breastfeeding women | |
| **Nitroglycerin** | 25–65 mcg PO q6–8 hr | PO | Angina | Hypersensitivity, acute MI, severe anemia, acute circulatory failure or shock, elevated ICP, pericardial tamponade | Hypotension, hypertrophic cardiomyopathy, hepatic disease, GI disease | |

**Indication: Hypertension and Preeclampsia**

| MEDICATION | DOSE | ROUTE | INDICATION | CONTRAINDICATIONS ABSOLUTE | CONTRAINDICATIONS RELATIVE | CONSIDERATIONS |
|---|---|---|---|---|---|---|
| **Diazepam** | 5–10 mg IV slowly | IV | Eclamptic seizure refractory to magnesium sulfate | Documented hypersensitivity Acute alcohol intoxication Acute narrow-angle glaucoma Severe respiratory depression Severe hepatic insufficiency Severe obstructive sleep apnea | Open-angle glaucoma in patients not receiving appropriate therapy Myasthenia gravis (allowable in limited circumstances) Shock, coma, depressed respiration, patients who recently received other respiratory depressants | |
| **Hydralazine** | 5–10 mg IV/IM initially, **then** 5–10 mg q20–30 min PRN | IV/IM | Acute hypertensive crisis | Hypersensitivity to hydralazine Coronary artery disease Mitral valve rheumatic heart disease | Severe tachycardia; porphyria; SLE | Max dose: 30 mg; switch to alternative anti-hypertensive |
| **Labetalol** | 20 mg IV over 2 minutes initially, then 40 mg in 10 minutes and then 80 mg in 10 min; repeat 80 mg in 10 minutes | IV | Acute hypertensive crisis | Asthma or obstructive airway disease, severe bradycardia, 2°/3° heart block (without pacemaker), cardiogenic shock, bronchial asthma, uncompensated cardiac failure, hypersensitivity, sinus bradycardia, sick sinus syndrome without permanent pacemaker; conditions associated with prolonged and severe hypotension; severe peripheral arterial circulatory disorder | 1st degree heart block, chronic heart failure, ischemic heart disease | Max dose: 300 mg |
| **Magnesium** | Bolus: 4–6 g (diluted in 250 mL NS/ D5W) (Maintenance: 1–2 g/hr IV<br><br>IM: Up to 10 g (20 mL of undiluted 50% solution) divided and administered into each buttock | IV or IM | Preeclampsia/ eclampsia/ HELLP syndrome | Hypersensitivity; Myocardial damage, diabetic coma, heart block; Hypermagnesemia; Hypercalcemia, Myasthenia gravis | | |

| Drug | Route | Indication | Contraindications | Comments |
|------|-------|-----------|-------------------|----------|
| **Nifedipine** | PO | Acute hypertensive crisis | Hypersensitivity to nifedipine or other calcium channel blockers Cardiogenic shock | 10 mg initially followed by repeated doses of 20 mg every 15 min (total 5 doses) to a maximum of 90 mg | Concomitant administration with strong CYP3A4 inducers (e.g., rifampin, rifabutin, phenobarbital, phenytoin, carbamazepine, St John's wort) significantly reduces nifedipine efficacy | Hypertensive emergency: use immediate release Can use extended release for maintenance BP control |

**Indication: Pulmonary Embolism**

| Drug | Route | Indication | Contraindications | Comments |
|------|-------|-----------|-------------------|----------|
| **Alteplase (rtPA)** | IV | Pulmonary embolism/ DVT | See Contraindications in Acute Ischemic Stroke section. | ≤67 kg: 15 mg IVP bolus over 1–2 minutes, **then** 0.75 mg/kg IV infusion over 30 minutes (not to exceed 50 mg), and **then** 0.5 mg/kg IV over next 60 minutes (not to exceed 35 mg over 1 hr) >67 kg (100 mg total dose infused over 1.5 hr): 15 mg IVP bolus over 1–2 minutes, **then** 50 mg IV infusion over next 30 minutes, and **then** remaining 35 mg over next 60 minutes | See Contraindications in Acute Ischemic Stroke section |
| **Enoxaparn (Low-molecular weight heparin)** | SC | Pulmonary embolism/ DVT | Active major bleeding, thrombocytopenia with antiplatelet antibody in presence of enoxaparin or heparin; hypersensitivity | 1 mg/kg SC q12 hr | Bleeding diathesis, uncontrolled arterial hypertension or a history of recent gastrointestinal ulceration, diabetic retinopathy, renal dysfunction, and hemorrhage |
| **Heparin** | IV | Pulmonary embolism/ DVT | Hypersensitivity; thrombocytopenia; history of heparin-induced thrombocytopenia, uncontrollable active bleeding, renal dysfunction, uncontrolled or severe hypertension | 5000 units IV bolus, **then** continuous infusion of 1300 units/hr | Hyperkalemia |
| **Potassium** | IV | Hypokalemia associated with hyperglycemia and insulin treatment | Hyperkalemia | Add 20–40 mEq/L of potassium chloride to each liter of fluid once the potassium level is less than 5.5 mEq/L | |

*(Continued)*

(Continued)

| MEDICATION | DOSE | ROUTE | INDICATION | CONTRAINDICATIONS ABSOLUTE | CONTRAINDICATIONS RELATIVE | CONSIDERATIONS |
|---|---|---|---|---|---|---|
| **Warfarin** | 2–5 mg PO/IV qDay for 2 days, OR 10 mg PO for 2 days in healthy individuals<br><br>Typical maintenance dose ranges between 2 and 10 mg/day. Initiate warfarin on day 1 or 2 of LMWH or unfractionated heparin therapy and overlap until desired INR, **then** discontinue heparin | PO or IV | Venous thrombosis | Large esophageal varices, major surgery within the last 72 hours, Platelet count less than 50 x 109/cu.mm, Hypersensitivity, clinically significant bleeding condition; coagulation defects at baseline such that the international normalized ratio (INR) is over 1.5, decompensated liver disease | | Previous history of intracranial hemorrhage, recent history of a major extracranial bleed without known cause, history of peptic ulceration within the past three months, alcoholism, poorly controlled or untreated hypertension |

### Indication: Resuscitative Cesarean Delivery

| MEDICATION | DOSE | ROUTE | INDICATION | CONTRAINDICATIONS ABSOLUTE | CONTRAINDICATIONS RELATIVE | CONSIDERATIONS |
|---|---|---|---|---|---|---|
| **Cefazolin** | Postoperatively: 2 g q 8 hr for 24 hr | IV | Prophylaxis against postoperative surgical infection | Hypersensitivity to cephalosporins or severe allergy to penicillins | | If BMI is >40, consider 3 g Q8 hr for 24 hr |
| **Clindamycin + gentamicin (use if penicillin allergic)** | Postoperatively: Clindamycin: 800 mg q 8 hr for 24 hr; Gentamicin: 5 mg/kg q24 hr | IV | Prophylaxis against postoperative surgical infection | Hypersensitivity or allergy to clindamycin and gentamicin | | |
| **Oxytocin** | 30 units/500 mL; set the infusion pump rate to 334 ml/hour for 30 minutes (10 units in 167 ml), then reduce the rate to 95 ml/hour (remaining 20 units) over 3.5 hours | IV | Postpartum hemorrhage | Hypersensitivity | None | Watch carefully in post-arrest setting—oxytocin can precipitate rearrest |

### Indication: Return of Spontaneous Circulation

| MEDICATION | DOSE | ROUTE | INDICATION | CONTRAINDICATIONS ABSOLUTE | CONTRAINDICATIONS RELATIVE | CONSIDERATIONS |
|---|---|---|---|---|---|---|
| **Betamethasone** | 12.5 mg and repeat in 24 hours | IM | Fetal lung maturity if patient remains pregnant | Hypersensitivity to betamethasone or bisulfite/metabisulfite, systemic fungal infection | | |
| **Magnesium** | See previous dosing | IV or IM | Preeclampsia/eclampsia/HELLP syndrome | Hypersensitivity Myocardial damage, diabetic coma, heart block Hypermagnesemia Hypercalcemia, Myasthenia gravis | | |

### Indication: Sepsis

| MEDICATION | DOSE | ROUTE | INDICATION | CONTRAINDICATIONS ABSOLUTE | CONTRAINDICATIONS RELATIVE | CONSIDERATIONS |
|---|---|---|---|---|---|---|
| **Ampicillin/sulbactam** | 3 g (2 g ampicillin and 1 g sulbactam) IV every 6 hours | IV | Sepsis | Hypersensitivity, previous history of cholestatic jaundice/hepatic dysfunction associated with ampicillin sulbactam | | |

| Drug | Dose | Route | Indication | Contraindication | Comments |
|---|---|---|---|---|---|
| **Clindamycin** | 600 mg IV or IM every 6 to 12 hours OR 900 mg IV every 8 to 12 hours | IV/IM | Sepsis | Hypersensitivity to clindamycin, lincomycin, or formulation components | For life-threatening infections, doses may be increased; doses up to 4,800 mg/day IV have been used |
| **Gentamicin** | 3–5 mg/kg/day IV/IM divided q8 hr; Monitor peak (4–12 mg/L) and trough (1–2 mg/L) Each regimen must be followed by at least trough level drawn on 3rd or 4th dose, 30 min before dosing unless renal toxicity suspected | IV/IM | Sepsis | Prior aminoglycoside toxicity or hypersensitivity | Monitor nephrotoxicity, neurotoxicity, and ototoxicity; assess at beginning of therapy and throughout |

**Indication: Return of Spontaneous Circulation (cont.)**

| Drug | Dose | Route | Indication | Contraindication | Comments |
|---|---|---|---|---|---|
| **Meropenem** | 1 g IV q8 hr | IV | Sepsis | Hypersensitivity to IV components, beta-lactams, or other drugs in this class | |
| **Penicillin** | 4 million units IV Q4 hr | IM | Group A Streptococcal infections | Hypersensitivity | To treat GAS, combine PCN with clindamycin 900 mg Q8 hr |
| **Vancomycin** | 15–20 mg/kg q8 h–q12 h (goal trough 15–20 mcg/mL) | IV | Sepsis | Hypersensitivity | |

Abbreviations: IV, intravenous; IM, intramuscular; IO, intraosseous; PRN, when necessary; PO, by mouth; PR, by rectum; PRBC, packed red blood cells; FFP, fresh frozen plasma; DIC, disseminated intravascular coagulation; INR, international normalized ratio; TID, three times a day; AV, atrioventricular; SC, subcutaneously; MI, myocardial infarction; PVD, peripheral vascular disease; VTE, venous thromboembolism; HELLP syndrome, hemolysis, elevated liver enzymes, and low platelets.

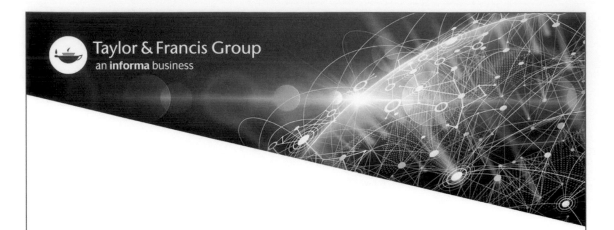
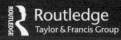
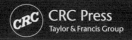